Biostatistics

2nd Edition

by Monika Wahi, MPH and John C. Pezzullo, PhD

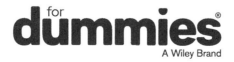

A Wiley Brand

Biostatistics For Dummies®, 2nd Edition

Published by: **John Wiley & Sons, Inc.**, 111 River Street, Hoboken, NJ 07030-5774, www.wiley.com

Contents at a Glance

Table of Contents

Introduction

Biostatistics is the practical application of statistical concepts and techniques to topics in the biology and life sciences fields. Because these are broad fields, biostatistics covers a very wide area. It is used when studying many types of experimental units, from viruses to trees to fleas to mice to people. Biostatistics involves designing research studies, safely conducting human research, collecting and verifying research data, summarizing and displaying the data, and analyzing the data to answer research hypotheses and draw meaningful conclusions.

It is not possible to cover all the subspecialties of biostatistics in one book, because such a book would have to include chapters on molecular biology, genetics, agricultural studies, animal research (both inside and outside the lab), clinical trials, and epidemiological research. So instead, we focus on the most widely applicable topics of biostatistics and on the topics that are most relevant to human research based on a survey of graduate-level biostatistics curricula from major universities.

About This Book

We wrote this book to be used as a reference. Our intention was for you to pull out this book when you want information about a particular topic. This means you don't have to read it from beginning to end to find it useful. In fact, you can jump directly to any part that interests you. We hope you'll be inclined to look through the book from time to time, open it to a page at random, read a page or two, and get a useful reminder or pick up a new fact.

Only in a few places does this book provide detailed steps about how to perform a particular statistical calculation by hand. Instruction like that may have been necessary in the mid-1900s. Back then, statistics students spent hours in a *computing lab*, which is a room that had an adding machine. Thankfully, we now have statistical software to do this for us (see Chapter 4 for advice on choosing statistical software). When describing statistical tests, our focus is always on the concepts behind the method, how to prepare your data for analysis, and how to interpret the results. We keep mathematical formulas and derivations to a minimum. We only include them when we think they help explain what's going on. If you really want to see them, you can find them in many biostatistics textbooks, and they're readily available online.

Because good study design is crucial for the success of any research, this book gives special attention to the design of both epidemiologic studies and clinical trials. We also pay special attention to providing advice on how to calculate the number of participants you need for your study. You will find easy-to-apply examples of sample-size calculations in the chapters describing significance tests in Parts 4, 5, and 6, and in Chapter 25.

Foolish Assumptions

We wrote this book to help several kinds of people. We assume you fall into one of the following categories:

>> Students at the undergraduate or graduate level who are taking a course in biostatistics and want help with the topics they're studying in class

>> Professionals who have had no formal biostatistical training, and possibly no statistical training at all, who now must analyze biological or research data as part of their work

>> Doctors, nurses, and other healthcare professionals who want to carry out human research

If you're interested in biostatistics, then you're no dummy! But perhaps you sometimes *feel* like a dummy when it comes to biostatistics, or statistics in general, or even mathematics. Don't feel bad. We both have felt that way many times over the years. In fact, we still feel like that whenever we are propelled into an area of biostatistics with which we are unfamiliar, because it is new to us. (If you haven't taken a basic statistics course yet, you may want to get *Statistics For Dummies* by Deborah J. Rumsey, PhD — published by Wiley — and read parts of that book first.)

What is important to keep in mind when learning biostatistics is that you don't have to be a math genius to be a good biostatistician. You also don't need any special math skills to be an excellent research scientist who can intelligently design research studies, execute them well, collect and analyze data properly, and draw valid conclusions. You just have to have a solid grasp of the basic concepts and know how to utilize statistical software properly to obtain the output you need and interpret it.

Icons Used in This Book

Icons are the little graphics in the margins of this book, and are used to draw your attention to certain kinds of material. Here's what they mean:

REMEMBER

This icon signals information especially worth keeping in mind. Your main take-aways from this book should be the material marked with this icon.

TECHNICAL STUFF

We use this icon to flag explanations of technical topics, such as derivations and computational formulas that you don't have to know to do biostatistics. They are included to give you deeper insight into the material.

TIP

This icon refers to helpful hints, ideas, shortcuts, and rules of thumb that you can use to save time or make a task easier. It also highlights different ways of thinking about a topic or concept.

WARNING

This icon alerts you to discussion of a controversial topic, a concept that is often misunderstand, or a pitfall or common mistake to guard against in biostatistics.

Beyond the Book

In addition to the abundance of information and guidance related to using biostatistics for analysis of research data that we provide in this book, you get access to even more help and information online at `Dummies.com`. Check out this book's online Cheat Sheet. Just go to `www.dummies.com` and search for "Biostatistics For Dummies Cheat Sheet."

Where to Go from Here

You're already off to a good start! You've read this introduction, so you have a good idea of what this book is all about. For a more detailed list of topics, take a look at the Contents at a Glance. This drills down into each part and shows you what each chapter is all about. Finally, skim through the full-blown Table of Contents, which drills further down into each chapter, showing you the headings for the sections and subsections of that chapter.

If you want to get the big picture of what biostatistics encompasses and the areas of biostatistics covered in this book, then read Chapter 1. This is a top-level overview of the book's topics. Here are a few other special parts of this book you may want to jump into first, depending on your interest:

>> If you're uncomfortable with mathematical notation, then Chapter 2 is the place to start.

>> If you want a quick refresher on basic statistics like what you would learn in a typical introductory course, then read Chapter 3.

>> You can get an introduction to human research and clinical trials in Chapters 5, 7, and 20.

>> If you want to learn about collecting, summarizing, and graphing data, jump to Part 3.

>> If you need to know about working with survival data, you can go right to Part 6.

>> If you're puzzled about a particular statistical distribution function, then look at Chapter 24.

>> And if you need to calculate some quick sample-size estimates, turn to Chapter 25.

1

Getting Started with Biostatistics

IN THIS PART . . .

Get comfortable with mathematical notation that uses numbers, special constants, variables, and mathematical symbols — a must for all you mathophobes.

Review basic statistical concepts you may have learned previously, such as probability, randomness, populations, samples, statistical inference, and more.

Chapter **1**

Biostatistics 101

Biostatistics deals with the design and execution of scientific studies involving biology, the acquisition and analysis of data from those studies, and the interpretation and presentation of the results of those analyses. This book is meant to be a useful and easy-to-understand companion to the more formal textbooks used in graduate-level biostatistics courses. Because most of these courses teach how to analyze data from epidemiologic studies and clinical trials, this book focuses on that as well. In this first chapter, we introduce you to the fundamentals of biostatistics.

Brushing Up on Math and Stats Basics

Chapters 2 and 3 are designed to bring you up to speed on the basic math and statistical background that's needed to understand biostatistics and give you supplementary information or context that you may find useful while reading the rest of this book.

» Many people feel unsure of themselves when it comes to understanding mathematical formulas and equations. Although this book contains fewer formulas than many statistics books, we include them when they help illustrate a concept or describe a calculation that's simple enough to do by hand. But if you're a real mathophobe, you probably dread looking at *any* chapter that has a math expression anywhere in it. That's why we include Chapter 2, "Overcoming Mathophobia" to show you how to read and understand the basic mathematical notation we use in this book. We cover everything from basic mathematical operations to functions and beyond.

» If you're in a graduate-level biostatistics course, you've probably already taken one or two introductory statistics courses. But that may have been a while ago, and you may feel unsure of your knowledge of the basic statistical concepts. Or you may have little or no formal statistical training but now find yourself in a work situation where you interact with clinical researchers, participate in the design of research projects, or work with the results from biological research. If so, read Chapter 3, which provides an overview of the fundamental concepts and terminology of statistics. There, you get the scoop on topics such as probability, randomness, populations, samples, statistical inference, accuracy, precision, hypothesis testing, nonparametric statistics, and simulation techniques.

Doing Calculations with the Greatest of Ease

For instructional purposes, some chapters in this book include step-by-step instructions for performing statistical tests and analyses by hand. We include such instruction only to illustrate the concepts that are involved in the procedure or to demonstrate calculations that are simple to do manually.

However, we demonstrate many of the statistical functions we talk about in this book using R, which is a free, open-source software package. If you are in a class and assigned a particular software package to use, you will have to use that software for the course, which may be commercial software associated with a fee. However, if you are learning on your own, you may choose to use open-source software, which is free. Chapter 4 provides guidance on both commercial and free software.

Concentrating on Epidemiologic Research

REMEMBER

This book covers topics that are applicable to all areas of biostatistics, concentrating on methods that are especially relevant to *epidemiologic research* — studies involving people. This includes *clinical trials,* which are experiments done to develop therapeutic interventions such as drugs. Because policy in healthcare is often based on the results from clinical trials, if you make mistake analyzing clinical trial data, it can have disastrous and wide-ranging human and financial consequences. Even if you don't expect to ever work in a domain that relies heavily on clinical trials (such as drug development research), ensuring that you have a working knowledge of how to manage the statistical issues seen in clinical trials is critical.

Three chapters discuss clinical trials:

>> Chapter 5 describes the statistical aspects of clinical trials as three phases. First, it covers the design phase, where a study protocol is written. Next, it describes the execution phase, where data are collected, and efforts are made to prevent invalid or missing data. In the final phase, data from the study are analyzed and interpreted to answer the hypotheses.

>> Chapter 7 presents epidemiologic study designs and explains the importance of the clinical trial as a study design.

>> Chapter 20 explains the role well-designed clinical trials play in accruing evidence of causal inference in biostatistics.

Much of the work in biostatistics is using data from samples to make inferences about the background population from which the sample was drawn. Now that we have large databases, it is possible to easily take samples of data. Chapter 6 provides guidance on different ways to take samples of larger populations so you can make valid population-based estimates from these samples. Sampling is especially important when doing observational studies. While clinical trials covered are experiments, where participants are assigned interventions, in observational studies, participants are merely observed, with data collected and statistics performed to make inferences. Chapter 7 describes these observational study designs, and the statistical issues that need to be considered when analyzing data arising from such studies.

Data used in biostatistics are often collected in online databases, but some data are still collected on paper. Regardless of the source of the data, they must be put into electronic format and arranged in a certain way to be able to be analyzed using statistical software. Chapter 8 is devoted to describing how to get your data into the computer and arrange it properly so it can be analyzed correctly. It also describes how to collect and validate your data. Then in Chapter 9, we show you how to summarize each type of data and display it graphically. We explain how to make bar charts, box-and-whiskers charts, and more.

Drawing Conclusions from Your Data

Most statistical analysis involves *inferring,* or drawing conclusions about the population at large based on your observations of a sample drawn from that population. The theory of *statistical inference* is often divided into two broad sub-theories: *estimation* theory and *decision* theory.

Statistical estimation theory

Chapter 10 deals with *statistical estimation theory,* which addresses the question of how accurately and precisely you can estimate a population parameter from the values you observe in your sample. For example, you may want to estimate the mean blood hemoglobin concentration in adults with Type II diabetes, or the true correlation coefficient between body weight and height in certain pediatric populations. Chapter 10 describes how to estimate these parameters by constructing a *confidence interval* around your estimate. The confidence interval is the range that is likely to include the true population parameter, which provides an idea of the precision of your estimate.

Statistical decision theory

Much of the rest of this book deals with *statistical decision theory,* which is how to decide whether some effect you've observed in your data reflects a real difference or association in the background population or is merely the result of random fluctuations in your data or sampling. If you measure the mean blood hemoglobin concentration in two different samples of adults with Type II diabetes, you will likely get a different number. But does this difference reflect a real difference between the groups in terms of blood hemoglobin concentration? Or is this difference a result of random fluctuations? Statistical decision theory helps you decide.

In Part 4, we cover statistical decision theory in terms of comparing means and proportions between groups, as well as understanding the relationship between two or more variables.

Comparing groups

In Part 4, we show you different ways to compare groups statistically.

>> In Chapter 11, you see how to compare *average values* between two or more groups by using t tests and ANOVAs. We also describe their nonparametric counterparts that can be used with skewed or other non-normally distributed data.

>> Chapter 12 shows how to compare *proportions* between two or more groups, such as the proportions of patients responding to two different drugs, using the chi-square and Fisher Exact tests on cross-tabulated (cross-tab) data.

>> Chapter 13 focuses on one specific kind of cross-tab called the *fourfold table,* which has exactly two rows and two columns. Because the fourfold table provides the opportunity for some particularly insightful calculations, it's worth a chapter of its own.

>> In Chapter 14, you discover how the terminology used in epidemiologic studies is applied to specifically formatted fourfold tables to calculate incidence and prevalence rates.

Looking for relationships between variables

Epidemiology and biostatistics are interested in *causal inference*, which means trying to figure out what causes particular outcomes in biological research. While it is possible to look at the relationship between two variables in a *bivariate analysis*, regression analysis is the part of statistics that enables you to explore the relationship between multiple variables and one outcome in the same model so you can evaluate their relative cause of the outcome. Here are some use-cases for regression:

>> You may want to know whether there's a *statistically significant association* between one or more variables and an outcome, even if there are other variables in the model. You may ask: Does being overweight increase the likelihood of getting liver cancer? Or: Is exercising fewer hours per week associated with higher blood pressure measurements? In answering both of those questions, you may want to control other variables known to influence the outcome.

>> You may want to develop a formula for predicting the value of a variable from the observed values of one or more other variables. For example, you may want to predict how long a newly diagnosed cancer patient may survive based on their age, obesity status, and medical history.

>> You may be fitting a theoretical formula to some data to estimate one of the parameters appearing in that formula. An example of such a problem is determining how fast the kidneys can remove a drug from the body, which is called a terminal elimination rate constant. This can be estimated from measurements of drug concentration in the blood taken at various times after taking a dose of the drug.

Regression analysis can manage all these tasks and many more. Regression is so important in biological research that all the chapters in Part 5 are focused on some aspect of regression.

TIP

If you have never learned correlation and regression analysis, read Chapter 15, which introduces these topics. We cover simple straight-line regression in Chapter 16, which includes one predictor variable. We extend that to cover multiple regression with more than one predictor variable in Chapter 17. These three chapters deal with ordinary linear regression, where you're trying to predict the value of a numerical outcome variable from one or more other variables. An example would be trying to predict mean blood hemoglobin concentration using variables like age, blood pressure level, and Type II diabetes status. Ordinary linear regression uses a formula that's a simple summation of terms, each of which consists of a predictor variable multiplied by a regression coefficient.

But in real-world biological and epidemiologic research, you encounter more complicated relationships. Chapter 18 describes *logistic regression,* where the outcome is the occurrence or non-occurrence of an event (such as being diagnosed with Type II diabetes), and you want to predict the probability that the event will occur. You also find out about several other kinds of regression in Chapter 19:

>> *Poisson regression,* where the outcome is the number of events that occur in an interval of time

>> *Nonlinear least-squares regression,* where the relationship between the predictors and numerical outcome can be more complicated than a simple summation of terms in a linear model

>> *LOWESS curve-fitting,* where you fit a custom function to describe your data

Finally, Part 5 ends with Chapter 20, which provides guidance on the mechanics of regression modeling, including how to develop a modeling plan, and how to choose variables to include in models.

A Matter of Life and Death: Working with Survival Data

Sooner or later, everyone dies, and in biological research, it becomes especially important to characterize that sooner-or-later part as accurately as possible using survival analysis techniques. But characterizing survival can get tricky. It's possible to say that patients may live an average of 5.3 years after they are diagnosed with a particular disease. But what is the exact survival experience? Imagine you do a study with patients who have this disease. You may ask: Do all patients tend to live around five or six years, or do half the patients die within the first few months, and the other half survive ten years or more? And what if some patients live longer than the observational period of your study? How do you include them in your analysis? And what about participants who stopped returning calls from your study staff? You do not know if these dropouts went on to live or die. How do you include their data in your analysis?

REMEMBER

The need to study survival with data like these led to the development of survival analysis techniques. But survival analysis is not only intended to study the outcome of death. You can use survival analysis to study the time to the first occurrence of non-death events as well, like remission or recurrence of cancer, the diagnosis of a particular condition, or the resolution of a particular condition. Survival analysis techniques are presented in Part 6.

Getting to Know Statistical Distributions

Statistics books always contain tables, so why should this one be any different? Back in the not-so-good old days, when analysts had to do statistical calculations by hand, they needed to use tables of the common statistical distributions to complete the calculation of the significance test. They needed tables for the normal distribution, Student t, chi-square, Fisher F, and others. Now, software does all this for you, including calculating exact p values, so these printed tables aren't necessary anymore.

But you should still be familiar with the common statistical distributions that may describe the fluctuations in your data, or that may be referenced in the course of performing a statistical calculation. Chapter 24 contains a list of commonly used distribution functions, with explanations of where you can expect to encounter those distributions and what they look like. We also include a description of some of their properties and how they're related to other distributions. Some of them are accompanied by a small table of critical values, corresponding to statistical significance at $\alpha = 0.05$.

Figuring Out How Many Participants You Need

Of all the statistical challenges a researcher may encounter, none seems to instill as much apprehension and insecurity as having to estimate the number of participants needed for a study. While smaller sample sizes mean less data collection work, you want to make sure your target sample size is large enough so that in the end, your study has sufficient power. You want to conduct a study with a high probability of yielding a statistically significant result if the hypothesized effect is truly present in the population.

TIP

Because sample-size estimation is such an important part of the design of any research project, this book shows you how to make those estimates for the situations you're likely to encounter when doing biological research. As we describe each statistical test in Parts 4, 5, 6, and 7, we explain how to estimate the number of participants needed to provide sufficient power for that test. In addition, Chapter 25 describes ten simple rules for getting a "quick and dirty" estimate of the required sample size.

Chapter **2**

Overcoming Mathophobia: Reading and Understanding Mathematical Expressions

L et's face it: Many people fear math, and statistical calculations require math. In this chapter, we help you become more comfortable with reading mathematical *expressions,* which are combinations of numbers, letters, math operations, punctuation, and grouping symbols. We also help you become more comfortable with *equations,* which connect two expressions with an equal sign. And we review *formulas,* which are equations designed for specific calculations. (For simplicity, for the rest of the chapter, we use the term *formula* to refer to expressions, equations, and formulas.) We also explain how to write formulas, which you need to know in order to tell a computer how to do calculations with your data.

We start the chapter by showing you how to interpret the mathematical formulas you encounter throughout this book. We don't deconstruct the intricacies of complicated mathematical operations. Instead, we explain how mathematical operations are indicated in this book. If you feel unsure of your grasp on algebra, consider reviewing *Algebra I For Dummies* and *Algebra II For Dummies,* which are both written by Mary Jane Sterling and published by Wiley.

Breaking Down the Basics of Mathematical Formulas

One way to think of a mathematical formula is as a shorthand way to describe how to do a certain calculation. Formulas are made up of numbers, constants, and variables interspersed with symbols that indicate mathematical operations, punctuation, and typographic effects. Formulas are constructed using relatively standardized rules that have evolved over centuries. In the following sections, we describe two different kinds of formulas that you encounter in this book: typeset and plain text. We also describe two of the building blocks from which formulas are created: constants and variables.

Displaying formulas in different ways

Formulas can be expressed *in print* in two different formats: *typeset format* and *plain text format*:

>> A **typeset format** utilizes special symbols, and when printed, the formula is spread out in a two-dimensional structure, like this:

$$SD = \sqrt{\frac{\sum_{i=1}^{n}(x_i - m)^2}{n-1}}$$

>> A **plain text format** prints the formula out as a single line, which is easier to type if you're limited to the characters on a keyboard:

$$SD = \text{sqrt}(\text{sum}((x[i] - m)\wedge 2, i, 1, n)/(n-1))$$

REMEMBER

You must know how to read both types of formula displays — typeset and plain text. The examples in this chapter show both styles. But you may never have to construct a professional-looking typeset formula (unless you're writing a book, like we're doing right now). On the other hand, you'll almost certainly have to write out plain text formulas as part of organizing, preparing, editing, and analyzing your data.

Checking out the building blocks of formulas

No matter how they're written, formulas are essentially recipes that tell you how to calculate a result, or how a value is defined. To cook up your own result, you need to know how to follow the recipe. When initially approaching a formula, it's helpful to start by examining the building blocks from which formulas are constructed. These include *constants,* which are numbers with specified values, and *variables,* which represent quantities that can take on different values at different times.

Constants

Constants are values that can be represented *explicitly* (using the numerals 0 through 9 with or without a decimal point), or *symbolically* (using a letter in the Greek or Roman alphabet). Symbolic constants represent a particular value important in mathematics, physics, or some other discipline, such as:

>> The Greek letter π usually represents 3.14159 (plus a zillion more digits). This Greek letter is spelled *pi* and pronounced *pie,* and represents the ratio of the circumference of any circle to its diameter.

>> The number 2.71828 (plus a zillion more digits) is represented by *e* (which is italicized when written, and is pronounced like the letter "e"). Later in this chapter, we describe one way *e* is used. You'll see *e* in statistical formulas throughout this book and in almost every other mathematical and statistical textbook. Whenever you see an italicized *e* in this book, it refers to the number 2.718 unless we explicitly say otherwise.

TECHNICAL STUFF

The official mathematical definition of *e* is: The value of the expression $(1 + 1/n)^n$, which approaches infinity as *n* gets larger and larger. Unlike π, *e* has no simple geometrical interpretation. Here is an example used to help learners envision *e*: Assume you put exactly one dollar in a bank account that's paying 100 percent annual interest, compounded continuously. After exactly one year, your account will have *e* dollars in it. That includes the interest on your original dollar, plus the interest on the interest — about $1.72 (to the nearest penny) — added to the original dollar for a total of $2.72. (This is just an example. We don't think there is a single bank out there advertising annual returns in terms of *e*!)

Mathematicians and scientists use lots of other specific Greek and Roman letters as symbols for specific constants, but you need only a few of them in your biostatistics work. π and *e* are the most common, and we define others in this book as they come up in topics we present.

Variables

The term *variable* has two slightly different meanings:

>> **In mathematics and engineering,** a variable is a symbol that represents some quantity in a formula. It is usually a letter of the alphabet. You are probably used to seeing variables like x and y in algebra, for example.

>> **In statistics and computer science,** a variable is a name referring to a single data value or an entire *field,* which is a column of data in a spreadsheet or database. The variable name is made up of letters (like SBP for systolic blood pressure), but may also contain numbers (such as SBP1, SBP2, and SBP3). Technically, the variable name refers to a place in the computer's memory where the data value or field is stored. For example, a computer programmer writing a statistical software program may ask if the variable SBP is greater than or equal to 120 mmHg.

The names of variables may be written in uppercase or lowercase letters depending upon typographic conventions or preferences, or on the requirements of the software being used.

REMEMBER

Variables are always italicized in typeset formulas, but not in plain text formulas.

Focusing on Operations Found in Formulas

A formula tells you how the building blocks of numbers, constants, and variables are to be combined. In other words, a formula is a recipe for the calculations you're supposed to carry out on these quantities. But formulas are not always easy to read. A particular symbol — such as the minus sign — can be interpreted differently, depending upon the context of the formula. Also, a particular mathematical operation like multiplication can be represented in different ways in a formula. In the following sections we explain the basic mathematical operations you see in formulas throughout this book and describe two types of equations you'll encounter in statistical books and articles.

Basic mathematical operations

The four basic mathematical operations are addition, subtraction, multiplication, and division (ah, yes — the basics you learned in elementary school). Different symbols are associated with these operations, as you discover in the following sections.

Addition and subtraction

Addition and subtraction are always indicated by the + and − symbols, respectively, placed between two numbers or variables. Compared to the plus sign, the minus sign can be tricky when it comes to interpreting it in a formula.

>> **A minus sign placed immediately before a number** indicates a negative quantity. For example, −5° indicates five degrees below 0, and −5 kg indicates a weight loss of 5 kilograms.

>> **A minus sign placed immediately before a variable** tells you to reverse the sign of the value of the variable. Therefore, −x means that if x is positive, you should now make it negative. But it also means that if x is negative, make it positive (so, if x was −5 kg, then −x would be 5 kg). Used this way, the minus sign is referred to as a *unary* operator because it's acting on only one variable.

Multiplication

The word *term* is generic for an individual item or element in a formula. Multiplication of terms is indicated in several ways, as shown in Table 2-1.

TABLE 2-1 **Multiplication Options**

What It Is	Example	Where It's Used
Asterisk	$2 * 5$	Plain text formulas, but almost never in typeset formulas
Cross	2×5	Typeset formula, between two variables or two constants being multiplied together
Raised dot	$2 \cdot 5$	Typeset formula
Term is immediately in front of a parenthesized expression	$2(5 + 3) = 16$	Typeset formula
Brackets and curly braces	$2[6 + (5 + 3)/2] = 20$	Typeset formula containing "nested" parentheses
Two or more terms running together	$2\pi r$ (versus $2 \times \pi \times r$)	In typeset formulas only

WARNING

You can put terms right next to each other to imply multiplication *only* when it's perfectly clear from the context of the formula that the authors are using only single-letter variable names (like x and y), and that they're describing calculations where it makes sense to multiply those variables together. In other words, you can't put numeric terms right after one another to imply multiplication, meaning you can't replace 5×3 with 53, because 53 is an actual number itself. And you shouldn't replace variables like length $\times$ width with *lengthwidth*, because it looks like you're referring to a single variable named *lengthwidth*.

Division

Like multiplication, division can be indicated in several ways:

>> With a **slash** (/) in plain text formulas: Distance/Time

>> With a **division symbol** ($\div$) in typeset formulas: Distance $\div$ Time

>> With a **long horizontal bar** in typeset formulas:

$$\frac{Distance}{Time}$$

Powers, roots, and logarithms

In the next section, we cover powers, roots, and logarithms, all three of which are related to the idea of repeated multiplication.

Raising to a power

Raising to a power is a shorthand way to indicate repeated multiplication by the same number. You indicate raising to a power by:

>> Superscripting in typographic formulas, such as 5^3

>> Using ** in plain text formulas, such as $5**3$

>> Using ^ in plain text formulas, such as 5^3

All the preceding expressions are read as "five to the third power," "five to the power of three," or "five cubed." It says to multiply three fives together: $5 \times 5 \times 5$, which gives you 125.

Here are some other features of power:

>> **A power doesn't have to be a whole number.** You can raise a number to a fractional power (such as 3.8). You can't visualize this in terms of repeated multiplications, but your scientific calculator can show you that $2.6^{3.8}$ is equal to approximately 37.748.

» **A power can be negative.** A negative power indicates the *reciprocal* of the quantity, which is when you divide the quantity by 1 (meaning $1/x$). So x^{-1} means 1 divided by x, and in general, x^{-n} is the same as $1/x^n$ (such as 2^{-3} = ½).

Remember the constant e (2.718. . .)? Almost every time you see e used in a formula, it's being raised to some power. This means you almost always see e with an exponent after it. Raising e to a power is called *exponentiating,* and another way of representing e^x in plain text is *exp(x).* Remember, x doesn't have to be a whole number. By typing *=exp(1.6)* in the formula bar in Microsoft Excel (or doing the equation on a scientific calculator), you see that exp(1.6) equals approximately 4.953. We talk more about exponentiating in other book sections, especially Chapters 18 and 24.

Taking a root

Taking a root involves asking the power question backwards. In other words, we ask: "What base number, when raised to a certain power, equals a certain number?" For example, "What number, when raised to the power of 2 (which is squared), equals 100?" Well, 10×10 (also expressed 10^2) equals 100, so the square root of 100 is 10. Similarly, the cube root of 1,000,000 is 100, because $100 \times 100 \times 100$ (also expressed 100^3) equals a million.

Root-taking is indicated by a *radical sign* ($\sqrt{}$) in a typeset formula, where the term from which we intend to take the root is located "under the roof" of the radical sign, as 25 is shown here: $\sqrt{25}$. If no numbers appear in the notch of the radical sign, it is assumed we are taking a square root. Other roots are indicated by putting a number in the notch of the radical sign. Because 2^8 is 256, we say 2 is the eighth root of 256, and we put 8 in the notch of the radical sign covering 256, like this: $\sqrt[8]{256}$. You also can indicate root-taking by expressing it different ways used in algebra: $\sqrt[n]{x}$ is equal to $x^{1/n}$ and can be expressed as $x \wedge (1/n)$ in plain text.

Looking at logarithms

In addition to root-taking, another way of asking the power question backwards is by saying, "What exponent (or power) must I raise a particular base number to in order for it to equal a certain number?" For root-taking, in terms of using a formula, we specify the power and request the base. With logarithms, we specify the base and request the power (or exponent).

For example, you may ask, "What power must I raise 10 to in order to get 1,000?" The answer is 3, because $10^3 = 1,000$. You can say that 3 is the *logarithm* of 1,000 (for base 10), or, in mathematical terms: $\text{Log}_{10}(1,000) = 3$. Similarly, because $2^8 = 256$, you say that $\text{Log}_2(256) = 8$. And because $e^{1.6} = 4.953$, then $\text{Log}_e(4.953) = 1.6$.

There can be logarithms to any base, but three bases occur frequently enough to have their own nicknames:

>> Base-10 logarithms are called *common logarithms.*

>> Base-*e* logarithms are called *natural logarithms.*

>> Base-2 logarithms are called *binary logarithms.*

WARNING

The logarithmic function naming is inconsistent among different authors, publishers, and software writers. Sometimes *Log* means natural logarithm, and sometimes it means common logarithm. Often *Ln* is used for natural logarithm, and *Log* is used for common logarithm. Names like *Log10* and *Log2* may also be used to identify the base.

REMEMBER

The most common kind of logarithm used in this book is the natural logarithm, so in this book we always use *Log* to indicate natural (base-*e*) logarithms. When we want to refer to common logarithms, we use Log_{10}, and when referring to binary logarithms, we use Log_2.

An *antilogarithm* (usually shortened to *antilog*) is the inverse of a logarithm. As an example of an antilog, if *y* is the log of *x*, then *x* is the antilog of *y*. For another example, the base-10 logarithm of 1,000 is 3, so the base-10 antilog of 3 is 1,000.

REMEMBER

Calculating an antilog is exactly the same as raising the base to the power of the logarithm. That is, the base-10 antilog of 3 is the same as 10 raised to the power of 3 (which is 10^3, or 1,000). Similarly, the natural antilog of any number is *e* (2.718) raised to the power of that number. As an example, the natural antilog of 5 is e^5, or approximately 148.41.

Factorials and absolute values

So far we've covered mathematical operators that are written either *between* the two numbers, which are the subject of the operation (such as the plus in 5 + 8), or *before* the number it operates on if there is only one number (like the minus sign used as a unary operator described earlier, as in −5°). Next we cover factorials and absolute values, which are mathematical operators that have a unique format in typeset expressions.

Factorials

Although a statistical formula may contain an exclamation point, that doesn't mean that you should sound excited when you read the formula aloud (although it may be tempting to do so!). An exclamation mark (!) *after* a number is shorthand for calculating that number's *factorial.* To do that, you write down all the whole numbers from 1 to the factorial number in a row, and then multiply them all together. For example, the expression 5!, which is read as *five factorial*, means to calculate $1 \times 2 \times 3 \times 4 \times 5$ (which equals 120).

Even though standard keyboards have a ! key, most computer programs and spreadsheets don't let you use ! to indicate factorials. For example, to do the calculation of 5! in Microsoft Excel, you use the formula =*FACT(5)*.

TECHNICAL
STUFF

Here are a few factorials fun facts:

>> Factorials can be very large. For example, 10! is 3,628,800, and 170! is about 7.3×10^{306}, which is close to the processing limits for many computers.

>> 0! isn't 0, but is actually 1. Actually, it's the same as 1!, which is also 1. That may not make obvious sense, but is true, so you can memorize it.

>> The definition of *factorial* can be extended to fractions and even to negative numbers. But good news! You don't have to deal with those kinds of factorials in this book.

Absolute values

The term *absolute value* refers to the value of a number when it is positive (meaning it has no minus sign before it). You indicate absolute value by placing vertical bars immediately to the left and right of the number. So |5.7| equals 5.7, and |−5.7| also equals 5.7. Even though most keyboards have the | (pipe) symbol, the absolute value is usually indicated in plain text formulas as abs(5.7).

Functions

In this book, a *function* is a set of calculations that accepts one or more numeric values (called *arguments*) and produces a numeric result. Regardless of typeset or plain text, a function is indicated in a formula by the function name followed by a set of parentheses that contain the argument or arguments. Here's an example of the function *square root of x*: sqrt(*x*).

The most commonly used functions have been given standard names. The preceding sections in this chapter covered some of these, including *sqrt* for square root, *exp* for exponentiate, *log* for logarithm, *ln* for natural log, *fact* for factorial, and *abs* for absolute value.

When writing formulas with functions using software, be aware that each software may have rules about case-sensitivity. It may require all caps, all lowercase, or first-letter capitalization. Make sure to check the software's documentation for guidance (Chapter 4 discusses different statistical software packages.)

Simple and complicated formulas

Simple formulas have one or two numbers and only one mathematical operator (for example, 5 + 3). But most statistical formulas you'll encounter are more complicated, with two or more operators and variables.

Whether doing calculations manually or using software, you need to ensure that you do your formula calculations in the correct order (called the *order of operation*). If you evaluate the terms and operations in the formula in the wrong order, you will get incorrect results. In a complicated formula, the order in which you evaluate the terms and operations is governed by the interplay of several rules arranged in a hierarchy. Most computer programs try to follow the customary conventions that apply to typeset formulas, but you need to check software's documentation to be sure.

Here's a typical set of operator hierarchy rules. Within each hierarchical level, operations are carried out from left to right:

1. **Evaluate any terms and operations within parentheses, brackets, curly braces, or absolute-value bars first,** including terms inside parentheses that follow the name of a function. Please note that nested functions are evaluated inside out, so additional parentheses may be needed to prevent any confusion.

2. **Evaluate negation, factorials, powers, and roots.**

3. **Evaluate multiplication and division.**

4. **Evaluate addition and subtraction.**

In a typeset fraction, evaluate terms and operations above the horizontal bar (the numerator) first, then terms and operations below the bar (the denominator) next. After that, divide the numerator by the denominator.

Equations

An *equation* has two expressions with an equal sign between them. Most equations appearing in this book have a single variable name to the left of the equal sign and a formula to the right, like this: $SEM = SD/\sqrt{N}$. This style of equation defines the variable appearing on the left in terms of the calculations specified on the right.

In doing so, it also provides the "cookbook" instructions for calculating the result, which in this case is the *SEM* for any values of *SD* and *N.*

The book also contains another type of equation that appears in algebra, asserting that the terms on the left side of the equation are equal to the terms on the right. For example, the equation $x + 2 = 3x$ asserts that x is a number that, when added to 2, produces a number that's 3 times as large as the original x. Algebra teaches you how to solve this expression for x, and it turns out that the answer is $x = 1$.

Counting on Collections of Numbers

A variable can refer to one value or to a collection of values called *arrays*. Arrays can come with one or more dimensions.

One-dimensional arrays

A one-dimensional array can be thought of as a list of values. For instance, you may record a list of fasting glucose values (in milligrams per deciliter, mg/dL) from five study participants as 86, 110, 95, 125, and 64. You could use the variable name *Gluc* to refer to this array containing five numbers, or *elements*. Using the term *Gluc* in a formula refers to the entire five-element array.

You can refer to one particular element of this array (meaning one glucose measurement) in several ways. You can use the *index* of the array, which is the number that indicates the position of the element to which you are referring in the array.

>> In a typeset formula, indices are typically indicated using subscripts. For example, Gluc_3 refers to the third element in the array (which would be 95 in our example).

>> In a plain text formula, indices are typically indicated using brackets (such as Gluc[3]).

The index can be a variable like I, so Gluc[i] would refer to the ith element of the array. The term ith means the variable would be allowed to take on any value between 1 and the maximum number of elements in the array (which in this case would be 5).

TIP

In some programming languages and statistical books and articles, the indices start at 0 for the first element, 1 for the second element, and so on, which can be confusing. In this book, all arrays are indexed starting at 1.

Higher-dimensional arrays

Two-dimensional arrays can be understood as a table of values with rows and columns, like a block of cells in a spreadsheet. There are also higher-dimensional arrays that can be thought of as a whole collection of tables. Suppose that you measure the fasting glucose on five participants on each of three treatment days. You could think of your 15 measurements being laid out in a table with five rows and three columns. If you want to represent this entire table with a single variable name like *Gluc*, you can use double-indexing, with the first index specifying the participant (1 through 5), and the second index specifying the day of the measurement (1 through 3). Under that system, *Gluc[3,2]* indicates the fasting glucose measurement for participant 3 on day 2. To express the array as a formula, we would use the expression *Gluc[i,j]*, which specifies the fasting glucose for the ith subject on the jth day.

Special terms may be used to refer to arrays with one or two dimensions:

» A one-dimensional array is also referred to as a *vector.* But this can be confusing, because the term *vector* is also used in mathematics, physics, and biology to refer to completely different concepts.

» A two-dimensional array is sometimes called a *matrix* (plural: *matrices*). To some, this term implies we are using a set of mathematical rules called *matrix algebra,* and that's not entirely incorrect. Mathematical descriptions of multiple regression (covered in Chapter 17 of this book) make extensive use of matrix algebra. Also, computer software may refer to tabular objects with the term matrix.

Arrays in formulas

If you see an array name in a formula without any subscripts, it usually means that you have to evaluate the formula for each element of the array, and the result is an array with the same number of elements. So, if *Gluc* refers to the array with the five elements 86, 110, 95, 125, and 64, then the expression $2 \times Gluc$ results in an array with each element in the same order multiplied by two: 172, 220, 190, 250, and 128.

When an array name appears in a formula with subscripts, the meaning depends upon the context. It can indicate that the formula is to be evaluated only for some elements of the array, or it can mean that the elements of the array are to be combined in some way before being used (as described in the next section).

Sums and products of the elements of an array

This Greek letter $\sum$ is known in English as capital *sigma*. Though harmless, $\sum$ strikes terror into the hearts of many learners as they encounter it statistics books and articles (not to mention its less common but even scarier cousin Π, also known as capital *pi*). Uppercase *sigma* and *pi* — namely $\sum$ and Π — correspond to the Roman letters S and P, which stand for *Sum* and *Product,* respectively. These symbols are almost always used in front of variables and expressions that represent arrays.

When you see $\sum$ in a formula, just think of it as saying "sum of." Assuming an array named *Gluc* that is comprised of the five elements 86, 110, 95, 125, and 64, you can read the expression $\sum Gluc$ as "the sum of the *Gluc* array" or "sum of *Gluc*." To evaluate it, add all five elements together to get $86 + 110 + 95 + 125 + 64$, which equals 480.

Sometimes the $\sum$ notation is written in a more complex form, where the index variable i is displayed under (or to the right of) the $\sum$ as a subscript of the array name, like this: $\sum_i Gluc_i$. Though its meaning is the same as $\sum Gluc$, you would read it as, "the sum of the *Gluc* array over all values of the index i" (which produces the same result as $\sum Gluc$, which is 480). The subscripted $\sum$ form is helpful in expressing multi-dimensional arrays, when you may want to sum over only one of the dimensions. For example, if Ai,j is a two-dimensional array:

10   15   33
25   8   1

then $\sum_i A_{i,j}$ means that you should sum over the *rows* (the i subscript) to get the one-dimensional array: 35, 23, and 34. Likewise, $\sum_i A_{i,j}$ means to sum across the *columns* (j') to get the one-dimensional array: 58, 34.

Finally, you may see the full-blown official mathematical $\sum$ in all its glory, like this:

$$\sum_{i=a}^{b} Gluc_i,$$

which reads "sum of the *Gluc* array over values of the index i going from a to b, inclusive." So if a was equal to 1, and b was equal to 5, the expression would become:

$$\sum_{i=1}^{5} Gluc_i,$$

which is just another way of summing all the elements, producing 480. But if you wanted to omit the first and last elements of the array from the sum, you could write:

$$\sum_{i=2}^{4} Gluc_i,$$

This expression says to add up only $Gluc_2 + Gluc_3 + Gluc_4$, to get $110 + 95 + 125$, which would equal 330.

$$\sum_{i=2}^{4} Gluc_i = Gluc_2 + Gluc_3 + Gluc_4 = 100 + 95 + 125 = 330$$

Π works just like Σ, except that you multiply instead of add:

$$\prod Gluc = \prod_i Gluc = \prod_{i=1}^{5} Gluc_i = 86 \times 110 \times 95 \times 125 \times 64 = 7,189,600,000$$

SCIENTIFIC NOTATION: THE EASY WAY TO WORK WITH REALLY BIG AND REALLY SMALL NUMBERS

Statistical analyses can generate extremely large as well as extremely small numbers, but humans are most comfortable working with numbers that are in the range of 10s, 100s or 1,000s. Numbers much smaller than 1 (like 0.0000000000005) or much larger than 1,000 (like 5,000,000,000,000) are difficult for humans to comprehend. So for humans, working with extremely large or extremely small numbers is difficult and error-prone (as is working with certain humans).

Fortunately, to make it easier on all of us, we have *scientific notation*, which is a way to represent very small or very large numbers to make the easier for humans to under-stand. Here are three different ways to express the same number in scientific notation: 1.23×10^7 or 1.23E7, or $1.23e + 7$. All three mean "take the number 1.23, and then slide the decimal point seven spaces to the *right* (adding zeros as needed)." To work this out by hand, you could start by adding extra decimal places with zeros, like 1.2300000000. Then, slide the decimal point seven places to the right to get 12300000.000 and clean it up to get 12,300,000.

For very small numbers, the number after the E (or e) is negative, indicating that you need to slide the decimal point to the *left*. For example, 1.23e–9 is the scientific notation for 0.00000000123.

Note: Don't be misled by the "e" that appears in scientific notation — it doesn't stand for the 2.718 constant. You should read it as "times ten raised to the power of."

Chapter **3**

Getting Statistical: A Short Review of Basic Statistics

This chapter provides an overview of basic concepts often taught in a one-term introductory statistics course. These concepts form a conceptual framework for the topics that we cover in greater depth throughout this book. Here, you get the scoop on probability, randomness, populations, samples, statistical inference, hypothesis testing, and nonparametric statistics.

Note: We only introduce the concepts here. They're covered in much greater depth in *Statistics For Dummies* and *Statistics II For Dummies*, both written by Deborah J. Rumsey, PhD, and published by Wiley. Before you proceed, you may want to skim through this chapter to review the topics we cover so you can fill any gaps in your knowledge you may need in order to understand the concepts we introduce.

Taking a Chance on Probability

Defining *probability* is hard to do without using another word that means the same thing (or almost the same thing). Probability is the degree of certainty, the chance, or the likelihood that an event will occur. Unfortunately, if you then try to define *chance* or *likelihood* or *certainty*, you may wind up using the word *probability* in the definition. No worries — we clear up the basics of probability in the following sections. We explain how to define probability as a number and provide a few simple rules of probability. We also define *odds*, and compare odds to probability (because they are not the same thing).

Thinking of probability as a number

Probability describes the *relative frequency* of the occurrence of a particular event, such as getting heads on a coin flip or drawing the ace of spades from a deck of cards. Probability is a number between 0 and 1, although in casual conversation, you often see probabilities expressed as percentages. Probabilities are usually followed by the word *chance* instead of *probability*. For example: If the probability of rain is 0.7, you may hear someone say that there's a 70 percent chance of rain.

Probabilities are numbers between 0 and 1 that can be interpreted this way:

>> **A probability of 0** (or 0 percent) means that the event definitely *won't* occur.

>> **A probability of 1** (or 100 percent) means that the event definitely *will* occur.

>> **A probability between 0 and 1** (such as 0.7) means that — on average, over the long run — the event will occur some predictable part of the time (such as 70 percent of the time).

The probability of one particular event happening out of N equally likely events that could happen is $1/N$. So with a deck of 52 different cards, the probability of drawing any one specific card (such as the ace of spades) compared to any of the other 51 cards is 1/52.

Following a few basic rules of probabilities

Here are three basic rules, or formulas, of probabilities. We call the first one the *not rule*, the second one the *and rule*, and the third one the *or rule*. In the formulas that follow, we use *Prob* as an abbreviation for *probability*, expressed as a fraction (between 0 and 1).

Don't use percentage numbers (0 to 100) in probability formulas.

Even though these rules of probabilities may seem simple when presented here, applying them together in complex situations — as is done in statistics — can get tricky in practice. Here are descriptions of the *not rule*, the *and rule*, and the *or rule*.

>> **The *not rule*:** The probability of some event *X not occurring* is 1 minus the probability of *X occurring*, which can be expressed in an equation like this:

$$\mathrm{Prob}(\mathrm{not}\,X) = 1 - \mathrm{Prob}(X)$$

So if the probability of rain tomorrow is 0.7, then the probability of no rain tomorrow is 1 – 0.7, or 0.3.

>> **The *and rule*:** For two independent events, *X* and *Y*, the probability of event *X* and event *Y* both occurring is equal to the product of the probability of each of the two events occurring independently. Expressed as an equation, the *and rule* looks like this:

$$\mathrm{Prob}(X \text{ and } Y) = \mathrm{Prob}(X) \times \mathrm{Prob}(Y)$$

As an example of the *and rule,* imagine that you flip a fair coin and then draw a card from a deck. What's the probability of getting heads on the coin flip *and also* drawing the ace of spades? The probability of getting heads in a fair coin flip is 1/2, and the probability of drawing the ace of spades from a deck of cards is 1/52. Therefore, the probability of having both of these events occur is 1/2 multiplied by 1/52, which is 1/104, or approximately 0.0096 (which is — as you can see — very unlikely).

>> **The *or rule*:** For two independent events, *X* and *Y*, the probability of *X* or *Y* (or both) occurring is calculated by a more complicated formula, which can be derived from the preceding two rules. Here is the formula:

$$\mathrm{Prob}(X \text{ or } Y) = 1 - (1 - \mathrm{Prob}(X)) \times (1 - \mathrm{Prob}(Y))$$

As an example, suppose that you roll a pair of six-sided dice. What's the probability of rolling a 4 on at least one of the two dice? For one die, there is a 1/6 chance of rolling a 4, which is a probability of about 0.167. (The chance of getting any particular number on the roll of a six-sided die is 1/6, or 0.167.) Using the formula, the probability of rolling a 4 on at least one of the two dice is $1 - (1 - 0.167) \times (1 - 0.167)$, which works out to $1 - 0.833 \times 0.833$, or 0.31, approximately.

The *and* and *or rules* apply only to *independent* events. For example, if there is a 0.7 chance of rain tomorrow, you may make contingency plans. Let's say that if it does not rain, there is a 0.9 chance you will have a picnic rather than stay in a read a book, but if it does rain, there is only a 0.1 chance you will have a picnic rather than stay in a read a book. Because the likelihood of having a picnic is conditional on whether or not it rains, raining and having a picnic are not independent events, and these probability rules cannot apply.

Comparing odds versus probability

You see the word *odds* used a lot in this book, especially in Chapter 13, which is about the fourfold cross-tab (contingency) table, and Chapter 18, which is about logistic regression. The terms *odds* and *probability* are linked, but they actually mean something different. Imagine you hear that a casino customer places a bet because the odds of losing are 2-to-1. If you ask them why they are doing that, they will tell you that such a bet wins — on average — one out of every three times, which is an expression of probability. We will examine how this works using formulas.

REMEMBER

The odds of an event equals the probability of the *event occurring* divided by the probability of that *event not occurring*. We already know we can calculate the probability of the event not occurring by subtracting the probability of the event occurring from 1 (as described in the previous section). With that in mind, you can express odds in terms of probability in the following formula:

$$Odds = Probability/(1 - Probability)$$

With a little algebra (which you don't need to worry about), you can solve this formula for probability as a function of odds:

$$Probability = Odds/(1 + Odds)$$

Returning to the casino example, if the customer says their odds of losing are 2-to-1, they mean 2/1, which equals 2. If we plug the odds of 2 into the second equation, we get 2/(1+2), which is 2/3, which can be rounded to 0.6667. The customer is correct — they will lose two out of every three times, and win one out of every three times, on average.

Table 3-1 shows how probability and odds are related.

REMEMBER

As shown in Table 3-1, for very low probabilities, the odds are very close to the probability. But as probability increases, the odds increase exponentially. By the time probability reaches 0.5, the odds have become 1, and as probability approaches 1, the odds become infinitely large! This definition of odds is consistent with its common-language use. As described earlier with the casino example, if the odds of a horse losing a race are 3:1, that means if you bet on this horse, you have three chances of losing and one chance of winning, for a 0.75 probability of losing.

TABLE 3-1

Probability	Odds	Interpretation
1.0	Infinity	The event will definitely occur.
0.9	9	The event will occur 90% of the time (it is nine times as likely to occur as to not occur).
0.75	3	The event will occur 75% of the time (it is three times as likely to occur as to not occur).
0.5	1.0	The event will occur about half the time (it is equally likely to occur or not occur).
0.25	0.3333	The event will occur 25% of the time (it is one-third as likely to occur as to not occur).
0.1	0.1111	The event will occur 10% of the time (it is 1/9th as likely to occur as to not occur).
0	0	The event definitely will not occur.

TABLE 3-1   **The Relationship between Probability and Odds**

Some Random Thoughts about Randomness

When discussing probability, it is also important to define the word *random*. Like the word *probability*, we use the word *random* all the time, and though we all have some intuitive concept of it, it is hard to define with precise language. In statistics, we often talk about random events and random variables. Random is a term that applies to sampling. In terms of a sequence of random numbers, *random* means the absence of any pattern in the numbers that can be used to predict what the next number will be.

REMEMBER

The important point about the term *random* is that you can't predict a *specific* outcome if a random element is involved. But just because you can't predict a specific outcome with random numbers doesn't mean that you can't make any predictions about these numbers. Statisticians can make reasonably accurate predictions about how a group of random numbers behave collectively, even if they cannot predict a specific outcome when any randomness is involved.

Selecting Samples from Populations

Suppose that we want to know the average systolic blood pressure (SBP) of all the adults in a particular city. Measuring an entire population is called doing a *census*, and if we were to do that and calculate the average SBP in that city, we would have calculated a population *parameter*.

But the idea of doing a census to calculate such a parameter is not practical. Even if we somehow had a list of everyone in the city we could contact, it would be not be feasible to visit all of them and measure their SBP. Nor would it be necessary. Using *inferential statistics*, we could draw a sample from this population, measure their SBPs, and calculate the mean as a sample *statistic*. Using this approach, we could estimate the mean SBP of the population.

But drawing a sample that is representative of the background population depends on probability (as well as other factors). In the following sections, we explain why samples are valid but imperfect reflections of the population from which they're drawn. We also describe the basics of probability distributions. For a more extensive discussion of sampling, see Chapter 6.

Recognizing that sampling isn't perfect

As used in epidemiologic research, the terms *population* and *sample* can be defined this way:

>> **Population:** All individuals in a defined target population. For example, this may be all individuals in the United States living with a diagnosis of Type II diabetes.

>> **Sample:** A subset of the target population actually selected to participate in a study. For example, this could be patients in the United States living with Type II diabetes who visit a particular clinic and meet other qualification criteria for the study.

Any sample, no matter how carefully it is selected, is only an imperfect reflection of the population. This is due to the unavoidable occurrence of random sampling fluctuations called *sampling error*.

To illustrate sampling error, we obtained a data set containing the number of private and public airports in each of the United States and the District of Columbia in 2011 from Statista (available at `https://www.statista.com/statistics/185902/us-civil-and-joint-use-airports-2008/`). We started by making a *histogram* of the entire data set, which would be considered a census because it contains the entire population of states. A histogram is a visualization to determine the distribution of numerical data, and is described more extensively in Chapter 9. Here, we briefly summarize how to read a histogram:

>> A histogram looks like a bar chart. It is specifically crafted to display a distribution.

>> The histogram's y-axis represents the number (or *frequency*) of individuals in the data that fall in the numerical ranges (known as *classes*) of the value being charted, which are listed across the x-axis. In this case, the y-axis would represent number of states falling in each class.

>> This histogram's x-axis represents classes, or numerical ranges of the value being charted, which is in this case is number of airports.

We first made a histogram of the census, then we took four random samples of 20 states and made a histogram of each of the samples. Figure 3-1 shows the results.

FIGURE 3-1:
Distribution of number of private and public airports in 2011 in the population (of 50 states and the District of Columbia), and four different samples of 20 states from the same population.

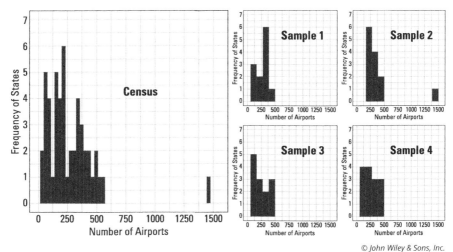

© John Wiley & Sons, Inc.

As shown in Figure 3-1, when comparing the sample distributions to the distribution of the population using the histograms, you can see there are differences. Sample 2 looks much more like the population than Sample 4. However, they are all valid samples in that they were randomly selected from the population. The samples are an approximation to the true population distribution. In addition, the mean and standard deviation of the samples are likely close to the mean and standard deviation of the population, but not equal to it. (For a refresher on mean and standard deviation, see Chapter 9.) These characteristics of sampling error — where valid samples from the population are almost always somewhat different than the population — are true of any random sample.

Digging into probability distributions

As described in the preceding section, samples differ from populations because of random fluctuations. Because these random fluctuations fall into patterns, statisticians can describe *quantitatively* how these random fluctuations behave using mathematical equations called *probability distribution functions.* Probability distribution functions describe how likely it is that random fluctuations will exceed any given magnitude. A probability distribution can be represented in several ways:

>> **As a mathematical equation** that calculates the chance that a fluctuation will be of a certain magnitude. Using calculus, this function can be *integrated,* which means turned into another related function that calculates the probability that a fluctuation will be at least as large as a certain magnitude.

>> **As a graph of the distribution,** which looks and works much like a histogram.

>> **As a table of values** indicating how likely it is that random fluctuations will exceed a certain magnitude.

In the following sections, we break down two types of distributions: those that describe fluctuations in your data, and those that you encounter when performing statistical tests.

Distributions that describe your data

Here are some common distributions that describe the random fluctuations found in data analyzed by biostatisticians:

>> **Normal:** The familiar, bell-shaped, *normal* distribution is probably the most common distribution you will encounter. As an example, systolic blood pressure (SBP) is found to follow a normal distribution in human populations.

>> **Log-normal:** The *log-normal* distribution is also called a *skewed* distribution. This distribution describes many laboratory results, such as enzymes and antibody titers, where most of the population tests on the low end of the scale. It is also the distribution seen for lengths of hospital stays, where most stays are 0 or 1 days, and the rest are longer.

>> **Binomial:** The *binomial* distribution describes proportions, and represents the likelihood that a value will take one of two independent values (as whether an event occurs or does not occur). As an example, in a class held regularly where students can only pass or fail, the proportion who fail will follow a binomial distribution.

>> **Poisson:** The *Poisson* distribution describes the number of occurrences of sporadic random events (rather than the binomial distribution, which is for more common events). Examples of where the Poisson distribution is used in biostatistics is where the events are not as common, such as deaths from specific cancers each year.

Chapter 24 describes these and other distribution functions in more detail, and you also encounter them throughout this book.

Distributions important to statistical testing

Some probability distributions don't describe fluctuations in *data values* but instead describe fluctuations in *calculated values* as part of a statistical test (when you are calculating what's called a *test statistic*). Distributions of test statistics include the Student t, chi-square, and Fisher F distributions. Test statistics are used to obtain the p values that result from the tests. See "Getting the language down" later in this chapter for a definition of p values.

Introducing Statistical Inference

Statistical inference is where you draw conclusions (or *infer*) about a population based on estimations from a sample from that population. The challenge posed by statistical inference theory is to extract real information from the *noise* in our data. This noise is made up of these random fluctuations as well as measurement error. This very broad area of statistical theory can be subdivided into two topics: statistical *estimation* theory and statistical *decision* theory.

Statistical estimation theory

Statistical estimation theory focuses how to improve the accuracy and precision of metrics calculated from samples. It provides methods to estimate how precise your measurements are to the true population value, and to calculate the range of values from your sample that's likely to include the true population value. The following sections review the fundamentals of statistical estimation theory.

Accuracy and precision

Whenever you make an estimation or measurement, your estimated or measured value can differ from the truth by being inaccurate, imprecise, or both.

>> **Accuracy** refers to how close your measurement tends to come to the *true value,* without being systematically biased in one direction or another. Such a bias is called a *systematic error*.

>> **Precision** refers to how close several replicate measurements come to *each other* — that is, how reproducible they are.

In estimation, both random and systematic errors reduce precision and accuracy. You cannot control random error, but you can control systematic error by improving your measurement methods. Consider the four different situations that can arise if you take multiple measurements from the same population:

>> **High precision and high accuracy** is an ideal result. It means that each measurement you take is close to the others, and all of these are close to the true population value.

>> **High precision and low accuracy** is not as ideal. This is where repeat measurements tend to be close to one another, but are not that close to the true value. This situation can when you ask survey respondents to self-report their weight. The average of the answers may be similar survey after survey, but the answers may be inaccurately lower than truth. Although it is easy to predict what the next measurement will be, the measurement is less useful if it does not help you know the true value. This indicates you may want to improve your measurement methods.

>> **Low precision and high accuracy** is also not as ideal. This is where the measurements are not that close to one another, but are not that far from the true population value. In this case, you may trust your measurements, but find that it is hard to predict what the next one will be due to random error.

>> **Low precision and low accuracy** shows the least ideal result, which is a low level of both precision and accuracy. This can only be improved through improving measurement methods.

Sampling distributions and standard errors

REMEMBER

The *standard error* (abbreviated SE) is one way to indicate the level of precision about an estimate or measurement from a sample. The SE tells you how much the estimate or measured value may vary if you were to repeat the experiment or the measurement many times using a different random sample from the same population each time, and recording the value you obtained each time. This collection of numbers would have a spread of values, forming what is called the *sampling distribution* for that variable. The SE is a measure of the width of the sampling distribution, as described in Chapter 9.

Fortunately, you don't have to repeat the entire experiment a large number of times to calculate the SE. You can usually estimate the SE using data from a single experiment by using confidence intervals.

Confidence intervals

An important application of statistical estimation theory in biostatistics is calculating confidence intervals. Confidence intervals provide another way to indicate the precision of an estimate or measurement from a sample. A *confidence interval* (CI) is an interval placed around an estimated value to represent the range in which you strongly believe the true value for that variable lies. How wide you make this interval is dependent on a numeric expression of how strongly you believe the true value lie within it, which is called the *confidence level* (CL). If calculated properly, your stated confidence interval should encompass the true value a percentage of the time at least equal to the stated confidence level. In fact, if you are indeed making an estimate, it is best practices to report that estimate along with confidence intervals. As an example, you could express the 95 percent CI of the mean ages of a sample of graduating master's degree students from a university this way: 32 years (95 percent CI 28 – 34 years).

At this point, you may be wondering how to calculate CIs. If so, turn to Chapter 10, where we describe how to calculate confidence intervals around means, proportions, event rates, regression coefficients, and other quantities you measure, count, or calculate.

Statistical decision theory

Statistical decision theory is a large branch of statistics that includes many subtopics. It encompasses all the famous (and many not-so-famous) statistical tests of significance, including the Student t tests and the analysis of variance (otherwise known as ANOVA). Both t tests and ANOVAs are covered in Chapter 11. Statistical decision theory also includes chi-square tests (explained in Chapter 12) and Pearson correlation tests (included in Chapter 16), to name a few.

REMEMBER

In its most basic form, statistical decision theory deals with using a sample to make a decision as to whether a real effect is taking place in the background population. We use the word *effect* throughout this book, which can refer to different concepts in different circumstances. Examples of effects include the following:

>> **The average value of a measurement may be different in one group compared to another.** For example, obese patients may have higher systolic blood pressure (SBP) measurements on average compared to non-obese patients. Another example is that the mean SBP of two groups of hypertensive patients may be different because each group is using a different drug — Drug A compared to Drug B. The difference between means in these groups is considered the *effect size*.

>> **The average value of a measurement may be different from zero** (or from some other specified value). For example, the average reduction in pain level measurement in surgery patients from post-surgery compared to 30 days later may have an effect that is different from zero (or so we would hope)!

>> **Two numerical variables may be associated** (also called *correlated*). For example, the taller people are on average, the more they weigh. When two variables like height and weight are associated in this way, the effect is called correlation, and is typically quantified by the Pearson correlation coefficient (described in Chapter 15).

Honing In on Hypothesis Testing

The theory of statistical hypothesis testing was developed in the early 20th century. Among other uses, it was designed to apply the scientific method to data sampled from populations. In the following sections, we explain the steps of hypothesis testing, the potential results, and possible errors that can be made when interpreting a statistical test. We also define and describe the relationships between power, sample size, and effect size in testing.

Getting the language down

Here are some of the most common terms used in hypothesis testing:

>> **Null hypothesis (abbreviated H_0):** The assertion that any apparent effect you see in your data is not evidence of a true effect in the population, but is merely the result of random fluctuations.

>> **Alternate hypothesis (abbreviated H_1 or H_{Alt}):** The assertion that there indeed is evidence in your data of a true effect in the population over and above what would be attributable to random fluctuations.

>> **Significance test:** A calculation designed to determine whether H_0 can reasonably explain what you see in your data or not.

>> **Significance:** The conclusion that random fluctuations alone can't account for the size of the effect you observe in your data. In this case, H_0 must be false, so you accept H_{Alt}.

>> **Statistic:** A number that you obtain or calculate from your sample.

>> **Test statistic:** A number calculated from your sample that is part of performing a statistical test. It can be for the purpose of testing H_0. In general, the test

statistic is usually calculated as the ratio of a number that measures the size of the effect (the signal) divided by a number that measures the size of the random fluctuations (the noise).

>> **p value:** The probability or likelihood that random fluctuations alone (in the absence of any true effect in the population) can produce the effect observed in your sample (or, at least as large as the effect you observe in your sample). The p value is the probability of random fluctuations making the test statistic at least as large as what you calculate from your sample (or, more precisely, at least as far away from H_0 in the direction of H_{Alt}).

>> **Type I error:** Choosing that H_{Alt} is correct when in fact, no true effect above random fluctuations is present.

>> **Alpha (α):** The probability of making a Type I error.

>> **Type II error:** Choosing that H_0 is correct when in fact there is indeed a true effect present that rises above random fluctuations.

>> **Beta (β):** The probability of making a Type II error.

>> **Power:** The same as $1 - \beta$, which is probability of choosing H_{Alt} as correct when in fact there is a true effect above random fluctuations present.

Testing for significance

REMEMBER

All the common statistical significance tests, including the Student t test, chi-square, and ANOVA, work on the same general principle. They compare the size of the effect seen in your sample against the size of the random fluctuations present in your sample. We describe individual statistical significance tests in detail throughout this book. Here, we describe the generic steps that underlie all the common statistical tests of significance.

1. **Reduce your raw sample data down into a single number called a *test statistic.***

    Each test statistic has its own formula, but in general, the test statistic represents the magnitude of the effect you're looking for relative to the magnitude of the random noise in your data. For example, the test statistic for the unpaired Student t test for comparing means between two groups is calculated as a fraction:

    $$\text{Student t statistic} = \frac{\text{Mean of Group 1} - \text{Mean of Group 2}}{\text{Standard Error of the Difference}}$$

    The numerator is a measure of the effect, which is the mean difference between the two groups. And the denominator is a measure of the random noise in your sample, which is represented by the spread of values within each group. Thinking about this fraction philosophically, you will notice that the larger the observed effect is (numerator) relative to the amount of random noise in your data (denominator), the larger the Student t statistic will be.

2. **Determine how likely (or unlikely) it is for random fluctuations to produce a test statistic as large as the one you actually got from your data.**

   To do this, you use complicated formulas to generate the test statistic. Once the test statistic is calculated, it is placed on a probability distribution. The distribution describes how much the test statistic bounces around if only random fluctuations are present (that is, if H_0 is true). For example, the Student T statistic is placed on the Student T distribution. The result from placing the test statistic on a distribution is known as the p value, which is described in the next section.

Understanding the meaning of "p value" as the result of a test

The end result of a statistical significance test is a *p value*, which represents the probability that random fluctuations alone could have generated results. If that probability is medium to high, the interpretation is that the null hypothesis, or H_0, is correct. If that probability is very low, then the interpretation is that we reject the null hypothesis, and accept the alternate hypothesis (H_{Alt}) as correct. If you find yourself rejecting the null, you can say that the effect seen in your data is *statistically significant*.

REMEMBER

How small should a p value be before we reject the null hypothesis? The technical answer is this is arbitrary and depends on how much of a risk you're willing to take of being fooled by random fluctuations (that is, of making a Type I error). But in practice, the value of 0.05 has become accepted as a reasonable criterion for declaring significance, meaning we fail to reject the null for p values of 0.05 or greater. If you adopt the criterion that p must be less than 0.05 to reject the null hypothesis and declare your effect statistically significant, this is known as setting alpha (α) to 0.05, and will establish your likelihood of making a Type I error to no more than 5 percent.

Examining Type I and Type II errors

The outcome of a statistical test is a decision to either accept the H_0, or reject H_0 in favor of H_{Alt}. Because H_0 pertains to the population's true value, the effect you see in your sample is either true or false for the population from which you are sampling. You may never know what that truth is, but an objective truth is out there nonetheless.

The truth can be one of two answers — the effect is there, or the effect is not there. Also, your conclusion from your sample will be one of two answers — the effect is there, or the effect is not there.

REMEMBER

These factors can be combined into the following four situations:

>> **Your test is not statistically significant, and H₀ is true.** This is an ideal situation because the conclusion of your test matches the truth. If you were testing the mean difference in effect between Drug A and Drug B, and in truth there was no difference in effect, if your test also was not statistically significant, this would be an ideal result.

>> **Your test is not statistically significant, but H₀ is false.** In this situation, the interpretation of your test is wrong and does not match truth. Imagine testing the difference in effect between Drug C and Drug D, where in truth, Drug C had more effect than Drug D. If your test was not statistically significant, it would be the wrong result. This situation is called *Type II error*. The probability of making a Type II error is represented by the Greek letter beta (β).

>> **Your test is statistically significant, and H_Alt is true.** This is another situation where you have an ideal result. Imagine we are testing the difference in effect between Drug C and Drug D, where in truth, Drug C has more of an effect. If the test was statistically significant, the interpretation would be to reject H₀, which would be correct.

>> **Your test is statistically significant, but H_Alt is false.** This is another situation where your test interpretation does not match the truth. If there was in truth no difference in effect between Drug A and Drug B, but your test was statistically significant, it would be incorrect. This situation is called Type I error. The probability of making a Type I error is represented by the Greek letter alpha (α).

TIP

We discussed setting $\alpha = 0.05$, meaning that you are willing to tolerate a Type I error rate of 5 percent. Theoretically, you could change this number. You can increase your chance of making a Type I error by increasing your α from 0.05 to a higher number like 0.10, which is done in rare situations. But if you reduce your α to number smaller than 0.05 — like 0.01, or 0.001 — then you run the risk of never calculating a test statistic with a p value that is statistically significant, even if a true effect is present. If α is set too low, it means you are being very picky about accepting a true effect suggested by the statistics in your sample. If a drug really is effective, you want to get a result that you interpret as statistically significant when you test it. What this shows is that you need to strike a balance between the likelihood of committing Type I and Type II errors — between the α and β error rates. If you make α too small, β will become too large, and vice versa.

At this point, you may be wondering, "Is there any way to keep both Type I and Type II error small?" The answer is yes, and it involves power, which is described in the next section.

Grasping the power of a test

REMEMBER

The power of a statistical test is the chance that it will come out statistically significant when it should — that is, when the alternative hypothesis is really true. Power is a probability and is very often expressed as a percentage. Beta (β) is the chance of getting a nonsignificant result when the alternative hypothesis is true, so you see that power and β are related mathematically: Power $= 1 - \beta$.

The power of any statistical test depends on several factors:

>> The α level you've established for the test — that is, the chance you're willing to accept making a Type I error (usually 0.05)

>> The actual magnitude of the effect in the population, relative to the amount of noise in the data

>> The size of your sample

Power, sample size, effect size relative to noise, and α level can't all be varied independently. They're interrelated, because they're connected and constrained by a mathematical relationship involving all four quantities.

This relationship between power, sample size, effect size relative to noise, and α level is often very complicated, and it can't always be written down explicitly as a formula. But the relationship does exist. As evidence of this, for any particular type of test, theoretically, you can determine any one of the four quantities if you know the other three. So for each statistical test, there are four different ways to do power calculations, with each way calculating one of the four quantities from arbitrarily specified values of the other three. (We have more to say about this in Chapter 5, where we describe practical issues that arise during the design of research studies.) In the following sections, we describe the relationships between power, sample size, and effect size, and briefly review how you can perform power calculations.

Power, sample size, and effect size relationships

REMEMBER

The α level of a statistical test is usually set to 0.05 unless there are special considerations, which we describe in Chapter 5. After you specify the value of α, you can display the relationship between α and the other three variables — power, sample size, and effect size — in several ways. The next three graphs show these relationships for the Student t test as an example, because graphs for other statistical tests are generally similar to these:

>> **Power versus sample size, for various effect sizes:** For all statistical tests, *power always increases as the sample size increases,* if the other variables including α level and effect size are held constant. This relationship is illustrated in Figure 3-2. "Eff" is the effect size — the between-group difference divided by the within-group standard deviation.

Small samples will not be able to produce significant results unless the effect size is very large. Conversely, statistical tests using extremely large samples including many thousands of participants are almost always statistically significant unless the effect size is near zero. In epidemiological studies, which often involve hundreds of thousands of subjects, statistical tests tend to produce extremely small (and therefore extremely significant) p values, even when the effect size is so small that it's of no practical importance (meaning it is clinically insignificant).

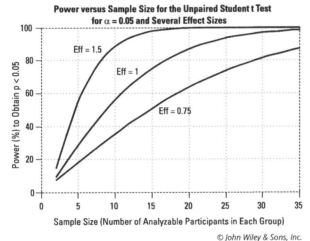

FIGURE 3-2:
The power of a statistical test increases as the sample size and the effect size increase.

>> **Power versus effect size, for various sample sizes:** For all statistical tests, *power always increases as the effect size increases,* if other variables including the α level and sample size are held constant. This relationship is illustrated in Figure 3-3. "N" is the number of participants in each group.

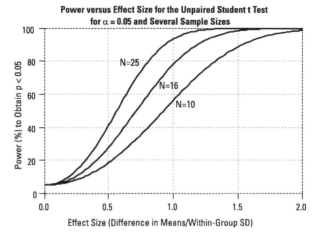

FIGURE 3-3:
The power of a statistical test increases as the effect size increases.

© John Wiley & Sons, Inc.

For very large effect sizes, the power approaches 100 percent. For very small effect sizes, you may think the power of the test would approach zero, but you can see from Figure 3-3 that it doesn't go down all the way to zero. It actually approaches the α level of the test. (Keep in mind that the α level of the test is the probability of the test producing a significant result when no effect is truly present.)

>> **Sample size versus effect size, for various values of power:** For all statistical tests, *sample size and effect size are inversely related,* if other variables including α level and power are held constant. Small effects can be detected only with large samples, and large effects can often be detected with small samples. This relationship is illustrated in Figure 3-4.

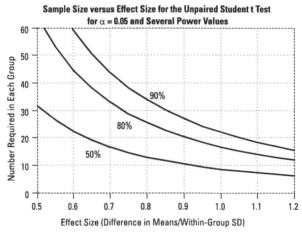

FIGURE 3-4:
Smaller effects need larger samples.

© John Wiley & Sons, Inc.

This inverse relationship between sample size and effect size takes on a very simple mathematical form (at least to a good approximation): The required sample size is inversely proportional to the square of the effect size that can be detected. Or, equivalently, the detectable effect size is inversely proportional to the square root of the sample size. So, quadrupling your sample size allows you to detect effect sizes only one-half as large.

How to do power calculations

TIP

Power calculations can be an important step in the design of a research study because they estimate how many individuals you will need in your sample to achieve the objectives of your study. You don't want your study to be underpowered, because then it will have a high risk of missing real effects. You also don't want your study to be overpowered, because then it's larger, costlier, and more time-consuming than necessary. You need to include a power/sample-size calculation for research proposals submitted for funding and for any protocol you submit to a human research ethical review board for approval. You can perform power calculations using several different methods:

» **Computer software:** The larger statistics packages such as SPSS, SAS, and R enable you to perform a wide range of power calculations. Chapter 4 describes these different packages. There are also programs specially designed for conducting power calculations, such as PS and G*Power, which are described in Chapter 4.

» **Web pages:** Many of the more common power calculations can be performed online using web-based calculators. An example of one of these is here: https://clincalc.com/stats/samplesize.aspx.

» **Rules of thumb:** Some approximate sample-size calculations are simple enough to do on a scrap of paper or even in your head! You find some of these in Chapter 25.

Going Outside the Norm with Nonparametric Statistics

All statistical tests are derived on the basis of some assumptions about your data. Most of the classical significance tests, including Student t tests, analysis of variance (ANOVA), and regression tests, assume that your data are distributed according to some classical sampling distribution, which is also called a *frequency distribution*. Most tests assume your data has a normal distribution (see

Chapter 24). Because the classic distribution functions are all written as mathematical expressions involving parameters (like means and standard deviation), they're called *parametric* distribution functions.

Parametric tests assume that your data conforms to a parametric distribution function. Because the normal distribution is the most common statistical distribution, the term *parametric test* is often used to mean a test that assumes normally distributed data. But sometimes your data don't follow a parametric distribution. For example, it may be very noticeably skewed, as shown in Figure 3-5a.

Sometimes, you may be able to perform a mathematical transformation of your data to make it more normally distributed. For example, many variables that have a skewed distribution can be turned into normally distributed numbers by taking logarithms, as shown in Figure 3-5b. If, by trial and error, you can find some kind of transformation that normalizes your data, you can run the classical tests on the transformed data, as described in Chapter 9.

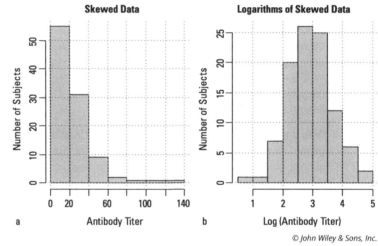

FIGURE 3-5: Skewed data (a) can sometimes be turned into normally distributed data (b) by taking logarithms.

© John Wiley & Sons, Inc.

WARNING If you transform your data to get it to assume a normal distribution, any analyses done on it will need to be "untransformed" to be interpreted. For example, if you have a data set of patients with different lengths of stay in a hospital, you will likely have skewed data. If you log-transform these data so that they are normally distributed, then generate statistics (like calculate a mean), you will need to do an inverse log transformation on the result before you interpret it.

But sometimes your data are not normally distributed, and for whatever reason, you give up on trying to do a parametric test. Maybe you can't find a good transformation for your data, or maybe you don't want to have to undo the transformation in order to do your interpretation, or maybe you simply have too small of a sample size to be able to perceive a clear parametric distribution when you make a histogram. Fortunately, statisticians have developed other tests that you can use that are not based on the assumption your data are normally distributed, or have any parametric distribution. Unsurprisingly, these are called *nonparametric tests*. Most of the common classic parametric tests have nonparametric counterparts you can use as an alternative. As you may expect, the most widely known and commonly used nonparametric tests are those that correspond to the most widely known and commonly used classical tests. Some of these are shown in Table 3-2.

TABLE 3-2

Nonparametric Counterparts of Classic Tests

Classic Parametric Test	Nonparametric Equivalent
One-group or paired Student t test (see Chapter 11)	Wilcoxon Signed-Ranks test
Two-group Student t test (see Chapter 11)	Mann-Whitney U test
One-way ANOVA (see Chapter 11)	Kruskal-Wallis test
Pearson Correlation test (see Chapter 15)	Spearman Rank Correlation test

Most nonparametric tests involve first sorting your data values, from lowest to highest, and recording the *rank* of each measurement. Ranks are like class ranks in school, where the person with the highest grade point average (GPA) is ranked number 1, and the person with the next highest GPA is ranked number 2 and so on. Ranking forces each individual to be separated from the next by one unit of rank. In data, the lowest value has a rank of 1, the next highest value has a rank of 2, and so on. All subsequent calculations are done with these ranks rather than with the actual data values. However, using ranks instead of the actual data loses information, so you should avoid using nonparametric tests if your data qualify for parametric methods.

Although nonparametric tests don't assume normality, they do make certain assumptions about your data. For example, many nonparametric tests assume that you don't have any *tied values* in your data set (in other words, no two participants have exactly the same values). Most parametric tests incorporate adjustments for the presence of ties, but this weakens the test and makes the results less exact.

TIP

Even in descriptive statistics, the common parameters have nonparametric counterparts. Although means and standard deviations can be calculated for any set of numbers, they're most useful for summarizing data when the numbers are normally distributed. When you don't know how the numbers are distributed, medians and quartiles are much more useful as measures of central tendency and dispersion (see Chapter 9 for details).

2

Examining Tools and Processes

Select statistical software to use from the commercial and free choices available, and discover other ways to do statistical calculations, such as using web-based programs and specialized software for sample-size calculations.

Understand human research — how biostatistics influences the design and execution of clinical trials and how treatments are developed and approved.

Grasp different ways of taking samples from populations to increase the accuracy of the statistical estimates you make.

Consider different study designs used in epidemiologic research and see how research design connects to the practice of biostatistics.

Chapter **4**

Counting on Statistical Software

B efore statistical software, complex regressions we could do in theory were too complicated to do manually using real datasets. It wasn't until the 1960s with the development of the SAS suite of statistical software that analysts were able to do these calculations. As technology advanced, different types of software were developed, including open-source software and web-based software.

As you may imagine, all these choices led to competition and confusion among analysts, students, and organizations utilizing this software. Organizations wonder what statistical packages to implement. Professors wonder which ones to teach, and students wonder which ones to learn. The purpose of this chapter is to help you make informed choices about statistical software. We describe and provide guidance regarding the practical choices you have today among the statistical software available. We discuss choosing between:

» Commercial software, such as SAS and SPSS

» Open-source software, such as R and Python

» Free software applications, such as G*Power and PS (Power and Sample Size Calculation)

We also provide guidance on how to choose between code-based and non–code-based software, and end by providing advice on cloud data storage.

Considering the Evolution of Statistical Software

The first widespread *commercial* statistical software invented is called SAS, and it is still used today. SAS was developed originally in the 1960s and 1970s to run on mainframe computers. Around 2000, SAS was adapted to personal computers (known as PC SAS), adding a user-friendly graphical user interface (GUI). During the growth of SAS, other commercial statistical packages appeared, the most popular being IBM's SPSS. SAS continues to be the go-to program for big data analysis, where analysts can easily access large datasets from servers. In contrast, SPSS continues to be used on a personal computer like PC SAS.

If you were to take a college statistics course in the year 2000, your course would have likely taught either SAS or SPSS. Professors would have made either SPSS or SAS available to you for free or for a nominal license fee from your college bookstore. If you take a college statistics course today, you may be in the same situation — or, you may find yourself learning so-called *open-source* statistical software packages. The most common are R and Python. This software is free to the user and downloadable online because it is built by the user community, not a company.

As the Internet evolved, more options became available for statistical software. In addition to the existing stand-alone applications described earlier, specialized statistical apps were developed that only perform one or a small collection of specific statistical functions (such as G*Power and PS, which are for calculating sample sizes). Similarly, web-based online calculators were developed, which are typically programmed to do one particular function (such as calculate a chi-square statistic and p value from counts of data, as described in Chapter 12). Some web pages feature a collection of such calculators.

Comparing Commercial to Open-Source Software

Before 2010, if an organization performed statistical analysis as part of its core function, it needed to purchase commercial statistical software like SAS or SPSS. Advantages of implementing commercial software include the ability to perform many statistical functions, technical support from the software company, and the expectation that the software will remain in use in the future as the company continues to support and upgrade it.

However, organizations today are hesitant to adopt commercial software when they can instead use open-source software like R or Python. Admittedly, even though it is free of charge, there are many downsides to open-source software. First, you need to hire analysts who know how to use it so well that they can figure out what to do when there's a problem because open-source software does not have tech support. Next, you need to hire a lot more analysts than you would with commercial software because a lot of their work will be in trying to customize the software for your use and keep it updated so that your organization runs smoothly.

So, why are new organizations today hesitant to adopt commercial software when open-source software has so many downsides? The main reason is that the old advantages of commercial software are not as true anymore. SAS and SPSS are expensive programs, but they have much of the same functionality as open-source R and Python, which are free. In some cases, analysts prefer the open-source application to the commercial application because they can customize it more easily to their setting. Also, it is not clear that commercial software is innovating ahead of open-source software. Organizations do not want to get entangled with expensive commercial software that eventually starts to perform worse than free open-source alternatives!

TIP

As a result, many organizations use both commercial and open-source statistical software in *integrated application pipelines*. Therefore, it is important to be comfortable evaluating and using various commercial software, even if open-source options are becoming more popular.

Checking Out Commercial Software

In the following sections, we discuss the most popular commercial statistical software available currently.

SAS

SAS is the oldest commercial software currently available. It started out as having two main components — *Base SAS* and *SAS Stat* — that provided the most used statistical calculations. However, today, it has grown to include many additional components and sublanguages. SAS has always been so expensive that only organizations with a significant budget can afford to purchase and use it. However, because individual learners need to be able to practice SAS even if they cannot afford it, SAS developed a free, online version called SAS OnDemand for Academics (ODA) that is available at `https://welcome.oda.sas.com`.

Originally, SAS ran as a command-prompt software without a guided user interface, or GUI, which came later in the 2000s when PC SAS was invented. In the original SAS, the user would gain access to datasets in SAS format that resided on a SAS server in the same environment. The user would write code files using SAS code and run these files against the SAS data. This action would produce a log file that explained how the code was executed and reported any errors. It would also produce output that provided the results of the statistical procedures.

Today, the experience of using SAS has been modernized. In PC SAS and SAS ODA, it is easy to view code, log, and output files in different windows and switch back and forth between them. It is also easier to import data into and out of the SAS environment and create integrated application pipelines involving the SAS environment. The new commercial cloud-based version of SAS called Viya is intended to be used with data stored in the cloud rather than on SAS servers (see the later section "Storing Data in the Cloud" for more).

SAS is entrenched in some industries, such as pharmaceutical, insurance, and banking, because SAS has historically been the only program powerful enough to handle the size of their datasets. Those settings traditionally used SAS servers for data storage. Now, this practice is being challenged because other analytic options may look more appealing than what SAS has to offer (see the section "Focusing on open-source and free software"). In addition, many companies are having trouble maintaining their old-fashioned SAS servers and want to move their data to cloud storage. These industries are looking for SAS users to help them modernize their operations.

TIP

Students often find that SAS is challenging to learn when compared to other statistical software, especially open-source software. Why learn legacy commercial software like SAS today, when it is so much harder to learn than other software? The answer is that SAS is still standard software in some domains, such as pharmaceutical research. This means that even if those organizations choose to eventually migrate away from SAS, they will need to hire SAS users to help with the migration.

SPSS

SPSS was invented more recently than SAS and runs in a fundamentally different way. SPSS does not expect you to have a data server the way SAS does. Instead, SPSS runs as a stand-alone program like PC SAS, and expects you to import data into it for analysis. Therefore, SAS is more likely to be used in a team environment, while SPSS tends to have individual users.

Like SAS, SPSS produces output, but unlike SAS, SPSS is typically manipulated by the user through selections in menus rather than through writing code and running it. SPSS produces one long output file that includes all the output from each SPSS session. In the output file, SPSS includes code it writes automatically from the way you manipulate the menu. Therefore, like with SAS, it is possible to save SPSS code files and output files and rerun the same code later. SPSS is available from IBM's website at www.ibm.com/products/spss-statistics/pricing.

Microsoft Excel

Microsoft Excel has been used in some domains for statistical calculations, but it is difficult to use with large datasets. Excel has built-in functions for summarizing data (such as calculating means and standard deviations talked about in Chapter 9). It also has common probability distribution functions such as Student t (Chapter 11) and chi-square (Chapter 12). You can even do straight-line regression (Chapter 16), as well as more extensive analyses available through add-ins.

WARNING

These functions can come in handy when doing quick calculations or learning about statistics, but using Excel for statistical projects evokes many challenges. Using a spreadsheet for statistics means your data are stored in the same place as your calculations, creating privacy concerns (and a mess!). So, while Excel can be helpful mathematically — especially when making extra calculations based on estimates in printed statistical output — it is not a good practice to use it for extensive statistical projects.

Microsoft Excel is available in different formats, including both downloadable and web based. Purchase it from Microsoft at www.microsoft.com.

Online analytics platforms

A more modern approach to statistical software is to create an online platform known as an *analytics suite* that allows you to connect to data sources and conduct analytics online. Here are a few popular online platforms:

>> **Tableau:** Tableau is known for being able to provide real-time data-driven graphical displays online, and organizations may adopt Tableau to develop customized dashboards. It is available at www.tableau.com.

>> **GraphPad:** This online platform provides analytics support, such as curve-fitting, and provides a graphical suite called Prism. It is available at www.graphpad.com.

REMEMBER

There are both advantages and disadvantages to using these online commercial platforms. Advantages include that online software tends to follow a cheaper subscription paid monthly or annually, and you get continuous upgrades because the software is web based. The main downside is these platforms have a high learning curve and require a lot of work to fully adopt, so you have to ask yourself if it makes sense with your project.

Focusing on Open-Source and Free Software

Open-source software refers to software that has been developed and supported by a user community. Although open-source software has licenses, they are typically free but require you to adhere to certain policies when using the software. In this section, we talk about the two most popular open-source statistical software packages: R and Python.

Open-source software

The two most popular and extensive open-source statistical programs are R and Python.

>> **R:** R is statistical software that has been developed and is maintained by the R user community. It has two interfaces: R GUI, which looks similar to PC SAS and SPSS, and RStudio, which is an integrated development environment (IDE). Analysts prefer to use RStudio when developing graphical displays for the web, while R GUI is fine for most statistical work. To run R, you download and install the base application. Then, for specified functions not included in the base application, you install additional R *packages*. Like with PC SAS, in R, you import or connect to datasets, develop and save code files to run on those datasets, and produce output you can save. Base R, R packages, and documentation are available on the Comprehensive R Archive Network (CRAN) server at https://cran.r-project.org.

>> **Python:** Python is an open-source programming language that is often used to analyze data. As with R, Python is developed and maintained by its own user community and runs in a similar way. Although you still develop code that runs against datasets in the Python environment, the Python and R code are different. Instead of packages as in R, Python has *libraries*. Python is available at www.python.org/downloads.

TIP

Students often wonder what the differences are between R and Python, and which one to learn. They are essentially the same, although scientific disciplines have leaned toward adopting R, and engineering disciplines have leaned toward Python. Many students find themselves easily learning both.

Other free statistical software

Other statistical software packages are free, but they are not technically open-source — meaning they were not developed by an open-source community, and they are not licensed the same way.

Software that performs many functions

This section provides examples of free software that performs many functions like SAS and R.

>> **OpenStat** and **LazStats** are free statistical programs developed by Dr. Bill Miller that use menus that resemble SPSS. Dr. Miller provides several excellent manuals and textbooks that support both programs. OpenStat and LazStats are available at `https://openstat.info`.

>> **Epi Info** was developed by the United States Centers for Disease Control to acquire, manage, analyze, and display the results of epidemiological research. What makes it different than other statistical software is that it contains modules for creating survey forms and collecting data. Epi Info is available at `https://www.cdc.gov/epiinfo/index.html`.

Software for calculating sample size

Biostatisticians frequently encounter the problem of estimating sample size. The following are two free applications we recommend for performing sample-size calculations:

>> **G*Power:** G*Power was developed at the Universität Düsseldorf and is used to estimate the sample size for many different types of tests. Throughout this book, when we discuss sample-size calculations, we give you advice on how to do them using G*Power. G*Power is available at `www.psychologie.hhu.de/arbeitsgruppen/allgemeine-psychologie-und-arbeitspsychologie/gpower`. To use the program, you download it from this website and install it on your computer.

>> **PS (Power and Sample Size Calculation):** The PS program was developed by W.D. Dupont and W.D. Plummer at Vanderbilt University. Like G*Power, you download the application from its website and install it on your computer. The PS interface is similar to that of G*Power. PS is available at https://biostat. app.vumc.org/wiki/Main/PowerSampleSize.

Choosing Between Code-based and Non–Code-Based Methods

Most of the software mentioned up to this point in this chapter — including SAS, SPSS, R and Python — use code files that can be saved and rerun on data at a later date. These programs run fundamentally differently from programs such as Microsoft Excel, where you can run statistics on data, but no code files are produced and saved. Also, when you use web-based calculators, specialized apps like G*Power and PS for sample-size calculations, or online commercial platforms, no code files are produced and saved.

WARNING

This is an important issue in statistics. When no code files are produced or saved, you have no record of the steps in your analysis. If you need to be able to reproduce your analysis, the only way to be sure of this is to use software that allows you to save the code so you can run it again.

Storing Data in the Cloud

Cloud-based storage refers to storing large data files on a set of Internet servers designed specifically for large data storage. Unlike old-fashioned stand-alone servers in server rooms, cloud-based servers share storage space across the Internet, providing instantaneous access and back-up capabilities. If you want to get rid of an old-fashioned server in your server room (that could be a SAS server), you will have to contract with a cloud-based storage company to use its space for your data. Then, you will have to find a way to move your data from your server into your new cloud storage. You will also have to make sure you want to have a long-term relationship with this company, so you don't have to move your data out anytime soon.

REMEMBER

Although moving data to the cloud may be an onerous task, you may not have any choice, because physical storage space may be running out. Many new organizations start with cloud data storage for that reason. Once your data are stored in the cloud, they are more easily accessed using online analytics platforms such as SAS Viya and Tableau.

Chapter **5**

Conducting Clinical Research

This chapter provides a closer look at a special kind of human research — the clinical trial. The purpose of a clinical trial is to test one or more *interventions*, such as a medication or other product or action thought to be therapeutic (such as drinking green tea or exercising). One of the important features of a clinical trial is that it is an *experimental* study design, meaning that participants in the study are assigned by the study staff which intervention to take. Therefore, there are serious ethical considerations around clinical trials. On the other hand, the clinical trial study design provides the highest quality evidence you can obtain to determine whether or not an intervention actually works, which is a form of causal inference. In this chapter, we cover approaches to designing and executing a high-quality clinical trial and explain the ethical considerations that go along with this.

Designing a Clinical Trial

Clinical trials should conform to the highest standards of scientific rigor, and that starts with the design of the study. The following sections note some aspects of good experimental design.

Identifying aims, objectives, hypotheses, and variables

The *aims* or *goals* of a clinical trial are short general statements (often just one statement) of the overall purpose of the experiment. For example, the aim of an experiment may be "to assess whether drinking green tea every day improves alertness in older adults."

The *objectives* are much more specific than the aims. In a clinical trial, the objectives usually refer to the effect of the *intervention* (treatment being tested) on specific outcome variables at specific points in time in a group of a specific type of study participants. In a drug trial, which is a type of experimental clinical research, an efficacy study may have many individual efficacy objectives, as well as one or two safety objectives, while a safety study may or may not have efficacy objectives.

REMEMBER

When designing a clinical trial, you should identify one or two *primary objectives* — those that are most directly related to the aim of the study. This makes it easier to determine whether the intervention meets the objectives once your analysis is complete. You may then identify up to several dozen *secondary objectives,* which may involve different variables or the same variables at different time points or in different subsets of the study population. You may also list a set of *exploratory objectives,* which are less important, but still interesting. Finally, if testing a risky intervention (such as a pharmaceutical), you should list one or more *safety objectives* (if this is an efficacy study) or some efficacy objectives (if this is a safety study).

TIP

The objectives you select will determine what data you need to collect, so you have to choose wisely to make sure all data related to those objectives can be collected in the timeframe of your study. Also, these data will be processed from various sources, including case report forms (CRFs), surveys, and centers providing laboratory data. These considerations may limit the objectives you choose to study!

Drug clinical trials are usually efficacy studies. Here is an example of each type of objectives you could have in an efficacy study:

>> **Primary efficacy objective:** To compare the effect of new hypertension (HTN) drug XYZ, relative to old drug ABC, on changes in systolic blood pressure (SBP) from baseline to week 12, in participants with HTN.

>> **Secondary efficacy objective:** To compare the effect of HTN drug XYZ, relative to drug ABC, on changes in serum total cholesterol and serum triglycerides from baseline to weeks 4 and 8, in participants with HTN.

>> **Exploratory efficacy objective:** To compare the effect of drug XYZ, relative to drug ABC, on changes in sexual function from baseline to weeks 4, 8, and 12, in male and female subsets of participants with HTN.

>> **Safety objective:** To evaluate the safety of drug XYZ, relative to drug ABC, in terms of the occurrence of adverse events, changes from baseline in vital signs such as temperature and heart rate, and changes in laboratory results of safety panels (including tests on kidney and liver function), in participants with HTN.

TIP

For each of these objectives, it is important to specify the time range of participation subject to the analysis (such as the first week of the trial compared to other time segments). Also, which groups are being compared for each objective should be specified.

Hypotheses usually correspond to the objectives but are worded in a way that directly relates to the statistical testing to be performed. So, the preceding primary objective may correspond to the following hypothesis: "The mean 12-week reduction in SBP will be greater in the XYZ group than in the ABC group." Alternatively, the hypothesis may be expressed in a more formal mathematical notation and as a null and alternate pair (see Chapters 2 and 3 for details on these terms and the mathematical notation used):

$$H_{\text{Null}} : \Delta_{\text{XYZ}} - \Delta_{\text{ABC}} = 0$$
$$H_{\text{Alt}} : \Delta_{\text{XYZ}} - \Delta_{\text{ABC}} > 0$$

where $\Delta = \text{mean of } (SBP_{\text{Week 12}} - SBP_{\text{Baseline}})$.

REMEMBER

In all types of human research, identifying the variables to collect in your study should be straightforward after you've selected a study design and enumerated all the objectives. In a clinical trial, you will need to *operationalize* the measurements you need, meaning you will need to find a way to measure each concept specified in the objectives. Measurements can fall into these categories:

>> **Administrative:** This information includes data related to recruitment, consent, and enrollment, as well as contact information for each participant. You need to keep track of study eligibility documentation, as well as the date of each visit, which study activities took place, and final status at end of study (such as whether participants completed the study, dropped out of the study, or any other outcome).

>> **Intervention-related:** This includes data related to the intervention for each participant, such as group assignment, dosing level, compliance, and adherence measures. If you plan to assign a participant to a particular group but they end up in another group, you need to keep track of both group assignments.

>> **Outcome-related:** This includes ensuring you are measuring both efficacy and safety outcomes on a regular schedule that is documented. You may be asking the participant to keep records, or they may need to be measured in person (to obtain laboratory values, X-rays, and other scans, ECGs, and so on).

>> **Potential confounding variables:** These variables are determined by way of what is known about participants' relationship with the intervention, outcome, and study eligibility criteria. Typically, potential confounding variables include basic demographic information such as date of birth, gender, and ethnicity. Confounders could also be measured with questions posed to the participant about health behaviors such as tobacco use, exercise patterns, and diet. There are also questions about medical history, including current conditions, past hospitalizations, family medical history, and current and past medication use. Measurements such as height and weight as well as other physical measurements can also be included.

REMEMBER

Values that do not change over time, such as birth date and medical history, only need to be recorded at the beginning of the study. In designs including follow-up visits, values that change over time are measured multiple times over the duration of data collection for the study. Depending on the research objectives, these could include weight, medication use, and test results. Most of this data collection is scheduled as part of study visits, and but some may be recorded only at unpredictable times, if at all (such as adverse events, and withdrawing from the study before it is completed).

Deciding who is eligible for the study

Because you can't examine the entire population for whom the intervention you're studying is intended, you must select a sample from that population. How you filter in the right sample for your study is by explicitly defining the criteria a potential participant has to meet to be eligible to be enrolled and maintained in the study as a participant.

>> **Inclusion criteria** are used during the screening process to identify potential participants who are members of the population about whom you want to draw conclusions. A reasonable inclusion criterion for a study of a lipid-lowering intervention would be, "Participant must have a documented diagnosis of hyperlipidemia, defined as total cholesterol > 200 mg/dL and LDL > 130 mg/dL at screening."

>> **Exclusion criteria** are used to identify potential participants who do not fall in the population being studied. They are also used to rule out participation by individuals who are otherwise in the population being studied but should not

participate for practical reasons (such as safety, or risk of privacy breach). A reasonable exclusion criterion for a study of a lipid-lowering treatment would be, "Participants who are not willing to change their medication during the study are not eligible to participate."

>> **Withdrawal criteria** apply to the follow-up portion of the study. They describe situations that could arise during the study that would put the participant in a state where participation should no longer take place. One example would be that the participant is diagnosed with Alzheimer's disease during the study and can no longer make decisions on their own. A typical withdrawal criterion may be, "If the participant no longer has decision-making capacity, they will be withdrawn."

Choosing the structure of a clinical trial

Many clinical trials include a comparison of two or more interventions. These types of clinical trials typically have one of the following *structures* (or *designs*), each of which has pros and cons:

>> **Parallel:** In this clinical trial design, each participant receives *one* of the interventions, and the groups are compared. Parallel designs are simpler, quicker, and easier for each participant than crossover designs, but you need more participants for the statistics to work out. Trials with very long treatment periods usually have to be parallel.

>> **Crossover:** In a crossover design, each clinical trial participant receives *all* the interventions in sequence during consecutive treatment periods (called *phases*) separated by *washout intervals* (lasting from several days to several weeks). Crossover designs can be more efficient because each participant serves their own control, eliminating inter-participant variability. But you can use crossover designs only if you're certain that at the end of each washout period, the participant will have been restored to the same condition as at the start of the study. This may be impossible for studies of progressive diseases, like cancer or emphysema, or for drugs that last a long time in the body and are hard to wash out, like SSRIs and marijuana.

Using randomization

Randomized controlled trials (RCTs) are the gold standard for clinical research (as described in Chapters 7 and 20). In an RCT, the participants are randomly allocated by intervention into treatment groups (in a parallel trial) or into treatment-sequence groups (in a crossover design). Randomization provides several advantages:

>> It helps in reducing bias. It specifically helps to eliminate *treatment bias,* which is where certain treatments are preferentially given to certain participants. A clinician may feel inclined to assign a drug with fewer side effects to healthier participants, but if participants are randomized, then this bias goes away. Another important bias reduced by randomization is *confounding,* where the treatment groups differ with respect to some characteristic that influences the outcome.

>> Randomization makes it easier to interpret the results of statistical testing.

>> It facilitates blinding. *Blinding* (also called *masking*) refers to concealing the identity of the intervention from both participants and researchers. There are two types of blinding:

- **Single-blinding:** Where participants don't know what intervention they're receiving, but the researchers do.

- **Double-blinding:** Where neither the participants nor the researchers know which participants are receiving which interventions.

- ***Note:*** In all cases of blinding, for safety reasons, it is possible to unblind individual participants, as at least one of the members of the research team has the authority to unblind.

Blinding eliminates bias resulting from the *placebo effect,* which is where participants tend to respond favorably to *any* treatment (even a placebo), especially when the efficacy variables are subjective, such as pain level. Double-blinding also eliminates deliberate and subconscious bias in the investigator's evaluation of a participant's condition.

The simplest kind of randomization involves assigning each newly enrolled participant to a treatment group by the flip of a coin or a similar method. But simple randomization may produce an unbalanced pattern, like the one shown in Figure 5-1 for a small study of 12 participants and two treatments: Drug (D) and Placebo (P).

FIGURE 5-1:
Simple randomization.

Participant	1	2	3	4	5	6	7	8	9	10	11	12
Treatment	P	D	P	P	D	P	P	P	D	P	P	P

© *John Wiley & Sons, Inc.*

If you were hoping to have six participants in each group, you won't be pleased if you end up with three participants receiving the drug and nine receiving the placebo, because it's unbalanced. But unbalanced patterns like this arise quite often from 12 coin flips. (Try it if you don't believe us.) A better approach is to require six participants in each group but shuffle those six Ds and six Ps around randomly, as shown in Figure 5-2.

FIGURE 5-2:
Random
shuffling.

Participant	1	2	3	4	5	6	7	8	9	10	11	12
Treatment	P	D	D	D	D	D	P	P	P	D	P	P

© John Wiley & Sons, Inc.

This arrangement is better because there are exactly six participants assigned to drug and placebo each. But this particular random shuffle happens to assign more drugs to the earlier participants and more placebos to the later participant (which is just by chance). If the recruitment period is short, this would be perfectly fine. However, if these 12 participants were enrolled over a period of five or six months, seasonal effects may be mistaken for treatment effects, which is an example of confounding.

To make sure that both treatments are evenly spread across the entire recruitment period, you can use *blocked randomization,* in which you divide your subjects into consecutive blocks and shuffle the assignments within each block. Often the block size is set to twice the number of treatment groups. For instance, a two-group study would use a block size of four. This is shown in Figure 5-3.

FIGURE 5-3:
Blocked
randomization.

Participant	1	2	3	4	5	6	7	8	9	10	11	12
Treatment	D	P	D	P	P	P	D	D	P	D	P	D

© John Wiley & Sons, Inc.

TIP

You can create simple and blocked randomization lists in Microsoft Excel using the RAND() built-in function to shuffle the assignments. You can also use the web page at `https://www.graphpad.com/quickcalcs/randomize1.cfm` to generate blocked randomization lists quickly and easily.

Selecting the analyses to use

You should select the appropriate analytic approach for each of your study hypotheses based on the type of data involved, the structure of the study, and the requirements of the hypothesis. The rest of this book describes statistical methods to analyze the kinds of data you're likely to encounter in human research. Your strategy is to apply them to a clinical trial design. In clinical trials, changes in values of variables over time, and differences between treatments in crossover studies are often analyzed by paired t tests and repeated-measures ANOVAs.

Differences between groups of participants in parallel studies are often analyzed by unpaired t tests and ANOVAs. Often, final regression models are developed for clinical trial interpretation because these can control for residual confounding (which are covered in the chapters in Part 5). In longer clinical trials, time until death (survival time) and the times to the occurrence of other endpoint events (besides death) are analyzed by survival methods (Part 6 focuses on survival analysis methods).

Determining how many participants to enroll in a clinical trial

Chapter 3 presents the concept of statistical power, and for a clinical trial, you should enroll enough participants to provide sufficient statistical power when testing the primary objective of the study. The specific way you calculate the required sample size depends on the statistical test that's used for the primary hypothesis. Each chapter of this book that describes hypothesis tests also shows how to estimate the required sample size for that test. To get quick sample-size estimates, you can use G*Power (an application for sample-size calculations described in Chapter 4), or you can use the formulas, tables, and charts in Chapter 25 and on the book's Cheat Sheet at www.dummies.com (just search for "Biostatistics For Dummies Cheat Sheet").

REMEMBER

You must also allow some extra space in your target sample-size estimate for some of the enrolled participants to drop out or otherwise not contribute the data you need for your analysis. For example, suppose that you need full data from 64 participants for sufficient statistical power to answer your main objective. If you expect a 15 percent attrition rate from the study, which means you expect only 85 percent of the enrolled participants to have analyzable data, then you need to plan to enroll 64/0.84, or 76, participants in the study.

Assembling the study protocol

A *study protocol* (or just *protocol*) is a document that lays out exactly what you plan to do to collect and analyze data in a research study. For ethical reasons, every research study involving human participants should have a protocol, and for other types of studies, having a protocol prepared before starting the research is considered best practices. In a clinical trial, the protocol is especially important because the participants are being assigned to interventions by the researcher, and there is often double-blinding and randomization.

In terms of standard elements, a formal drug clinical trial protocol typically contains these components:

>> **Title:** A title conveys as much information about the trial as you can fit into one sentence, including the protocol ID, name of the study, clinical phase, type and structure of trial, type of randomization and blinding, name of the drug or drugs being tested, treatment regimen, intended effect, and the population being studied (which could include a reference to individuals with a particular medical condition). A title can be quite long — this example title has all the preceding elements:

   Protocol BCAM521-13-01 (ASPIRE-2) — a Phase-IIa, double-blind, placebo-controlled, randomized, parallel-group study of the safety and efficacy of three different doses of AM521, given intravenously, once per month for six months, for the relief of chronic pain, in adults with knee osteoporosis.

>> **Background information:** This section includes information about the disease for which the drug is an intended treatment. It includes the epidemiology (the condition's prevalence and impact), and its known physiology down to the molecular level. It also includes a review of treatments currently available (if any), and information about the drug or drugs being tested, including mechanism of action, the results of prior testing, and known and potential risks and benefits to participants.

>> **Rationale:** The rationale for the study states why it makes sense to do this study at this time and includes a justification for the choice of doses, how the drug is administered (such as orally or intravenously), duration of drug administration, and follow-up period.

>> **Aims, objectives, and hypotheses:** We discuss these items in the earlier section "Identifying aims, objectives, hypotheses, and variables."

>> **Detailed descriptions of all inclusion, exclusion, and withdrawal criteria:** See the earlier section "Deciding who is eligible for the study" for more about these terms.

>> **Design of the clinical trial:** As described in the earlier section "Choosing the structure of a clinical trial," the clinical trial's design defines its structure. This includes the number of treatment groups as well as consecutive stages of the study. These stages could include eligibility screening, washout, treatment, follow-up, and so on. This section often includes a schematic diagram of the structure of the study.

- » **Drug description:** This description details each drug that will be administered to the participants. This includes the chemical composition with the results of chemical analysis of the drug, if available. It also includes instructions about how to store, prepare, and administer the drug correctly.

- » **Blinding and randomization schemes:** These schemes include descriptions of how and when the study will be unblinded. This includes the emergency unblinding of individual participants if necessary. See the earlier section "Using randomization" for more information.

- » **Procedural descriptions:** This section describes every procedure that will be performed at every visit. These include administrative procedures, such as enrollment and informed consent, and diagnostic procedures, such as physical exams and measuring vital signs. It covers all activities where data are collected from participants in the study.

- » **Safety considerations:** These factors include the known and potential side effects of each drug included. This section also includes the known and potential side effects of each procedure in the study, including X-rays, MRI scans, and blood draws. It also describes steps taken to minimize the risk to the participants.

- » **Handling of adverse events:** This section describes how adverse events will be addressed should they occur during the study. It includes a description of the data that will be recorded, including the nature of the adverse event, severity, dates and times of onset and resolution, any medical treatment given for the event, and whether or not the investigator thinks the event was related to the study drug. It also explains how the research study will support the participant after the adverse event.

- » **Definition of safety, efficacy, and other analytical populations:** This section includes definitions of safety and efficacy variables and endpoints. In other words, this section defines variables or changes in variables that serve as indicators of safety or efficacy.

- » **Planned enrollment and analyzable sample size:** Justification for these numbers must also be provided.

- » **Proposed statistical analyses:** Some protocols describe, in detail, every analysis for every objective. Others include only a summary and refer to a separate *Statistical Analysis Plan* (SAP) document for details of the proposed analysis. This section should also include descriptions of how missing data will be handled analytically, adjustments for multiple testing to control Type I errors (see Chapter 3), and whether any interim analyses are planned. If a separate SAP is used, it typically contains a detailed description of all the calculations and analyses that will be carried out on the data, including the descriptive summaries of all data and the testing of all the hypotheses specified in the protocol. The SAP also usually contains mock-ups called *shells* of all the tables, listings, and figures (referred to as TLFs) that will be generated from the data.

It will also contain administrative details, like names and contact information for the research team, a table of contents, a list of abbreviations, description of policies of data handling, and financing and insurance agreements.

Carrying Out a Clinical Trial

After you've designed your clinical trial and have described it in the protocol document, it's time to move on to the next step. The operational details will, of course, vary from one study to another, but a few aspects apply to all clinical trials. In any study involving human participants, the most important consideration is protecting those participants from harm.

TIP

Since the end of World War II, international agreements have established ethical guidelines for human research all over the world. Regardless of the country in which you are conducting research, prior to beginning a human research study, your protocol will need to be approved by at least one ethics board. Selection of ethics boards for human research depends upon where the research is taking place and what institutions are involved (see the later section "Working with Institutional Review Boards").

Protecting clinical trial participants

REMEMBER

In any research involving humans, two issues are of utmost importance:

>> **Safety:** Minimizing the risk of physical harm to the participant from the drug or drugs being tested and from the procedures involved in the study

>> **Privacy/confidentiality:** Ensuring that data collected during the study are not breached (stolen) and are not made public in a way that identifies a specific participant without the participant's consent

The following sections describe some of the *infrastructure* that helps protect human subjects.

Surveying regulatory agencies

In the United States, several government organizations oversee human subjects' protection:

>> Commercial pharmaceutical research is governed by the Food and Drug Administration (FDA).

>> Most academic biological research is sponsored by the National Institutes of Health (NIH) and is governed by the Office for Human Research Protections (OHRP).

TECHNICAL STUFF

Because research ethics are international, other countries have similar agencies, so international clinical trial oversight can get confusing. An organization called the International Conference on Harmonization (ICH) works to establish a set of consistent standards that can be applied worldwide. The FDA and NIH have adopted many ICH standards (with some modifications).

Working with Institutional Review Boards

For all protocols that describe research that could potentially be considered human research, in the United States, an ethics board called an Institutional Review Board (IRB) must review the protocol and approve it (or find it exempt from human research laws) before you can start the research. You have to submit an application along with the protocol and your plans for gaining informed consent of potential participants to an IRB with jurisdiction over your research and ensure that you are approved to proceed before you start.

Most medical centers and academic institutions (as well as some industry partners) run their own IRBs with jurisdiction over research conducted at their institution. If you're not affiliated with one of these centers or institutions (for example, if you're a freelance biostatistician or clinician), you may need the services of a *consulting* or *free-standing* IRB. The sponsor of the research may recommend or insist you use a particular IRB for the project.

Getting informed consent

An important part of protecting human participants is making sure that they're aware of the risks of a study before agreeing to participate in it. They also need to be fully informed as to what will happen in the study before they can give consent to participate. You must prepare an *Informed Consent Form* (ICF) describing, in simple language, the nature of the study, why it is being conducted, what is being tested, what procedures participants will undergo, and the risks and benefits of participation. The ICF is used to guide study staff when they explain the study to potential participants, who are then expected to sign it if they want to participate in the study.

Potential participants must be told that they can refuse to participate with no penalty to them, and if they join the study, they can withdraw at any time for any reason without fear of retribution or the withholding of regular medical care. The IRB can provide ICF templates with examples of their recommended or required wording.

REMEMBER

Prior to performing any procedures on a potential participant (including screening tests involved in determining eligibility), study staff must go through an approved ICF document with the potential participant and give them time to read it and decide whether or not they want to participate. If they choose to participate, the ICF must be signed and witnessed. The signed ICFs must be retained as part of the official documentation for the project, along with all data collected (including laboratory reports, ECG tracings, and records of all test products administered to the participants), as well as records of all procedures performed on participants. The sponsor, the regulatory agencies, the IRB, and other entities may ask to review these documents at any time as part of oversight.

Considering data safety monitoring boards and committees

For clinical trials of interventions that are likely to be of low risk (such as drinking green tea), investigators are usually responsible for ensuring participant safety by tracking unexpected adverse events, abnormal laboratory tests, and other red flags during the course of the study. But for studies involving high-risk treatments (like cancer chemotherapy trials), a separate *data safety monitoring board* or *committee* (DSMB or DSMC) should be arranged. A DSMB is typically required by the sponsor, the investigator, the IRB, or a regulatory agency. A DSMB typically has about six members, including expert clinicians in the relevant area of research and a statistician, who are external to the study staff. A DSMB meets at regular intervals during the clinical trial to review the unblinded safety data acquired up to that point. The committee is authorized to modify, suspend, or even terminate a study if it has serious concerns about the safety of the participants.

Getting certified in human subjects protection

WARNING

As you may have surmised from the preceding sections, clinical research involves regulatory requirements that include penalties for noncompliance. Therefore, you shouldn't try to guess how to write a research protocol, obtain IRB approval, or engage in any other research methods with which you are unfamiliar, and just hope that everything goes well. You should ensure that you, along with any others who may be assisting you, are properly trained in matters relating to human subjects protection.

Fortunately, such training is readily available. Most hospitals and medical centers provide training in the form of online courses, workshops, lectures, and other resources. As you comply with ongoing IRB training, you receive a certification in human subjects protection. Most IRBs and funding agencies require proof of certification from study staff. If you don't have access to that training at your institution, you can get certified by taking an online tutorial offered by the NIH (`https://grants.nih.gov/policy/humansubjects/research/training-and-resources.htm`).

Collecting and validating data

Data in a clinical trial are typically collected digitally and manually. Examples of data collected digitally include a participant filling out an online survey or a blood pressure monitor collecting data from a participant. Data are collected manually when they are written down on paper first, then undergo data entry to become digital. Either way, some paper forms may be included, and many digital forms are created for data entry in a clinical trial. These forms are for data entry of data collected from various parts of the study, but in clinical trial lingo, they are all referred to as *case report forms*, or CRFs.

>> In the case of digitally collected data, the central analytic team will run routines for validating the data. They will communicate with study staff if they find errors and work them out.

>> In the case of manually collected data, data entry into a digital format will be required. Study staff typically are expected to log into an online database with CRFs and do data entry from data collected on paper.

>> The sponsor of the study will provide detailed data entry instructions and training to ensure high-quality data collection and validation of the data collected in the study.

Analyzing Your Data

In the following sections, we describe some general situations that come up in all clinical research, regardless of what kind of analysis you use.

Dealing with missing data

Most clinical trials have incomplete data for one or more variables, which can be a real headache when analyzing your data. The statistical aspects of missing data are quite complicated, so you should consult a statistician if you have more than just occasional, isolated missing values. Here we describe some commonly used approaches for coping with missing data:

>> **Exclusion:** Exclude a case from an analysis if any of the required variables for that analysis is missing. This seems simple, but the downside to this approach is it can reduce the number of analyzable cases, sometimes quite severely. And if the result is missing for a reason that's related to treatment efficacy, excluding the case can bias your results.

>> **Imputation:** Imputation is where you replace a missing value with a value you *impute,* or create yourself. When analysts impute in a clinical trial, they typically take the mean or median of all the available values for that variable and fill that in for the missing variable. In reality, you have to keep the original variable, and then save a separate, imputed variable so that you can document the type of imputation applied. There are a lot of downsides to imputation. If you are imputing a small number of values, it's not worth it because it adds bias. You may as well just exclude those cases. But if you impute a large number of values, you are basically making up the data yourself, adding more bias.

>> **Last Observation Carried Forward (LOCF):** LOCF is a special case of imputation. Sometimes during follow-up, one of a series of sequential measurements on a particular participant is missing. For example, imagine that there were supposed to be four weekly glucose values measured, and you were missing a measurement only on week three. In that case, you could use the most recent previous value in the series, which is the week two measurement, to impute the week three measurement. This technique is called *Last Observation Carried Forward* (LOCF) and is one of the most widely used strategies. Although imputation adds bias, LOCF adds bias in the *conservative* direction, making it more difficult to demonstrate efficacy. This approach is popular with regulators, who want to put the burden of proof on the drug and study sponsor.

Handling multiplicity

Every time you perform a statistical significance test, you run a chance of being fooled by random fluctuations into thinking that some real effect is present in your data when, in fact, none exists (review Chapter 3 for a refresher on statistical testing). If you declare the results of the test are statistically significant, and in reality they are not, you are committing *Type I error.* When you say that you require $p < 0.05$ to declare statistical significance, you're testing at the 0.05 (or 5 percent) alpha (α) level. This is another way of saying that you want to limit your Type I error rate to 5 percent. But that 5 percent error rate applies to each and every statistical test you run. The more analyses you perform on a data set, the more your overall α level increases. If you perform two tests at $\alpha = 0.05$, your chance of at least one of them coming out falsely significant is about 10 percent. If you run 40 tests, the overall α level jumps to 87 percent! This is referred to as the problem of *multiplicity,* or as *Type I error inflation.*

Chapter 11 covers dealing with multiplicity when making multiple comparisons. One approach discussed in Chapter 11 is performing post-hoc tests following an ANOVA for comparing several groups. Post-hoc tests incorporate a built-in adjustment to keep the overall α at only 5 percent across all comparisons. This can be especially important when conducting *an interim analysis,* or an analysis done before the official end of study data collection. But when you're testing different hypotheses — like when comparing different variables at different time points between different groups — you are faced with some difficult decisions to make about reducing Type I error inflation.

TIP

In sponsored clinical trials, the sponsor and DSMB will weigh in on how they want to see Type I error inflation controlled. If you are working on a clinical trial without a sponsor, you should consult with another professional with experience in developing clinical trial analyses to advise you on how to control your Type I error inflation given the context of your study.

TIP

Each time an interim analysis is conducted, a process called *data close-out* must occur. This creates a *data snapshot,* and the last data snapshot from a data close-out process produces the final *analytic dataset,* or dataset to be used in all analyses. Data close-out refers to the process where current data being collected are copied into a research environment, and this copy is edited to prepare it for analysis. These edits could include adding imputations, unblinding, or creating other variables needed for analysis. The analytic dataset prepared for each interim analysis and for final analysis should be stored with documentation, as decisions about stopping or adjusting the trial are made based on the results of interim analyses.

Chapter **6**

Taking All Kinds of Samples

S ampling — or taking a sample — is an important concept in statistics. As described in Chapter 3, the purpose of taking a sample — or a group of individuals from a population — and measuring just the sample is so that you do not have to conduct a census and measure the whole population. Instead, you can measure just the sample and use statistical approaches to make inferences about the whole, which is called *inferential statistics*. You can estimate a measurement of the entire population, which is called a *parameter*, by calculating a statistic from your sample.

Some samples do a better job than others at representing the population from which they are drawn. We begin this chapter by digging more deeply into some important concepts related to sampling. We then describe specific sampling approaches and discuss their pros and cons.

Making Forgivable (and Non-Forgivable) Errors

A central concept in statistics is that of error. In statistics, the term *error* sometimes means what you think it means — that a mistake has been made. In those cases, the statistician should take steps to avoid the error. But other times in statistics, the term *error* refers to a phenomenon that is unavoidable, and as statisticians, we just have to cope with it.

For example, imagine that you had a list of all the patients of a particular clinic and their current ages. Suppose that you calculated the average age of the patients on your list, and your answer was 43.7 years. That would be a population parameter. Now, let's say you took a random sample of 20 patients from that list and calculated the mean age of the sample, which would be a sample statistic. Do you think you would get exactly 43.7 years? Although it is certainly possible, in all likelihood, the mean of your sample — the statistic — would be a different number than the mean of your population — the parameter. The fact that most of the time a sample statistic is not equal to the population parameter is called *sampling error*. Sampling error is unavoidable, and as statisticians, we are forced to accept it.

Now, to describe the other type of error, let's add some drama. Suppose that when you went to take a sample of those 20 patients, you spilled coffee on the list so you could not read some of the names. The names blotted out by the coffee were therefore ineligible to be selected for your sample. This is unfair to the names under the coffee stain — they have a zero probability of being selected for your sample, even though they are part of the population from which you are sampling. This is called *undercoverage,* and is considered a type of *non-sampling error*. Non-sampling error is essentially a mistake. It is where something goes wrong during sampling that you should try to avoid. And unlike sampling error, undercoverage is definitely a mistake you should avoid making if you can (like spilling coffee).

Framing Your Sample

In the previous example, the patient list is considered your *sampling frame*. A sampling frame represents the practical representation of the population from which you are literally drawing your sample. We described this list as a printout of patient names and their ages. Suppose that after the list was printed, a few more patients joined the clinic, and a few patients stopped using the clinic because they moved away. This situation means that your sampling frame — your list — is not a perfect representation of the actual population from which you are drawing your sample.

REMEMBER

If you omit population members from your sampling frame, you get undercoverage, which is a form of non-sampling error (the type of error you want to avoid). Also, if you accidentally include members in your sampling frame who are not part of the population (such as patients who moved away from the clinic after you printed your list), and they actually get sampled, you have another form of non-sampling error. Non-sampling error can also creep in from making sloppy measurements during data collection, or making poor choices when designing your study. Chapter 8 provides guidance on how to minimize errors during data collection, and Chapters 5 and 7 provide advice on study design.

Another sampling-related vocabulary word is *simulation*. When talking about sampling, a simulation refers to pretending to have data from an entire population from which you can take samples, and then taking different samples to see what happens when you analyze the data. That way, you can make sample statistics while peeking at what the population parameters actually are behind the scenes to see how they behave together.

One simulation you could do to illustrate sampling error in Microsoft Excel is to create a column of 100 values that represent ages of imaginary patients at a clinic as an entire population.

>> If you calculated the mean of these 100 values, you would be doing a simulation of the population parameter.

>> If you randomly sampled 20 of these values and calculated the mean, you would be doing a simulation of a sample statistic.

>> If you compared your parameter to the statistic to see how close they were to each other, you would be doing a simulation of sampling error.

So far we've reviewed several concepts related to the act of sampling. However, we haven't yet examined different sampling strategies. It matters how you go about taking a sample from a population; some approaches provide a sample that is more *representative* of the population than other approaches. In the next section, we consider and compare several different sampling strategies.

Sampling for Success

As mentioned earlier, the purpose of taking measurements from a sample of a population is so that you can use it to perform inferential statistics, which enables you to make estimates about the population without having to measure the entire population. Theoretically, you want the statistics from your sample to be as close as possible to the population parameters you are trying to estimate. To increase the likelihood that this happens, you should try your best to draw a sample that is representative of the population.

You may be wondering, "What is the best way to draw a sample that is representative of the background population?" The honest answer is, "It depends on your resources." If you are a government agency, you can invest a lot of resources in conducting representative sampling from a population for your studies. But if you are a graduate student working on a dissertation, then based on resources available, you probably have to settle for a sample that is not as representative of the population as a government agency could afford. Nevertheless, you can still use your judgment to make the wisest decisions possible about your sampling approach.

Taking a simple random sample

Taking a simple random sample (SRS) is considered a representative approach to sampling from a background population. In an SRS, every member of the population has an equal chance of being selected randomly and included in the sample. As an example, recall the printout of the current patient list from a clinic discussed in the previous section. Considering that list a clinical population, imagine that you used scissors to cut the list up so that each name was on its own slip of paper, and then you put all the slips of paper into a hat. If you want to take an SRS of 20 patients, you could randomly remove 20 names from the hat. The SRS would be seen as a highly representative sample.

TECHNICAL STUFF

In practice, an SRS is usually taken using a computer so that you can take advantage of a *random number generator* (RNG) (and do not have to cut up all that paper). Imagine that the patient list from which you were sampling was not printed on paper, but was instead stored in a column in a spreadsheet in Microsoft Excel. You could use the following steps to take an SRS of 20 patients from this list using the computer:

1. **Create a column containing random numbers.**

   You could create another column in the spreadsheet called "Random" and enter the following formula into the top cell in the column: =*RAND()*. If you drag that cell down so that the entire column contains this command, you will see that Excel populates each cell with a random number between 0 and 1. Each time Excel evaluates, the random number gets recalculated.

2. **Sort the list by the random number column.**

3. **Select the top 20 rows from the list.**

This process ensures that your sample of 20 patients was taken completely at random. Statistical packages like those described in Chapter 4 have RNG commands similar to the one in Excel.

WARNING

Learners sometimes think that as long as they sort a spreadsheet of data by a column containing *any* value and then select a sample of rows from the top, that they have automatically obtained an SRS. This is not correct! If you think about it more carefully, you will realize why. If you sort names alphabetically, you will see patterns in names (such as religious names, or names associated with certain languages, countries, or ethnicities). If you sort by another identifying column, such as email address or city of residence, you will again see patterns in the data. If you attempt to take an SRS from such data, it will be *biased,* not random, and not be representative. That is why it is important to use a column with an RNG in it for sorting if you are taking an SRS electronically.

WARNING

Taking an SRS intuitively seems like the optimal way to draw a representative sample. However, there are caveats. In the previous example, you started with a clinical population in the form of a printed or electronic list of patients from which you could draw a sample. But what if you want to sample from patients presenting to the emergency department during a particular period of time in the future? Such a list does not exist. In a situation like that, you could use systematic sampling, which is explained later in the section "Engaging in systematic sampling."

Another caveat of SRS is that it can miss important subgroups. Imagine that in your list of clinic patients, only 10 percent were pediatric patients (defined as patients under the age of 18 years). Because 10 percent of 20 is two, you may expect that a random sample of 20 patients from a population where 10 percent are pediatric would include two pediatric patients. But in practice, in a situation like this, it would not be unusual for an SRS of 20 patients to include zero pediatric patients. If your SRS needs to ensure representation by certain subgroups, then you should consider using stratified sampling instead.

Taking a stratified sample

In the previous section, we discussed a scenario where 10 percent of the patients of a clinic are pediatric patients, and taking a sample of 20 using an SRS from a list of the clinic population runs the risk of not including any pediatric patients. If pediatric patients were important to the study, then this problem can be solved with stratified sampling. The word *stratum* refers to a layer (as you see in a layer cake), and the word *strata* is the plural of stratum. Stratified sampling can be seen as sampling from strata, or layers.

In our scenario, if you choose to draw a stratified sample by age groups, you would first have to separate the list into a pediatric list and a list of everyone else. Then, you could take an SRS from each. Because you are concerned about each stratum, you could make a rule that even though pediatric patients make up only 10 percent of the background population, you want them to make up 50 percent of your sample. If you did that, then when you took your SRS, you would *oversample* from the pediatric list and select 10, while also taking an SRS of 10 from the list of everyone else.

REMEMBER

Drawing a stratified sample requires you to weight your overall estimate, or else it will be biased. As an example, imagine that 15 percent of pediatric patients had an oral health condition, and 50 percent of the rest of the patients had an oral health condition. In a stratified sample of 20 patients where you draw 10 from the pediatric population and 10 from the rest of the population, because the pediatric population is oversampled (because they only make up 10 percent of the background population but make up 50 percent of our sample), if weights are not applied, the estimate of the percentage of the population with an oral health condition would be artificially reduced. That is why it is necessary to apply weights to overall estimates derived from a stratified sample.

TECHNICAL STUFF

If you are familiar with large epidemiologic surveillance studies such as the National Health and Nutrition Examination Survey (NHANES) in the United States, you may be aware that extremely complex stratified sampling is used in the design and execution of such studies. Stratified sampling in these studies is unlike the simple example described earlier, where the stratification involves only two age groups. In surveillance studies like NHANES, there may be stratified sampling based on many characteristics, including age, gender, and location of residence. If you need to select factors on which to stratify, trying looking at what factors were used for stratification in historical studies of the same population. The kind of stratified sampling used in large-scale surveillance studies is reviewed later in this chapter in the section "Sampling in multiple stages."

Engaging in systematic sampling

Earlier you considered a scenario where a clinic had a printed list of the entire population of patients from which an SRS could be drawn. But what if you want to sample from the population of patients who present to a particular emergency department tonight between 6 p.m. and midnight? There is no convenient list from which to draw such a sample. In a scenario like this, even though you can't draw an SRS, you want to use a system for obtaining a sample such that it would be representative of the underlying population. To do that, you could use systematic sampling.

Imagine you are surveying a sample of patients about their opinions of waiting times at a particular emergency department, and you are doing this in the time window of between 6 p.m. and midnight tonight. To take a systematic sample of this population, follow these steps:

1. **Select a small number.**

   This is your starting number. If you select three, this means that — starting at 6 p.m. — the first patient to whom you would offer your survey would be the third one presenting to the emergency department.

2. **Select another small number.**

   This is your sampling number. If you select five, then after the first patient to whom you offered the survey, you would ask every fifth patient presenting to the emergency department to complete your survey.

3. **Continue sampling until you have the size sample you need (or the time window expires).**

   Chapter 4 describes the software G*Power that can be used for making sample-size calculations.

TECHNICAL STUFF

In systematic sampling, you are technically starting at a random individual, then selecting every *kth* member of the population, where *k* stands for the sampling number you selected.

WARNING

Systematic sampling is not representative if there are any time-related cyclic patterns that could confer *periodicity* onto the underlying data. For example, suppose that it was known that most pediatric patients present to the emergency department between 6 p.m. and 8 p.m. If you chose to collect data during this time window, even if you used systematic sampling, you would undoubtedly oversample pediatric patients.

Sampling clusters

Another challenge you may face as a biostatistician when it comes to sampling from populations occurs when you are studying an environmental exposure. The term *exposure* is from epidemiology and refers to a factor hypothesized to have a causal impact on an outcome (typically a health condition). Examples of environmental exposures that are commonly studied include air pollution emitted from factories, high levels of contaminants in an urban water system, and environmental pollution and other dangers resulting from a particular event (such as a natural disaster).

Consider the scenario where parents in a community are complaining that a local factory is emitting pollutants that they believe is resulting in a higher rate of leukemia being diagnosed in the community's youth. To study whether the parents are correct or not, you need to sample members of the population based on their proximity to the factory. This is where *cluster sampling* comes in.

Planning to do cluster sampling geographically starts with getting an accurate map of the area from which you are sampling. In the United States, each state is divided up into counties, and each county is further subdivided into smaller regions determined by the U.S. census. Other countries have similar ways their maps can be divided along official geographic boundaries. In the scenario described where a factory is thought to be polluting, the factory could be placed on the map and lines drawn around the locations from which a sample should be drawn. Different methodologies are used depending upon the specific study, but they usually involve taking an SRS of regions and from the sampled regions known as *clusters*, taking an SRS of community members for study participation.

REMEMBER

But cluster sampling is not only done geographically. As another example, clusters of schools may be selected based on school district, rather than geography, and an SRS drawn from each school. The important takeaway from cluster sampling is that it is a sampling strategy optimized for drawing a representative sample when studying an exposure known to be uneven across the population.

Sampling at your convenience

If you have read this chapter from the beginning until now, you may be feeling a little exasperated. And that may be because all the sampling strategies we have discussed so far — SRS, stratified sampling, systematic sampling, and cluster sampling — involve a lot of work for the researcher. In an SRS, you need to have a list of the population from which to draw, and in stratified sampling, you have to know the value of the characteristics on which you want to stratify your sample. Each of these features makes designing your sampling frame more complicated.

Thinking this way, both systematic sampling and cluster sampling also add complexity to your sampling frame. In systematic sampling, whether you use a static list or you sample in real time, you need to keep track of the details of your sampling process. In cluster sampling, you may be using a map or system of groupings from which to sample, and that also involves a lot of recordkeeping. You may be asking by now, "Isn't there an easier way?"

Yes! There is an easier and more convenient way: *convenience sampling*. Convenience sampling is what you probably think it is — taking a sample from a population based on convenience. For example, when statistics professors want to know what students think about a new policy on campus, they can just ask whoever is in their classes, as those students are a convenient sample of the student population.

The problem is that the answer they get may be very biased. Most of the students in their classes may come from the sciences, and those studying art or literature may feel very differently about the same policy. Although our convenience sample would be a *valid* sample of the background population of students, it would be such a *biased* sample that the results would probably be rejected by the rest of the faculty — especially those from the art and literature departments!

TIP

Given that the results from convenience samples are usually biased, you may think that convenience sampling is not a good strategy. In actuality, convenience sampling comes in handy if you have a relatively low-stakes research question. Customer satisfaction surveys are usually done with convenience samples, such as those placing an order on a restaurant's app. It is simple to program such a survey into an app, and if the food quality is terrific and the service terrible, it will be immediately evident even from a small convenience sample of app users completing the survey.

WARNING

While low-stakes situations are fine for convenience sampling, high-stakes situations — like studying whether a new drug is safe and/or effective — require study designs and sampling approaches completely focused on minimizing bias. As with SRS, convenience sampling is prone to omitting important subgroups from the sample. Minimizing bias through sampling and other strategies is covered in detail in Chapter 5, which examines clinical research and describes how researchers must present a well-defined protocol that includes selection criteria, a sampling plan, and an analytic plan that undergoes regulatory approval prior to the commencement of research activities. Other strategies for minimizing bias are presented in Chapters 7 and 20, which cover study designs and causal inference.

Sampling in multiple stages

When conducting large, epidemiologic surveillance studies, it is necessary to do an especially good job of sampling, because governments use results from these studies on which to base public policy. As an example, because being obese puts community members at risk for serious health conditions, government public health agencies have a vested interest in making accurate estimates of the rates of obesity in their communities.

For this reason, to strive to obtain a representative sample, researchers designing large epidemiologic surveillance studies use *multi-stage sampling*. Multi-stage sampling is a general term for using multiple sampling approaches at different stages as part of a strategy to obtain a representative sample. Figure 6-1 provides a schematic describing the multi-stage sampling in the U.S. surveillance study mentioned earlier, NHANES.

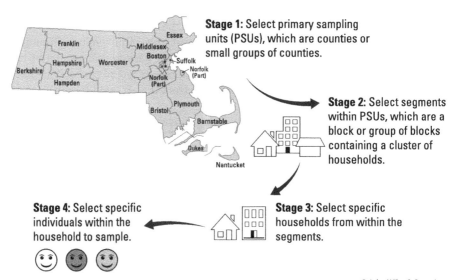

FIGURE 6-1: Example of multi-stage sampling from the National Health and Nutrition. Examination Survey (NHANES).

As shown in Figure 6-1, in NHANES, there are four stages of sampling. In the first stage, primary sampling units, or PSUs, are randomly selected. The PSUs are made up of counties, or small groups of counties together. Next, in the second stage, segments — which are a block or group of blocks containing a cluster of households — are randomly selected from the counties sampled in the first stage. Next, in the third stage, households are randomly selected from segments. Finally, in stage four, to select each actual community member who will be offered participation in NHANES, an individual is randomly selected from each household sampled in the third stage.

That is how a sample of 8,704 individuals participating in NHANES in 2017–2018 was selected to represent the population of the approximately 325 million people living in the United States at that time. The good news is that biostatisticians work on teams to develop a multi-stage sampling strategy — no one is expected to set up something so complicated all by themselves.

Chapter **7**

Having Designs on Study Design

Biostatistics can be seen as the application of a set of tools to answer questions posed through human research. When studying samples, these tools are used in conjunction with epidemiologic study designs in such a way as to facilitate *causal inference,* or the ability to determine cause and effect. Some study designs are better than others at facilitating causal inference. Nevertheless, regardless of the study design selected, an appropriate sampling strategy and statistical analysis that complements the study design must be used in conjunction with it.

In this chapter, we provide an overview of epidemiologic study designs and present them in a hierarchy so that you can relate them to the biostatistical approaches described in the different chapters of this book. We start by looking at broad study design categories such as observational, experimental, descriptive, and analytic, and move into descriptive study designs including expert opinion, case studies and case series, ecological (correlational) studies, and cross-sectional studies. We present analytic study designs next — case-control studies and longitudinal cohort studies — which are superior to descriptive designs in terms of developing evidence for causal inference, and then move into the highest-level designs: systematic reviews and meta-analyses.

TIP

For a deeper dive into epidemiologic study designs, we encourage you to read *Epidemiology For Dummies* by Amal K. Mitra (Wiley) and pay special attention to Chapters 16 and 17, which are about causal inference and study design.

Presenting the Study Design Hierarchy

Figure 7-1 illustrates the epidemiologic study designs in terms of their relationship with each other in a hierarchy as they apply to human health research (not animal research or other domains of human research like psychology). As shown in Figure 7-1, human health research may be split into two types: observational and experimental.

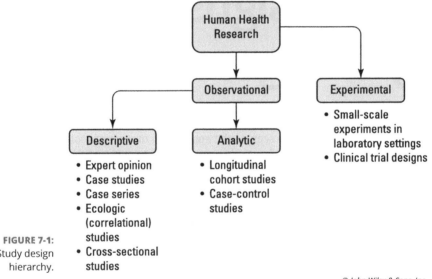

FIGURE 7-1: Study design hierarchy.

© John Wiley & Sons, Inc.

Observational research is where humans are studied in terms of their health and behavior, but they are not assigned to do any particular behavior as part of the study — they are just observed. For example, imagine that a sample of women were contacted by phone and asked about their use of birth control pills. In this case, researchers are observing their behavior with regard to birth control pills.

This is in contrast to *experimental research,* which is where the researcher assigns research participants to engage in certain behaviors as part of an intervention being studied. Imagine that you were studying a new birth control pill on the market and you wanted to know whether taking it changed a woman's lipid profile, which is determined by a laboratory test. You may do an experiment where you assign research participants to take the pill and then evaluate their lipid profiles.

REMEMBER

The difference between observational and experimental research is important because there is a heavier ethical obligation in experimental research when the researcher is assigning an intervention. Also, because of such ethical considerations in addition to time, cost, and other limitations, there are far more observational studies than experimental studies.

Note that there are only two entries under the experimental category in Figure 7-1 — small-scale experiments in laboratory settings and clinical trial designs. The example of assigning research participants to take a new birth control pill and then testing their lipid profiles is an example of a small-scale experiment in a laboratory setting. We describe clinical trials later in this chapter in "Advancing to the clinical trial stage."

Observational studies, on the other hand, can be further subdivided into two types: descriptive and analytic. Descriptive study designs include expert opinion, case studies, case series, ecologic (correlational) studies, and cross-sectional studies. These designs are called descriptive study designs because they focus on describing health in populations. (We explain what this means in "Describing What We See.") In contrast to descriptive study designs, there are only two types of analytic study designs: longitudinal cohort studies and case-control studies. Unlike descriptive studies, analytic studies are designed specifically for causal inference. These are described in more detail in the section, "Getting Analytical."

Describing what we see

As shown in Figure 7-1, there are two types of observational studies: descriptive and analytic. Descriptive study designs focus on describing patterns of human health and disease in populations, usually as part of *surveillance,* which is the act of quantifying patterns of health and disease in populations. Cross-sectional is one descriptive study design used in surveillance to produce incidence and prevalence rates of conditions or behaviors (see Chapter 14). For example, results from cross-sectional surveillance studies tell us that approximately 25 percent of women aged 15 to 44 who currently use contraception in the United States choose the birth control pill as their method of choice. While descriptive study designs are necessary in a practical sense, they are poor at developing evidence for causal inference, so they are considered inferior to analytic study designs.

Getting analytical

Analytic designs include longitudinal cohort studies and case-control studies. These are the strongest observational study designs for causal inference. Longitudinal cohort studies are used to study causes of more common conditions, like hypertension (HTN). It is called *longitudinal* because follow-up data are collected over years to see which members of the sample, or *cohort*, eventually get the outcome, and which members do not. (In a cohort study, none of the participants has the condition, or outcome, when they enter the study.) The cohort study design is described in more detail under the section, "Following a cohort over time."

Case-control studies are used when the outcome is not that common, such as liver cancer. In the case of rare conditions, first a group of individuals known to have the rare condition (cases) is identified and enrolled in the study. Then, a comparable group of individuals known to not have the rare condition is enrolled in the study as controls. The case-control study design is described in greater detail under the section "Going from case series to case-control."

Going from observational to experimental

You may notice in Figure 7-1 that observational studies (which are either descriptive or analytic) comprise most of the figure. Experimental studies — where participants are assigned to engage in certain behaviors or interventions — are less common than observational studies because they have ethical concerns, and are often expensive and complex. However, experimental studies benefit from generating the highest level of evidence for causal inference — much higher than observational studies.

Climbing the Evidence Pyramid

Each of the study designs discussed in the previous sections generates a particular level of evidence for causal inference. These levels of evidence may be arranged in a pyramid. As shown in Figure 7-2, the study designs with the strongest evidence for causal inference are at the top of the pyramid, and those with the weakest are at the bottom.

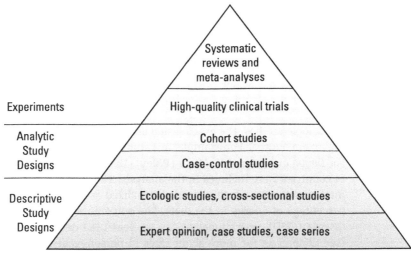

FIGURE 7-2: Levels of evidence in study designs.

© John Wiley & Sons, Inc.

Starting at the base: Expert opinion

At the base of the study design evidence pyramid shown Figure 7-2 is a descriptive study design: *expert opinion*. When the condition of dementia was first identified, few clinicians had seen patients with dementia. These clinicians served as experts who would write about the dementia patients they treated and share their experiences at medical conferences. This is what is meant by expert opinion, and while it is helpful when conditions are first identified, expert opinion is considered a very weak descriptive study design.

Making the case with case studies

Also at the base of Figure 7-2 are case studies and case series. To develop an understanding of dementia when it was first identified, clinicians treating patients needed to study them. They would write up *case studies* or *case reports* on individual patients describing their symptoms and providing the best descriptive evidence as possible. If the clinician was able to identify more than one patient, they could write about a series of patients, which is known as a *case series*. While case studies and case series are helpful for researchers when a condition is first identified, they are considered as providing very weak evidence to use for causal inference.

Making statements about the population

REMEMBER

Ecologic studies (also called correlational studies) and cross-sectional studies appear in the next level up from expert opinion and case studies and case series. Though ecologic studies are still descriptive designs that provide weak evidence, they have the advantage of having potentially very large samples.

In ecologic studies, the *experimental units* are often entire populations (such of a region or country). For example, in a study presented in Chapter 16 of *Epidemiology For Dummies* by Amal K. Mitra (Wiley), the experimental unit is a country, and 15 countries were included in the analysis. The exposure being investigated is fat intake from diet (which was operationalized as average saturated fat intake as a percentage of energy in the diet). The outcome was deaths from coronary heart disease (CHD), operationalized as 50-year CHD deaths per 1,000 person-years (see Chapter 15 for more about rates in person-years). Figure 7-3 presents the results in the form of a scatter plot.

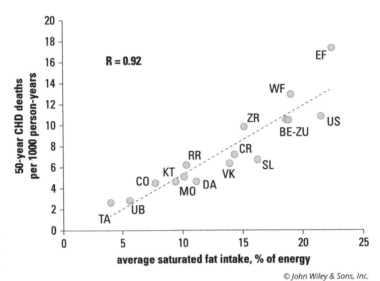

FIGURE 7-3:
Ecologic study
results.

© John Wiley & Sons, Inc.

As shown in Figure 7-3, the country's average value of the outcome (rate of CHD deaths) is plotted on the y-axis because it's the outcome. The exposure, average dietary fat intake for the country, is plotted on the x-axis. The 15 countries in the study are plotted according to their x-y coordinates. Notice that the United States is in the upper-right quadrant of the scatter plot because it has high rates of both the exposure and outcome. The strong, positive value of correlation coefficient *r* (which is 0.92) indicates that there is a strong positive bivariate association between the exposure and outcome, which is weak evidence for causality (flip to Chapter 15 for more on correlation).

But the problem with ecologic studies is that the experimental unit is a whole population — not an individual. What if the individuals in the United States who ate low-fat diets were actually the ones to die of CHD? And what if the ones who ate high-fat diets were more likely to die of something else? Attributing the behavior of a group to an individual is called the *ecologic fallacy,* and can be a problem with interpreting results like the ones shown in Figure 7-3.

That is why we also have cross-sectional studies, where the experimental unit is an individual, not a population. A cross-sectional study takes measurements of individuals at one point in time — either through an in-person hands-on examination, or by survey (over the phone, Internet, or in person). The National Health and Nutrition Examination Survey (NHANES) is a cross-sectional surveillance effort done by the U.S. government on a sample of residents every year. NHANES makes many measurements relevant to human health in the United States, including dietary fat intake as well as status of many chronic diseases including CHD. If an analysis of cross-sectional data like NHANES found that there was a strong positive association between high dietary fat intake and a CHD diagnosis in the individuals participating, it would still be weak evidence for causation, but would be stronger than what was found in the ecologic study presented in Figure 7-3.

Going from case series to case-control

The reason that there are two types of analytic study designs — case-control studies and cohort studies — is that cohort study designs do not work for statistically rare conditions. We use the term *statistically rare* because if someone you love gets cancer, cancer does not seem very rare. Yet, if you enroll a cohort of thousands of individuals including your loved one (who is free of cancer) in a cohort study and measure this cohort yearly to see who is diagnosed with cancer, it would take many years to get enough outcomes to be able to develop the regression models (like the ones described in Chapters 16 through 23) that would be necessary for causal inference. So for statistically rare conditions like the various cancers, you use the case-control design.

You can use a fourfold, or 2x2, table to better understand how case-control studies are different from cohort studies. (Refer to Chapters 13 and 14 for more about 2x2 tables.) As shown in Figure 7-4, the 2x2 table cells are labeled relative to exposure status (the rows) and outcome or disease status (the columns). For the columns, D+ stands for having the disease (or outcome), and D− means not having the disease or outcome. Also, for the rows, E+ means having the exposure, and E− means not having the exposure. Cell *a* includes the counts of individuals in the study who were positive for both the exposure and outcome, and cell *d* includes the counts of individuals who were negative for both the exposure and outcome (*a* and *d* are concordant cells because the exposure and outcome statuses agree). In the discordant cells, where the exposure and outcome do not agree, is *b*, which represents the count of those positive for the exposure but negative for the outcome, and *c*, which represents the count of those negative for the exposure but positive for the outcome.

Disease (Outcome) Status

		D+	D–	Total Exposed
Exposure Status	E+	a	b	(a + b)
	E–	c	d	(c + d)
	Total Disease (Outcome)	(a + c)	(b + d)	(a + b + c + d)

FIGURE 7-4:
2x2 table cells.

© *John Wiley & Sons, Inc.*

REMEMBER

The 2x2 table shown in Figure 7-4 is generic — meaning it can be filled in with data from a cross-sectional study, a case-control study, a cohort study, or even a clinical trial (if you replace the E+ and E– entries with intervention group assignment). How the results are interpreted from the 2x2 table depend upon the underlying study design. In the case of a cross-sectional study, an odds ratio (OR) could be calculated to quantify the strength of association between the exposure and outcome (see Chapter 14). However, any results coming from a 2x2 table do not control for *confounding*, which is a bias introduced by a nuisance variable associated with the exposure and the outcome, but not on the causal pathway between the exposure and outcome (more on confounding in Chapter 20).

TIP

Imagine that you were examining the cross-sectional association between having the exposure of obesity (yes/no), and having the outcome of HTN (yes/no). Household income may be a confounding variable, because lower income levels are associated with barriers to access to high-quality nutrition that could prevent both obesity and HTN. However, in a bivariate analysis like is done in a 2x2 table, there is no ability to control for confounding. To do that, you need to use a regression model like the ones described in Chapters 15 through 23.

So how would you use a 2x2 table for a case-control study on a statistically rare condition like liver cancer? Suppose that patients thought to have liver cancer are referred to a cancer center to undergo biopsies. Those with biopsies that are positive for liver cancer are placed in a registry. Suppose that in 2023 there were 30 cases of liver cancer found at this center that were placed in the registry. This would be a case series. Imagine that you had a hypothesis — that high levels of alcohol intake may have caused the liver cancer. You could interview the cases to determine their exposure status, or level of alcohol intake before they were diagnosed with liver cancer. Imagine that 10 of the 30 reported high alcohol intake. You will see that as some evidence for your hypothesis.

But you could not do causal inference unless you had a comparable comparison group without liver cancer so that you could fill out your 2x2 table. Imagine that you went back to the cancer center and were able to contact and enroll 30 patients who had liver biopsies but were found not to have liver cancer to serve as controls. Suppose that you interviewed this group and discovered that only two of them reported high levels of alcohol intake. You could develop the 2x2 table like the one shown in Figure 7-5.

Outcome

		Liver Cancer	No Liver Cancer	Total Exposed
Exposure	**High Alcohol Intake**	10	2	12
	Low Alcohol Intake	20	28	48
	Total Outcome	30	30	60

© John Wiley & Sons, Inc.

FIGURE 7-5: Example of a typical case-control study 2x2 table.

As shown in Figure 7-5, what is important is not the 2x2 table itself, but the order in which the counts are filled in. Notice that at the beginning of the study, you already knew the case total was 30, and you had determined that your control total would be 30 (although you are allowed to sample more controls if you want in a case-control study).

TIP

The correct measure of *relative risk* to present for a case-control study is the OR (as described in Chapter 14). It is important to acknowledge that when you present an OR from a case-control study, you interpret it as an *exposure OR*, not an outcome or disease OR. (It is also acceptable to present an OR in a cross-sectional study, but in that case, you are presenting an outcome or disease OR.)

REMEMBER

In a case-control study, because the condition is rare, you are sampling on the outcome and calculating the likelihood that the cases compared to controls were exposed. This study design is seen as extremely biased, which is why cohort studies are preferred, and are at a higher level of evidence. However, case-control study designs are necessary for rare diseases.

Following a cohort over time

In the previous section, we pointed out that case-control studies are used for rare diseases. Therefore, case-control studies do not have large sample sizes, which is evident in Figure 7-5 where the total sample size is 60. In contrast, cohort studies are used for studying common conditions, such as HTN, so they include very large sample sizes — but they still use the same 2x2 table for interpretation. Figure 7-6 offers an example of what a 2x2 table for a cohort study might look like where the exposure is high alcohol intake and the outcome is HTN.

Outcome

Exposure		Hypertension	No Hypertension	Total
	High Alcohol Intake	140	70	210
	Low Alcohol Intake	120	270	390
	Total	260	340	600

FIGURE 7-6: Example of a typical cohort study 2x2 table.

As shown in Figure 7-6, the total number of participants is large. This cohort of 600 participants could have been naturally sampled from the population, or they could be stratified by exposure, meaning that the study design could require a certain number of participants to be exposed and to be unexposed. Imagine that you insisted that 300 of your participants have high alcohol intake, and 300 have low alcohol intake. It may be harder to recruit for the study, but you would be sure to have enough exposed participants for your statistics to work out. In the case of Figure 7-6, 210 exposed and 390 unexposed participants were enrolled.

In cohort studies, all the participants are examined upon entering the study, and those with the outcome are not allowed to participate. Therefore, at the beginning of the study, all 600 of the participants did not have the outcome, which is HTN. A cohort study is essentially a series of cross-sectional studies on the same cohort called *waves*. The first wave is *baseline*, when the participants enter the study (all of whom do not have the outcome). Baseline values of important variables are measured (and criteria about baseline values may be used to set inclusion criteria, such as minimum age for the study). Subsequent waves of cross-sectional data collection take place at regular time intervals (such as every year or every two years). Changes in measured baseline values are tracked over time, and subgroups of the cohort are compared in terms of outcome status. Figure 7-6 shows the exposure status from baseline, and the outcome status from the first wave.

REMEMBER

Because the exposure is measured in a cohort study before any participants get the outcome, it is considered the highest level of evidence among the observational study designs. It is far less biased than the case-control study design. Several measures of relative risk can be used to interpret a cohort study, including the OR, risk ratio, and incidence rate (see Chapter 14).

Advancing to the clinical trial stage

Higher up the pyramid of evidence shown in Figure 7-2 are experiments. Not all experiments are at such a high level of evidence — only high-quality clinical trials. These are experiments, not observational studies. This is where the researcher assigns the participants to engage in a particular behavior or intervention during the study. There are different types of clinical trials as described in Chapter 5; however, the highest-quality trials use both double-blinding and randomization. *Double-blinding* is where both the researcher and the participant do not know whether the participant was assigned to an active intervention (one being studied), or a control intervention. *Randomization* is where participants are randomly assigned to groups (so there is no bias in selecting participants for each group).

TIP

It is possible to use a 2x2 table to analyze the results of a high-quality clinical trial as long as the rows are replaced with the intervention groups. You can report the same measure of relative risk as for a cohort study; however, the difference is that the high-quality clinical trial would be seen as having much less bias than the cohort study — and stronger causal evidence.

Reaching the top: Systematic reviews and meta-analyses

Imagine a scenario where a new drug for HTN was developed, and several clinical trials were conducted to see whether this drug was better than the most popular current drug used for HTN. How would we be able to know whether, on balance, the new drug was actually better when we have so many different clinical trials on the same drug with different results?

We could ask a similar question about observational studies as well. Imagine that multiple case-control studies were conducted to determine whether having liver cancer was associated with the exposure of having high prediagnosis alcohol intake. What is the overall answer? Does high alcohol intake cause liver cancer or not? You could also imagine that multiple cohort studies could be conducted examining association between the exposure of high alcohol intake and developing the outcome of HTN. How would the results of these cohort studies be taken together to answer the question of whether high alcohol intake actually causes HTN?

The answer to this question are systematic reviews and meta-analyses. In a systematic review, researchers set up inclusion and exclusion criteria for reports of studies. Included in those criteria are requirements for a certain study design. For interventions, randomized clinical trials containing a control group (called *randomized controlled trials*, or RCTs) are usually required, but for other exposures, either case-control or cohort study designs are required. With respect to medications, RCTs are required as part of regulatory approval for distribution (see Chapter 5), so expect to see meta-analyses arising from results from clinical trials. In a systematic review, the studies included are compared and summarized in a table, but their numerical estimates coming from their results are not combined. The meta-analysis is the same as a systematic review except the numerical estimates coming from the results reported are combined statistically to produce an overall estimate based on the studies included. Systematic reviews and meta-analyses are described in more detail in Chapter 20.

TIP

If you are looking for the highest quality of evidence right now about a current treatment or exposure and outcome, read the most recent systematic reviews and meta-analyses on the topic. If there aren't any, it may mean that the treatment, exposure, or outcome is new, and that there are not a lot of high quality observational or experimental studies published on the topic yet.

3

Getting Down and Dirty with Data

IN THIS PART . . .

Collect and validate your data, avoiding common pitfalls up front that can cause trouble later on.

Summarize your data in informative tables and display them in easy-to-understand graphs.

Understand the concepts of *accuracy,* which is how close a sample statistic is to the corresponding population parameter, and *precision,* which refers to how close replicate values of the sample statistic are to each other.

Calculate standard errors and confidence intervals for the sample estimates you can calculate from your data.

interval, and ratio)

» **Defining and entering different kinds of data into your research database**

» **Making sure your data are accurate**

» **Creating a data dictionary to describe the data in your database**

Chapter **8**

Getting Your Data into the Computer

efore you can analyze data, you have to collect it and get it into the computer in a form that's suitable for analysis. Chapter 5 describes this process as a series of steps — figuring out what data you need and how they are structured, creating data entry forms and computer files to hold your data, and entering and validating your data.

In this chapter, we describe a crucially important component of that process, which is storing the data properly in your research database. Different kinds of data can be represented in the computer in different ways. At the most basic level, there are numerical values and classifications, and most of us can immediately tell the two apart — you don't have to be a math genius to recognize "age" as numerical data, and "occupation" as categorical information.

So why are we devoting a whole chapter to describing, entering, and checking different types of data? It turns out that the topic of data storage is not quite as trivial as it may seem at first. You need to be aware of some important details or you may wind up collecting your data the wrong way and finding out too late that you can't run the appropriate analysis. This chapter starts by explaining the different levels of measurement, and shows you how to define and store different types of data. It also suggests ways to check your data for errors, and explains how to formally describe your database so that others are able to work with it if you're not available.

Looking at Levels of Measurement

Around the middle of the 20th century, the idea of levels of measurement caught the attention of biological and social-science researchers and, in particular, psychologists. One classification scheme, which has become widely used (at least in statistics textbooks), recognizes four levels at which variables can be measured: *nominal*, *ordinal*, *interval*, and *ratio*:

>> **Nominal variables** are expressed as mutually exclusive categories, like country of origin (United States, China, India, and so on), type of care provider (nurse, physician, social worker, and so on), and type of bacteria (such as coccus, bacillus, rickettsia, mycoplasma, or spirillum). Nominal indicates that the sequence in which you list the different categories is purely arbitrary. For example, listing type of care provider as nurse, physician, and social worker is no more or less natural than listing them as social worker, nurse, and physician.

>> **Ordinal data** have categorical values (or levels) that fall naturally into a logical sequence, like the severity of cancer (Stages I, II, III, and IV), or an agreement scale (often called a *Likert scale*) with levels of strongly disagree, somewhat disagree, neither agree nor disagree, somewhat agree, or strongly agree. Note that the levels are not necessarily equally spaced with respect to the conceptual difference between levels.

>> **Interval data** represents numerical measurements where, unlike with ordinal classifications, the difference (or interval) between two numbers *is* a meaningful measure in terms of being equally spaced, but the zero point is completely arbitrary and does *not* denote the complete absence of what you're measuring. For example, a change from 20 to 25 degrees Celsius represents the same amount of temperature increase as a change from 120 to 125 degrees Celsius. But 0 degrees Celsius is purely arbitrary — it does *not* represent the total absence of temperature; it's simply the temperature at which water freezes (or, if you prefer, ice melts).

>> **Ratio data,** unlike interval data, *does* have a true zero point. The numerical value of a ratio variable is directly proportional to how much there is of what you're measuring, and a value of zero means there's nothing at all. Income and systolic blood pressure are good examples of ratio data; an individual without a job may have zero income, which is not as bad as having a systolic blood pressure of 0 mmHg, because then that individual would no longer be alive!

REMEMBER

Statisticians may pontificate about *levels of measurement* excessively, pointing out cases that don't fall neatly into one of the four levels and bringing up various counterexamples. Nevertheless, you need to be aware of the concepts and terminology in the preceding list because you'll see them in statistics textbooks and articles, and because teachers love to include them on tests. The level of measurement of variables impacts how and to what precision data are collected. Other level-of-measurement considerations include minimizing the data collected to only what is needed, which also reduces data-privacy concerns and cost. And, more practically, knowing the level of measurement of a variable can help you choose the most appropriate way to analyze that variable.

Classifying and Recording Different Kinds of Data

Although you should be aware of the four levels of measurement described in the preceding section, you also need to be able to classify and deal with data in a more pragmatic way. The following sections describe various common types of data you're likely to encounter in the course of clinical and other research. We point out some considerations you need to think through before you start collecting your data.

WARNING

Making bad decisions (or avoiding making decisions) about exactly how to represent the data values in your research database can mess it up, and quite possibly doom the entire study to eventual failure. If you record the values to your variables the wrong way in your data, it may take an enormous amount of additional effort to go back and fix them, and depending upon the error, a fix may not even be possible!

Dealing with free-text data

REMEMBER

It's best to limit *free-text* variables that are difficult to box into one of the four levels of measurement, such as participant comments or write-in fields for *Other* choices in a questionnaire. Basically, you should only collect free-text variables when you need to record verbatim what someone said or wrote. Don't use free-text fields as a lazy-person's substitute for what should be precisely defined categorical data. Doing any meaningful statistical analysis of free-text fields is generally very difficult, if not impossible.

You should also be aware that most software has field-length limitations for text fields. Although commonly used statistical programs like Microsoft Excel, SPSS, SAS, R, and Python may allow for long data fields, this does not excuse you from designing your study so as to limit collection of free-text variables. Flip to Chapter 4 for an introduction to statistical software.

Assigning participant study identification (ID) numbers

Every participant in your study should have a unique *participant study identifier* (typically called a study ID). The study ID is present in the participant's data and is used for identifying the participant on study materials (for example, laboratory specimens sent for analysis). You may need to combine two variables to create a unique identifier. In a *single-site study* that is carried out at only one geographical location, the study ID can be a whole number that is two- to four-digits long. It doesn't have to start at 1; it can start at 100 if you want all the ID numbers to be three-digits long without leading zeros. In *multi-site studies* that are carried out at several locations (such as different clinics or labs), the number often follows some logic. For example, it could have two parts, such as a site number and a local study ID number separated by a hyphen (for example, 03-104), which is where you need two variables to get a unique ID.

Organizing name and address data in the study ID crosswalk

TIP

A research database should not include private identifying information for the participant, such as the participant's full name and home address. Yet, these data need to be accessible to study staff to facilitate the research. Private data like this is typically stored in a spreadsheet called a *study ID crosswalk*. This spreadsheet keeps a link (or crosswalk) between the participant's study ID and their private data not to be stored in the research database. When you store names in the study ID crosswalk, choose one of the following formats so that you can easily sort participants into alphabetical order, or use the spreadsheet to facilitate study mailings:

>> **A single variable:** Last, First Middle (like Smith, John A)

>> **Two columns:** One for Last, another for First and Middle

You may also want to include separate fields to hold prefixes (Mr., Mrs., Dr., and so on) and suffixes (Jr., III, PhD, and so forth).

Addresses should be stored in separate fields for street, city, state (or province), ZIP code (or comparable postal code).

Collecting categorical data in your research database

Setting up your data collection forms and database tables for categorical data requires more thought than you may expect. You may assume you already know how to record and enter categorical data. You just type in the values — such as "United States," "nurse," or "Stage I" — right? Wrong! (But wouldn't it be nice if it were that simple?) The following sections look at some of the issues you have to address when storing categorical values as research data.

Carefully coding categories

The first issue you need to decide is how to code the categories. How are you going to store the values in the research database? Do you want to enter the type of care provider as *nurse, physician,* or *social worker*; or as *N, P,* or *SW*; or as *1 = nurse, 2 = physician,* and *3 = social worker*; or in some other manner? Most modern statistical software can analyze categorical data with any of these representations, but it is easiest for the analyst if you code the variables using numbers to represent the categories. Software like SPSS, SAS, and R lets you specify a connection between number and text (for example, attaching a label to *1* to make it display *Nurse* on statistical output) so you can store categories using a numerical code while also displaying what the code means on statistical output. In general, best practices are to set conventions and be consistent, and make sure the content and meaning of each variable is documented. You can also attach variable labels.

Nothing is worse than having to deal with a data set in which a categorical variable has been stored with numerical codes, but there is no key to the codes and the person who created the data set is no longer available. This is why maintaining a data dictionary — described later in this chapter in "Creating a File that Describes Your Data File" — is a critical step for ensuring you analyze your research data properly.

Microsoft Excel doesn't care whether you type a word or a number in a cell, which can create problems when storing data. You can enter *Type of Caregiver* as *N* for the first subject, *nurse* for the second, *NURSE* for the third, *1* for the fourth, and *Nurse* for the fifth, and Excel won't stop you or throw up an error. Statistical programs like R would consider each of these entries as a separate, unique category. Even worse, you may inadvertently add a blank space in the cell before or after the text, which will be considered yet another category. Details such as case-sensitivity of character values (meaning patterns of being upper or lowercase) can impact queries. In Excel, avoid using autocomplete, and enter all levels of categorical variables as numerical codes (which can be decoded using your data dictionary).

Dealing with more than two levels in a category

When a categorical variable has more than two levels (like the *Type of Caregiver* or *Likert agreement scale* examples we describe in the earlier section "Looking at Levels of Measurement"), data storage gets even more interesting. First, you have to ask yourself, "Is this variable a *Choose only one* or *Choose all that apply* variable?" The coding is completely different for these two kinds of multiple-choice variables.

You handle the *Choose only one* situation just as we describe for *Type of Caregiver* in the preceding section — you establish numeric code for each alternative. For the *Likert scale* example, if the item asked about patient satisfaction, you could have a categorical variable called *PatSat*, with five possible values: 1 for strongly disagree, 2 for somewhat disagree, 3 for neither agree nor disagree, 4 for somewhat agree, and 5 for strongly agree. And for the *Type of Caregiver* example, if only one kind of caregiver is allowed to be chosen from the three choices of nurse, physician, or social worker, you can have a categorical variable called *CaregiverType* with three possible values: 1 for nurse, 2 for physician, and 3 for social worker. Depending upon the study, you may also choose to add a 4 for other, and a 9 for unknown (9, 99, and 999 are codes conventionally reserved for unknown). If you find unexpected values, it is important to research and document what these mean to help future analysts encountering the same data.

But the situation is quite different if the variable is *Choose all that apply.* For the *Type of Caregiver* example, if the patient is being served by a team of caregivers, you have to set up your database differently. Define separate variables in the database (separate columns in Excel) — one for each possible category value. Imagine that you have three variables called *Nurse, Physician,* and *SW* (the *SW* stands for *social worker*). Each variable is a two-value category, also known as a *two-state flag,* and is populated as 1 for having the attribute and 0 for not having the attribute. So, if participant 101's care team includes only a physician, participant 102's care team includes a nurse and a physician, and participant 103's care team includes a social worker and a physician, the information can be coded as shown in the following table.

Subject	Nurse	Physician	SW
101	0	1	0
102	1	1	0
103	0	1	1

If you have variables with more than two categories, missing values theoretically can be indicated by leaving the cell blank, but blanks are difficult to analyze in statistical software. Instead, categories should be set up for missing values so they can be part of the coding system (such as using a numerical code to indicate *unknown, refused,* or *not applicable*). The goal is to make sure that for every categorical variable, a numerical code is entered and the cell is not left blank.

Never try to cram multiple choices into one column! For example, don't enter 1, 2 into a cell in the *CaregiverType* column to indicate the patient has a nurse and physician. If you do, you have to painstakingly split your single multi-valued column into separate two-state flag columns (described earlier) before you analyze the data. Why not do it right the first time?

Recording numerical data

For numerical data (meaning interval and ratio data), the main issue is how much precision to record. Recording a numeric value to as many decimals as you have available is usually best. For example, if a scale can measure body weight to the nearest tenth of a kilogram, record it in the database to that degree of precision. You can always round off to the nearest kilogram later if you want, but you can never "unround" a number to recover digits you didn't record. So it's best to record values in your data from measurement instruments to the degree of precision provided.

Along the same lines, don't group numerical data into intervals when recording it. If you know the age to the nearest year, don't record *Age* in 10-year intervals (such as 20 to 29, 30 to 39, 40 to 49, and so on). You can always have the computer do that kind of grouping later, but you can never recover the age in years if all you record is the decade.

Some statistical programs let you store numbers in different formats. The program may refer to these different *storage modes* using arcane terms for short, long, or very long *integers* (whole numbers) or *single-precision* (short) or *double-precision* (long) *floating point* (fractional) numbers. Each type has its own limits, which may vary from one program to another or from one kind of computer to another. For example, a short integer may be able to represent only whole numbers within the range from $-32,768$ to $+32.767$, whereas a double-precision floating-point number could easily handle a number like $1.23456789012345 \times 10^{250}$. Excel has no trouble storing numerical data in any of these formats, so to make these choices, it is best to study the statistical program you will use to analyze the data. That way, you can make rules for storing the data in Excel that make it easy for you to analyze the data once it is imported into the statistical program.

Following are issues to consider with respect to numerical variables in Excel:

» Don't put two numbers (such as a blood pressure reading of 135 / 85 mmHg) into one column of data. Excel won't complain about it, but it will treat it as text because of the embedded "/", rather than as numerical data. Instead, create two separate variables and enter each number into the appropriate variable.

>> When recording multiple types of measurements (such as days, weeks, months, and years), use two columns to record the data (such as *time* and *type*). In the first column, store the value of the variable, and in the second column, store a code to indicate the type (such as *1 = days, 2 = weeks, 3 = months,* and *4 = years*). As an example, "3 weeks" would be entered as a *3* in the *time* column and *2* in the *type* column.

WARNING

Missing numerical data requires a little more thought than missing categorical data. Some researchers use 99 (or 999, or 9999) to indicate a missing value in categorical data, but this approach should not be used for numeric data (because the statistical program will see these values as actual measured values, and not codes for missing data). The simplest technique for indicating missing numerical data is to leave it blank. Most software treats blank cells as missing data in a calculation, but this changes depending on the software, so it's important to confirm missing values handling in your analysis.

Entering date and time data

Now we're going to tell you something that sounds like we're contradicting the advice we just gave you (but, of course, we're not!). Most statistical software (including Microsoft Excel) can represent dates and times as a single variable (an "instant" on a continuous timeline), so take advantage of that if you can. In Excel, you can enter the date and time as one variable (for example, 07/15/2020 08:23), not as a separate date variable and a time variable. This method is especially useful when dealing with events that take place over a short time interval (like events occurring during a surgical procedure). It is important to collect all potential start and end dates so any duration during the study can be calculated.

Some programs may store a date and time as a *Julian Date*, whose zero occurred at noon, Greenwich Mean Time, on Jan. 1, 4713 BC. (Nothing happened on that date; it's purely a numerical convenience.)

TIP

What if you don't know the day of the month? This happens a lot with medical history items; a participant may say, "I got the flu in September 2021." Most software (including Excel) insists that a date variable be a complete date, and won't accept just a month and a year. In this case, a business rule is created to set the day (as either the 1st, 15th, or last day of the month). Similarly, if both the month and day are missing, you can set up a business rule to estimate both.

If you impute a date, just create a new column with the imputed date, because you want to be cautious. Make sure to keep the original partial date for traceability. Any date imputation should be consistent with the study protocol, and not bias the results. Completely missing dates should be left blank, as statistical software treats blank cells as missing data.

TIP

Because of the way most statistics programs store dates and times, they can easily calculate intervals between any two points in time by simple subtraction. It is best practices to store raw dates and times, and let the computer calculate the intervals later (rather than calculate them yourself). For example, if you create variables for date of birth (*DOB*) and a visit date (*VisDt*) in Excel, you can calculate an accurate age at the time of the visit with this formula:

$$Age = (VisDt - DOB) / 365.25$$

Checking Your Entered Data for Errors

REMEMBER

After you've entered all your data into the computer, there are a few things you can do to check for errors:

>> **Examine the smallest and largest values in numerical data:** Have the software show you the smallest and largest values for each numerical variable. This check can often catch decimal-point errors (such as a hemoglobin value of 125 g/dL instead of 12.5 g/dL) or transposition errors (for example, a weight of 517 pounds instead of 157 pounds).

>> **Sort the values of variables:** If your program can show you a sorted list of all the values for a variable, that's even better — it often shows misclassified categories as well as numerical outliers.

>> **Search for blanks and commas:** You can have Excel search for blanks in category values that shouldn't have blanks, or for commas in numeric variables. Make sure the "Match entire cell contents" option is deselected in the Find and Replace dialog box (you may have to click the Options button to see the check box). This operation can also be done using statistical software. Be wary if there a large number of missing values, because this could indicate a data collection problem.

>> **Tabulate categorical variables:** You can have your statistics program tabulate each categorical variable (showing you the frequency each different category occurred in your data). This check usually finds misclassified categories. Note that blanks and special characters in character variables may cause incorrect results when querying, which is why it is important to do this check.

>> **Spot-checking data entry:** If doing data entry from forms or printed material, choose a percentage to double-check (for example, 10 percent of the forms you entered). This can help you tell if there are any systematic data entry errors or missing data.

Creating a File that Describes Your Data File

Every research database, large or small, simple or complicated, should include a *data dictionary* that describes the variables contained in the database. It is a necessary part of study documentation that needs to be accessible to the research team. A data dictionary is usually set up as a table (often in Excel), where each row provides documentation for each variable in the database. For each variable, the dictionary should contain the following information (sometimes referred to as *metadata*, which means "data about data"):

>> **A variable name** (usually no more than ten characters) that's used when telling the software what variables you want it to use in an analysis

>> **A longer verbal description of the variable** in a human-readable format (in other words, a person reading this description should be able to understand the content of the variable)

>> **The type of data** (text, categorical, numerical, date/time, and so on)

- **If numeric:** Information about how that number is displayed (how many digits are before and after the decimal point)

- **If date/time:** How it's formatted (for example, 12/25/13 10:50pm or 25Dec2013 22:50)

- **If categorical:** What codes and descriptors exist for each level of the category (these are often called *picklists,* and can be documented on a separate tab in an Excel data dictionary)

>> **How missing values are represented** in the database (99, 999, "NA," and so on)

Database programs like SQL and statistical programs like SAS often have a function that can output information like this about a data set, but it still needs to be curated by a human. It may be helpful to start your data dictionary with such output, but it is best to complete it in Excel. That way, you can add the human curation yourself to the Excel data dictionary, and other research team members can easily access the data dictionary to better understand the variables in the database.

Chapter **9**

Summarizing and Graphing Your Data

A large study can involve thousands of participants, hundreds of variables, and millions of individual data points. You need to summarize this ocean of individual values for each variable down to a few numbers, called *summary statistics,* that give readers an idea of what the whole collection of numbers looks like — that is, how they're *distributed.*

When presenting your results, you usually want to arrange these summary statistics into tables that describe how the variables change over time or differ between categories, or how two or more variables are related to each other. And, because a picture really is worth a thousand words, you will want to display these distributions, changes, differences, and relationships graphically. In this chapter, we show you how to summarize and graph both categorical and numerical data. *Note:* This chapter doesn't cover *time-to-event* (survival) data, which is the topic of Chapter 22.

Summarizing and Graphing Categorical Data

A categorical variable is summarized by tallying the number of participants in each category and expressing this number as a count. You might also compute a percentage of the total number of participants in all categories combined. So a sample of 422 participants can be summarized by health insurance type, as shown in Table 9-1.

TABLE 9-1

Study Participants Categorized by Health Insurance Type

Health Insurance Type	Count	Percent of Total
Commercial	128	30.3%
Public	141	33.4%
Military	70	16.6%
Other	83	19.7%
Total	**422**	**100%**

The joint distribution of participants between two categorical variables is summarized by a *cross-tabulation* (or *cross-tab*). Table 9-2 shows an example of a cross-tab of the same participants in our example with type of health insurance on one axis, and urban-rural classification of their residence on the other.

TABLE 9-2

Cross-Tabulation of Participants by Two Categorical Variables

		Health Insurance Type				
		Commercial	Public	Military	Other	Total
Urban-Rural Classification of Residence	*Rural*	60	60	34	42	196
	Urban	68	81	36	41	226
	Total	128	141	70	83	422

After looking at the frequencies in Table 9-2, you may be curious about the percentages, which would make these numbers more comparable. But a cross-tab can get very cluttered if you try to include them, as there are different types: the column percentage, the row percentage, and the total percentage. For example, the 60 rural residents with commercial health insurance in Table 9-2 comprise 46.9 percent of all participants with commercial health insurance, because 60 divided by the total number with commercial health insurance, which is 128 (the column total), equals 46.9 percent.

Groups are often compared across columns, and if that is the intention, column percentages should be displayed. But if you divide these same 60 rural residents with commercial insurance by their row total of 169 rural residents, you find they make up 30.6 percent of all rural residents, which is a row percentage. And if you go on to divide these 60 participants by the total sample size of the study, which is 422, you find that they make up 14.2 percent of all participants in the study.

Categorical data are typically displayed graphically as frequency bar charts and as pie charts:

>> **Frequency bar charts:** Displaying the spread of participants across the different categories of a variable is commonly done by a bar chart (see Figure 9-1a). Generally, statistical programs are used to make bar charts. To create a bar chart manually from a tally of participants in each category, you draw a graph containing one vertical bar for each category, making the height proportional to the number of participants in that category.

>> **Pie charts:** Pie charts indicate the relative number of participants in each category by the angle of a circular wedge, which can also be considered more deliciously as a piece of the pie. To create a pie chart manually, you multiply the percentage of participants in each category by 360, which is the number of degrees of arc in a full circle, and then divide by 100. By doing that, you are essentially figuring out what proportion of the circle to devote to that pie piece. Next, you draw a circle with a compass, and then split it up into wedges using a *protractor* — remember from high school math? Trust us, it's easier to use statistical software.

TIP

Most scientific writers recommend the usage of bar charts over pie charts. They express more information in a smaller space, and allow for more accurate visual comparisons.

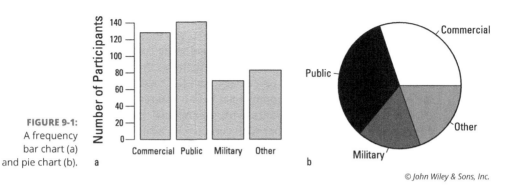

FIGURE 9-1:
A frequency
bar chart (a)
and pie chart (b).

© John Wiley & Sons, Inc.

Summarizing Numerical Data

Summarizing a numerical variable isn't as simple as summarizing a categorical variable. The summary statistics for a numerical variable should convey how the individual values of that variable are distributed across your sample in a concise and meaningful way. These summary statistics should give you some idea of the shape of the true distribution of that variable in the population from which you draw your sample (read Chapter 3 and Chapter 6 to refresh your memory about sampling). That true population distribution can have almost any shape, including the typical shapes shown in Figure 9-2: normal, skewed, pointy-topped, and bimodal (two-peaked).

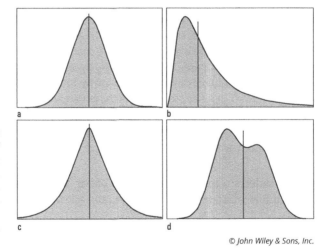

FIGURE 9-2:
Four different
shapes of
distributions:
normal (a),
skewed (b),
pointy-topped (c),
and bimodal
(two-peaked) (d).

© John Wiley & Sons, Inc.

How can you convey a visual picture of what the true distribution may look like by using just a few summary numbers? By reporting values of measures of some important characteristics of these distributions, so that the reader can infer the shape. This is similar to learning that one Olympic ice skater scored an average of 9.0 compared to another who scored an average of 5.0. You will not know what the skate routines looked like unless you watch them, but the score will already tell you that if you were to watch them, you would expect to see that the one that scored 9.0 was executed in a more visually pleasing way than the one that scored 5.0.

Frequency distributions have names for their important characteristics, including:

» **Center:** Where along the distribution of the values do the numbers tend to center?

» **Dispersion:** How much do these numbers spread out?

» **Symmetry:** If you were to draw a vertical line down the middle of the distribution, does the distribution shape appear as if the vertical line is a mirror, reflecting an identical shape on both sides? Or do the sides look noticeably different — and if so, how?

» **Shape:** Is the top of the distribution nicely rounded, or pointier, or flatter?

Like using average skating scores to describe the visual appeal of an Olympic skate routine, to describe a distribution you need to calculate and report numbers that measure each of these four characteristics. These characteristics are what we mean by summary statistics for numerical variables.

Locating the center of your data

When you start exploring a set of numbers, an important first step is to determine what value they tend to center around. This characteristic is called, intuitively enough, *central tendency.* Many statistical textbooks describe three measures of central tendency: *mean* (which is the same as *average*), *median,* and *mode.* You may assume these are the three optimal measures to describe a distribution (because they all begin with *m* and are easy to remember). But all three have limitations, especially when dealing with data obtained from samples in human research, as described in the following sections.

Arithmetic mean

The *arithmetic mean,* also commonly called the *mean* (or the *average*), is the most familiar and most often quoted measure of central tendency. Throughout this book, whenever we use the two-word term *the mean,* we're referring to the arithmetic mean. (There are several other kinds of means besides the arithmetic mean, which we describe later in this chapter.)

REMEMBER

The mean of a sample is often denoted by the symbol m or by placing a horizontal bar over the name of the variable, like $\overline{X}$. The mean is obtained by adding up the values and dividing by the sample size — meaning how many there are. (If you are using software for this, make sure missing values are excluded, or the equation will not compute.) Here's a small sample of numbers — the diastolic blood pressure (DBP) values of seven study participants (in mmHg) arranged in increasing numerical order: 84, 84, 89, 91, 110, 114, and 116. For the DBP sample:

$$\text{Arithmetic Mean} = (\ 84 + 84 + 89 + 91 + 110 + 114 + 116\ ) / 7$$
$$= 688 / 7 = 98.3 (\text{approximately})$$

You can write the general formula for the arithmetic mean of N number of values contained in the variable X in several ways:

$$\text{Arithmetic Mean} = m = \overline{X} = \frac{\sum_{i=1}^{N} X_i}{N} = \frac{\sum_i X_i}{N} = \frac{\sum X}{N}$$

See Chapter 2 for a refresher on mathematical notation and formulas, including how to interpret the various forms of the summation symbol Σ (the Greek capital sigma). In the rest of this chapter, we use the simplest form, meaning the form without the i subscripts that refer to specific elements of an array, whenever possible.

TIP

Some statistical books use the notation such that capital $\overline{X}$ and capital N refer to census parameters, and lowercase versions of those to refer to sample statistics. In this book, we make it clear each time we present this notation whether we are talking about a census or a sample.

Median

Like the mean, the *median* is a common measure of central tendency. In fact, it could be argued that the median is the only one of the three that really takes the word *central* seriously.

REMEMBER

The median of a sample is the middle value in the sorted (ordered) set of numbers. By definition, half of the numbers are smaller than the median, and half are larger. The median of a *population* frequency distribution function (like the curves shown in Figure 9-2) divides the total area under the curve into two equal parts: Half of the *area under the curve* (AUC) lies to the left of the median, and half lies to the right.

Consider the sample of diastolic blood pressure (DBP) measurements from seven study participants from the preceding section. If you arrange the values in order from lowest to highest mmHg, you can list them as 84, 84, 89, 91, 110, 114, and 116. There are seven values, and 91 is the fourth of the seven sorted values, so that is the median. Three DBPs in the sample are smaller than 91 mmHg, and three are larger than 91 mmHg. If you have an even number of values, the median is the average of the two middle values. So imagine that you add a value of 118 mmHg to the top of your list, so you now have eight values. To get the median, you would make an average of the fourth and fifth value, which would be (91 + 110)/2 = 100.5 mmHg (don't be thrown off by the 0.5).

Statisticians often say that they prefer the median to the mean because the median is much less strongly influenced by extreme outliers than the mean. For example, if the largest value for DBP had been very high — such as 150 mmHg instead of 116 mmHg — the mean would have jumped from 98.3 mmHg up to 103.1 mmHg. But in the same case, the median would have remained unchanged at 91. Here's an even more extreme example: If a multibillionaire were to move into a certain state, the *mean* family net worth in that state might rise by hundreds of dollars, but the *median* family net worth would probably rise by only a few cents (if it were to rise at all). This is why you often hear the median rather than mean income in reports comparing income across regions.

Mode

REMEMBER

The *mode* of a sample of numbers is the most frequently occurring value in the sample. One way to remember this is to consider that mode means *fashion* in French, so the mode is the most popular value in the data set. But the mode has several issues when it comes to summarizing the centrality of observed values for continuous numerical variables. Often there are no exact duplicates, so there is no mode. If there are any exact duplicates, they usually are not in the center of the data. And if there is more than one value that is duplicated the same number of times, you will have more than one mode.

So the mode is not a good summary statistic for sampled data. But it's useful for characterizing a *population* distribution, because it's the value where the peak of the distribution function occurs. Some distribution functions can have two peaks (a *bimodal* distribution), as shown earlier in Figure 9-2d, indicating two distinct subpopulations, such as the distribution of age of death from influenza in many populations, where we see a mode in young children, and another mode in older adults.

Considering some other "means" to measure central tendency

Several other kinds of means are useful measures of central tendency in certain circumstances. They're called *means* because they all calculated using the same approach. The difference is that each type of mean adds a slightly different twist to the basic mathematical process.

INNER MEAN

REMEMBER

The *inner mean* (also called the *trimmed mean*) of N numbers is calculated by removing the lowest value (the *minimum*) and the highest value (the *maximum*), and calculating the arithmetic mean of the remaining N − 2 *inner* values. For the sample of seven values of DBP from study participants from the example used earlier in this chapter (which were 84, 84, 89, 91, 110, 114, and 116 mmHg), you would drop the minimum and the maximum to compute the inner mean: $(84 + 89 + 91 + 110 + 114)/5 = 488/5 = 97.6$.

An inner mean that is even more inner can be calculated by making an even stricter rule. The rule could be to drop the two (or more) of the highest and two (or more) of the lowest values from the data, and then calculate the arithmetic mean of the remaining values. In the interest of fairness, you should always chop the same number of values from the low end as from the high end. Like the median (discussed earlier in this chapter), the inner mean is more resistant to extreme values called *outliers* than the arithmetic mean.

GEOMETRIC MEAN

REMEMBER

The *geometric mean* (often abbreviated GM) can be defined by two different-looking formulas that produce exactly the same value. The basic definition has this formula:

$$\text{Geometric Mean} = GM = \sqrt[N]{\Pi X}$$

We describe the product symbol Π (the Greek capital pi) in Chapter 2. This formula is telling you to multiply the values of the N observations together, and then take the Nth root of the product. Using the numbers from the earlier example (where you had DBP data on seven participants, with the values 84, 84, 89, 91, 110, 114, and 116 mmHg), the equation looks like this:

$$GM = \sqrt[7]{84 \times 84 \times 89 \times 91 \times 110 \times 114 \times 116} = \sqrt[7]{83,127,648,746,160,} = 93.4$$

Even with technology, this formula is computationally challenging. By using log-arithms (which turn multiplications into additions and roots into divisions), you can develop a *numerically stable* alternative formula, which is:

$$\log(GM) = \frac{\sum \log(X)}{N}, \text{or } GM = \text{antilog}\left(\frac{\sum \log(X)}{N} \right)$$

This formula may look complicated, but it really just says, "The geometric mean is the *antilog* of the *mean* of the *logs* of the values in the sample." In other words, to calculate the GM using this formula, you take the log of each value in your sample, then average all those logs together, and then take the antilog of that average. You can choose to use either natural or common logarithms, but make sure that whatever you choose, you use same type of antilog. (Flip to Chapter 2 for the basics of logarithms.)

Describing the spread of your data

After central tendency (described earlier in "Locating the center of your data"), the second most important set of summary statistics for numerical values refers to how tightly or loosely they tend to cluster around a central value, meaning how they are *dispersed*. There are several common measures of dispersion, as you find out in the following sections.

Standard deviation, variance, and coefficient of variation

The *standard deviation* (usually abbreviated SD, sd, or just s) of a set of numerical values tells you how much the individual values tend to differ from the mean in either direction (see "Locating the center of your data" for a discussion of the mean). The SD is calculated as follows:

$$SD = sd = s = \sqrt{\frac{\sum_i (d_i)^2}{N-1}} \text{ where } d_i = X_i - \overline{X}$$

REMEMBER

This formula is saying that you calculate the SD of a set of N numbers by first subtracting the mean from each value (X_i) to get the *deviation* (d_i) of each value from the mean. Then, you take the square each of these deviations and add up the d_i^2 terms. After that, you divide that number by $N - 1$, and finally, you take the square root of that number to get your answer, which is the SD.

For the sample of diastolic blood pressure (DBP) measurements for seven study participants in the example used earlier in this chapter, where the values are 84, 84, 89, 91, 110, 114, and 116 mmHg and the mean is 98.3 mmHg, you calculate the SD as follows:

$$SD = \sqrt{\frac{(84-98.3)^2 + (84-98.3)^2 + \dots + (116-98.3)^2}{7-1}} = 14.4$$

Several other useful measures of dispersion are related to the SD:

>> **Variance:** The *variance* is just the square of the SD. For the DBP example, the variance $14.4^2 = 207.36$.

>> **Coefficient of variation:** The *coefficient of variation* (CV) is the SD divided by the mean. For the DBP example, $CV = 14.4 / 98.3 = 0.1465$, or 14.65 percent.

Range

REMEMBER

The *range* of a set of values is the minimum value subtracted from the maximum value:

Range = maximum value – minimum value

Consider the example from the preceding section, where you had DBP measurements from seven study participants (which were 84, 84, 89, 91, 110, 114, and 116 mmHg). The minimum value is 84, the maximum value is 116, and the range is 32 (equal to $116 - 84$).

Centiles

The basic idea of the median is that ½ (half) of your numbers are less than the median, and the other ½ are greater than the median. This concept can be extended to other fractions besides ½.

REMEMBER

A *centile* (also referred to as *percentile*) is a value that a certain percentage of the values are less than. For example, ¼ of the values are less than the 25th centile (and ¾ of the values are greater). The median is just the 50th centile. The 25th, 50th, and 75th centiles are called the first, second, and third *quartiles,* respectively, and are used often. There are other sets of centiles, such as *deciles*, which break at every ten percentiles, that are used less often.

As we explain in the earlier section "Median," if the sorted sequence of your numerical variable has no middle value, you have to calculate the median as the average of the two middle numbers. The same situation comes up in calculating centiles, but there are different ways that statistical software does the calculation. Fortunately, the different formulas they use give nearly the same result.

TIP

The *inter-quartile range* (IQR) is the difference between the 25th and 75th centiles (the first and third quartiles).

Numerically expressing the symmetry and shape of the distribution

In the following sections, we discuss two summary statistics used to describe aspects of the symmetry and shape of the distribution of values of numerical variables (pictured earlier in Figure 9-2).

Skewness

Skewness refers to the left-right symmetry of the distribution. Figure 9-3 illustrates some examples.

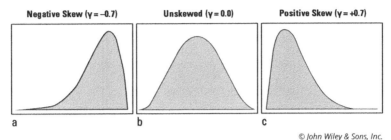

Negative Skew (γ = –0.7)   **Unskewed (γ = 0.0)**   **Positive Skew (γ = +0.7)**

a   b   c

© *John Wiley & Sons, Inc.*

FIGURE 9-3: Distributions can be left-skewed (a), symmetric (b), or right-skewed (c).

Figure 9-3b shows a symmetrical distribution. If you look back to Figures 9-2a and 9-2c, which are also symmetrical, they look like the vertical line in the center is a mirror reflecting perfect symmetry, so these have no skewness. But Figure 9-2b has a long tail on the right, so it is considered *right skewed* (and if you flipped the shape horizontally, it would have a long tail on the left, and be considered *left-skewed*, as in Figure 9-3a).

How do you express skewness in a summary statistic? The most common skewness coefficient, often represented by the Greek letter γ (lowercase gamma), is calculated by averaging the cubes (third powers) of the deviations of each point from the mean and scaling by the SD. Its value can be positive, negative, or zero.

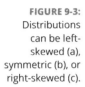

REMEMBER

Here is how to interpret the skewness coefficient (γ):

>> A negative γ indicates *left-skewed* data (Figure 9-3a).

>> A zero γ indicates *unskewed* data (Figures 9-2a and 9-2c, and Figure 9-3b).

>> A positive γ indicates *right-skewed* data (Figures 9-2b and 9-3c).

Notice that in Figure 9-3a, which is left-skewed, the γ = –0.7, and for Figure 9-3c, which is right-skewed, the γ = 0.7. And for Figure 9-3b — the symmetrical distribution — the γ = 0, but this almost never happens in real life. So how large does γ have to be before you suspect real skewness in your data? A rule of thumb for large samples is that if γ is greater than $4 / \sqrt{N}$, your data are probably skewed.

Kurtosis

Kurtosis is a less-used summary statistic of numerical data, but you still need to understand it. Take a look at the three distributions shown in Figure 9-4, which all have the same mean and the same SD. Also, all three have perfect left-right symmetry, meaning they are unskewed. But their shapes are still very different. *Kurtosis* is a way of quantifying these differences in shape.

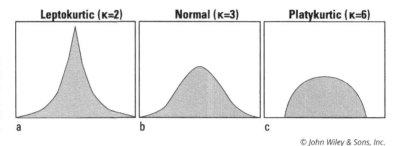

FIGURE 9-4:
Three distributions: leptokurtic (a), normal (b), and platykurtic (c).

A good way to compare the kurtosis of the distributions in Figure 9-4 is through the *Pearson kurtosis index*. The Pearson kurtosis index is often represented by the Greek letter k (lowercase kappa), and is calculated by averaging the fourth powers of the deviations of each point from the mean and scaling by the SD. Its value can range from 1 to infinity and is equal to 3.0 for a normal distribution. The *excess kurtosis* is the amount by which k exceeds (or falls short of) 3.

REMEMBER

One way to think of kurtosis is to see the distribution as a body silhouette. If you think of a typical distribution function curve as having a *head* (which is near the center), *shoulders* on either side of the head, and *tails* out at the ends, the term kurtosis refers to whether the distribution curve tends to have

>> A pointy head, fat tails, and no shoulders, which is called *leptokurtic,* and is shown in Figure 9-4a (where $k < 3$).

>> An appearance of being normally distributed, as shown in Figure 9-4b (where $k = 3$).

>> Broad shoulders, small tails, and not much of a head, which is called *platykurtic*. This is shown in Figure 9-4c (where k > 3).

TIP

A *very rough* rule of thumb for large samples is that if k differs from 3 by more than $8 / \sqrt{N}$, your data have abnormal kurtosis.

Structuring Numerical Summaries into Descriptive Tables

Now you know how to calculate the basic summary statistics that convey the general idea of how a set of numerical values is distributed. So which summary statistics do you report? Generally, you select a few of the most useful summary statistics in summarizing your particular data set, and arrange them in a concise way. Many biostatisticians choose to report N, mean, SD, median, minimum, and maximum, and arrange them something like this:

$$\text{mean} \pm \text{SD} \, (\text{N})$$

$$\text{median} \, (\text{minimum} - \text{maximum})$$

Consider the example used earlier in this chapter of seven measures of diastolic blood pressure (DBP) from a sample of study participants (with the values of 84, 84, 89, 91, 110, 114, and 116 mmHg), where you calculated all these summary statistics. Remember not to display decimals beyond what were collected in the original data. Using this arrangement, the numbers would be reported this way:

$$98.3 \pm 14.4 \, (7)$$

$$91 \, (84 - 116)$$

The real utility of this kind of compact summary is that you can place it in each cell of a table to show changes over time and between groups. For example, a sample of systolic blood pressure (SBP) measurements taken from study participants before and after treatment with two different hypertension drugs (Drug A and Drug B) can be summarized concisely, as shown in Table 9-3.

TABLE 9-3   **Systolic Blood Pressure Treatment Results**

	Before Treatment		After Treatment		Change	
	Mean ± SD (N)	Median (min – max)	Mean ± SD (N)	Median (min – max)	Mean ± SD (N)	Median (min – max)
Drug A	138.7 ± 10.3 (40)	139.5 (117 – 161)	121.1 ± 13.9 (40)	121.5 (85 – 154)	-17.6 ± 8.0 (40)	–17.5 (–34 – 4)
Drug B	141.0 ± 10.8 (40)	143.5 (111 – 160)	141.0 ± 15.4 (40)	142.5 (100 – 166)	-0.1 ± 9.9 (40)	1.5 (–25 – 18)

Table 9-3 shows that Drug A tended to lower blood pressure by about 18 mmHg. For Drug A, mean SBP changed from 139 to 121 mmHg from before to after treatment, whereas the Drug B group produced no noticeable change in blood pressure because it stayed around 141 mmHg from pretreatment to post-treatment. All that's missing are some p values to indicate the *significance* of the changes over time within each group and of the differences between the groups. We show you how to calculate those in Chapter 11.

Graphing Numerical Data

Displaying information graphically is a central part of interpreting and communicating the results of scientific research. You can easily spot subtle features in a graph of your data that you'd never notice in a table of numbers. Entire books have been written about graphing numerical data, so we only give a brief summary of some of the more important points here.

Showing the distribution with histograms

REMEMBER

Histograms are bar charts that show what fraction of the participants have values falling within specified intervals called *classes*. The main purpose of a histogram is to show you how the values of a numerical value are distributed. This distribution is an approximation of the true population frequency distribution for that variable, as shown in Figure 9-5.

Population: Mean = 100 mmHg, SD = 15 mmHg

60 Participants: Mean = 98.2 mmHg, SD = 13.7 mmHg

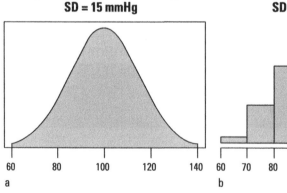
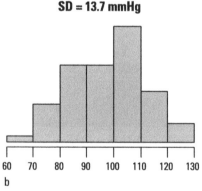

FIGURE 9-5: Population distribution of systolic blood pressure (SBP) measurements in mmHg (a) and distribution of a sample from that population (b).

© John Wiley & Sons, Inc.

The smooth curve in Figure 9-5a shows how SBP values are distributed in an infinitely large population. The height of the curve at any SBP value is proportional to the fraction of the population in the immediate vicinity of that SBP. This curve has the typical *bell* shape of a normal distribution.

The histogram in Figure 9-5b indicates how the SBP measurements of 60 study participants randomly sampled from the population might be distributed. Each bar represents an interval or class of SBP values with a width of ten mmHg. The height of each bar is proportional to the number of participants in the sample whose SBP fell within that class.

Log-normal distributions

Because a sample is only an imperfect representation the population, determining the precise shape of a distribution can be difficult unless your sample size is very large. Nevertheless, a histogram usually helps you spot skewed data, as shown in Figure 9-6a. This kind of shape is typical of a *log-normal* distribution (Chapter 25), which is a distribution you often see when analyzing biological measurements, such as lab values. It's called log-normal because if you take a logarithm (of any type) of each data value, the resulting logs will have a normal distribution, as shown in Figure 9-6b.

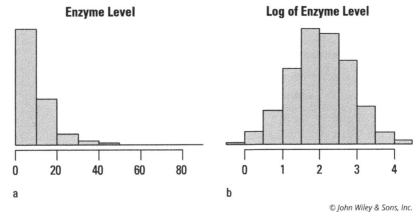

FIGURE 9-6:
Log-normal data are skewed (a), but the logarithms are normally distributed (b).

© John Wiley & Sons, Inc.

Because distributions are so important to biostatistics, it's a good practice to prepare a histogram for every numerical variable you plan to analyze. That way, you can see whether it's noticeably skewed and, if so, whether a logarithmic transformation makes the distribution normal enough so you can use statistics intended for normal distributions on your data.

If you can't find any transformation that makes your data look even approximately normal, then you have to analyze your data using *nonparametric* methods, which don't assume that your data are normally distributed.

Summarizing grouped data with bars, boxes, and whiskers

Sometimes you want to show how a numerical variable differs from one group of participants to another. For example, blood levels of a certain cardiovascular enzyme vary among the cardiology patients at four different clinics: Clinic A, B, C, and D. Two types of graphs are commonly used for this purpose: bar charts and box-and-whiskers plots.

Bar charts

One simple way to display and compare the means of several groups of data is with a bar chart, like the one shown in Figure 9-7a. Here, the bar height for each group of patients equals the mean (or median, or geometric mean) value of the enzyme level for patients at the clinic represented by the bar. And the bar chart becomes even more informative if you indicate the spread of values for each clinical sample by placing lines representing one SD above and below the tops of the bars, as shown in Figure 9-7b. These lines are always referred to as *error bars,* which is an unfortunate choice of words that can cause confusion when error bars are added to a bar chart. In this case, error refers to statistical error (described in Chapter 6).

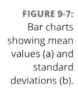

FIGURE 9-7:
Bar charts showing mean values (a) and standard deviations (b).

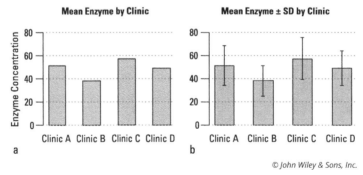

© *John Wiley & Sons, Inc.*

But even with error bars, a bar chart still doesn't provide a picture of the *distribution* of enzyme levels within each group. Are the values skewed? Are there outliers? Imagine that you made a histogram for each subgroup of patients — Clinic A, Clinic B, Clinic C, and Clinic D. But if you think about it, four histograms would take up a lot of space. There is a solution for this! Keep reading to find out what it is.

Box-and-whiskers charts

The *box-and-whiskers plot* (or *B&W*, or just *box plot*) plot uses very little space to display a lot of information about the distribution of numbers in one or more groups of participants. A box plot of the same enzyme data used in Figure 9-7 is shown in Figure 9-8a.

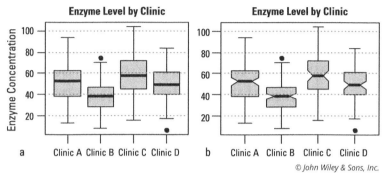

FIGURE 9-8: Box-and-whiskers charts: no-frills (a) and with variable width and notches (b).

Looking at Figure 9-8a, you notice the box plot for each group has the following parts:

>> A box spanning the interquartile range (IQR), extending from the first quartile of the variable to the third quartile, thus encompassing the middle 50 percent of the data.

>> A thick horizontal line, drawn at the median, which is also the 50th centile. If this falls in the middle of the box, your data are not skewed, but if it falls on either side, be on the lookout for skewness.

>> Lines called whiskers extending out to the farthest data point that's not more than 1.5 times the IQR away from the box, and terminate with a horizontal bar on each side.

>> Individual points lying outside the whiskers, which are considered outliers.

Box plots provide a useful visual summary of the distribution of each subgroup for comparison, as shown in Figure 9-8a. As mentioned earlier, a median that's not located near the middle of the box indicates a skewed distribution.

WARNING

Some software draws the different parts of a box plot according to different rules, so you should always check your software's documentation before you present a box plot so you can describe your box plot accurately.

TIP

Software can provide various enhancements to the basic box plot. Figure 9-8b illustrates two such embellishments you may consider using:

>> **Variable width:** The widths of the bars can be scaled to indicate the relative size of each group.

>> **Notches:** The box can have notches that indicate the uncertainty in the estimation of the median. If two groups have non-overlapping notches, they probably have significantly different medians.

Depicting the relationships between numerical variables with other graphs

We started this chapter by developing summary statistics and making graphs of one numeric variable at a time. One example was where we took seven measurements of diastolic blood pressure (DBP) from a group of study participants and developed summary statistics. This is called a *univariate analysis* because it only concerns one variable. But in the example of box plots in the preceding section, we conducted a *bivariate analysis* because we were looking at the relationship between two variables in a sample of patients from four different clinics. The two variables were enzyme levels, and source clinic (Clinic A, B, C, or D). We could have done another bivariate analysis looking at two continuous variables (such as two different enzyme levels in participants) using a scatter plot, which is covered thoroughly in Chapter 16.

This chapter focused on univariate and bivariate summary statistics and graphs that can be developed to help you and others better understand your data. But many research questions are actually answered using *multivariate analysis,* which allows for the control of confounders. Being able to control for confounders is one of the main reasons biostatisticians opt for regression analysis, which we describe in Part 5 and Chapter 23. In these chapters, we cover the appropriate summary statistics and graphical techniques for showing relationships between variables when setting up multivariate regression models.

Chapter **10**

Having Confidence in Your Results

I n Chapter 3, we describe how statistical inference relies on both accuracy and precision when making estimates from your sample. We also discuss how the standard error (SE) is a way to indicate the level of precision of your sample statistic, but that SE is only one way of expressing the preciseness of your statistic. In this chapter, we focus on another way — through the use of a *confidence interval* (CI).

REMEMBER

We assume that you're familiar with the concepts of populations, samples, and statistical estimation theory (see Chapters 3 and 6 if you're not), and that you know what SEs are (read Chapter 3 if you don't). Keep in mind that when you conduct a human research study, you're typically enrolling a *sample* of study participants drawn from a hypothetical *population*. For example, you may enroll a sample of 50 adult diabetic patients who agree to be in your study as participants, but they represent the hypothetical population of all adults with diabetes (for details about sampling, turn to Chapter 6). Any numerical estimate you observe from your sample is a *sample statistic.* A statistic is a valid but imperfect estimate of the corresponding *population parameter,* which is the true value of that quantity in the population.

Feeling Confident about Confidence Interval Basics

The main part of this chapter is about how to calculate confidence intervals (CIs) around the sample statistics you get from research samples. But first, it's important for you to be comfortable with the basic concepts and terminology related to CIs.

Defining confidence intervals

REMEMBER

Informally, a *confidence interval* indicates a range (or interval) of numerical values that's likely to encompass the true value. More formally, the CI around your sample statistic is calculated in such a way that it has a specified likelihood of including or containing the value of the corresponding population parameter.

The SE is usually written after a sample mean with a ± (read "plus or minus") symbol followed by the number representing the SE. As an example, you may express a mean and SE blood glucose level measurement from a sample of adult diabetics as 120 ± 3 mg/dL. By contrast, the CI is written as a pair of numbers — known as *confidence limits* (CLs) — separated by a dash. The CI for the sample mean and SE blood glucose could be expressed like this: 114 – 126 *mg/dL*. Notice that 120 mg/dL — the mean — falls in the middle of the CI. Also, note that the lower confidence limit (LCL) is 114 mg/dL, and the upper confidence limit (UCL) is 126 mg/dL. Instead of LCL and UCL, sometimes abbreviations are used, and are written with a subscript L or U (as in CL_L or CL_U) indicating the lower and upper confidence limits, respectively.

REMEMBER

Although SEs and CIs are both used as indicators of the precision of a numerical quantity, they differ in what they are intending to describe (the sample or the population):

>> A SE indicates how much your observed sample statistic may fluctuate if the same study is repeated a large number of times, so the SE intends to describe the *sample*.

>> A CI indicates the range that's likely to contain the true population parameter, so the CI intends to describe the *population*.

If you want to have a more precise estimate of your population parameter from your sample statistic, it's best if the SEs are small and the CIs narrow. One important property of both CIs and SEs is that how big they are varies inversely with the square root of the sample size. For example, if you were to blow up your sample size — let's pretend to quadruple it — it would cut the size of the SE and the width of the CI in half! This *square root law* is one of the most widely applicable rules in all of statistics, and is the reason why you often hear researchers trying to find ways to increase the sample size in their studies. In practice, a reasonable sample size is reached based on budget and historical studies, because including the whole population is usually not possible (or necessary).

Understanding and interpreting confidence levels

The probability that the CI encompasses the true value of the population parameter is called the *confidence level* of the CI. You can calculate a CI for any confidence level, but the most commonly seen value is 95 percent. Whenever you report a CI, you must state the confidence level. As an example, let's restate our CI from the analysis of mean blood glucose levels in a sample of adult diabetics to express that we used the 95 percent confidence level: 95 percent CI = 114 – 126 *mg/dL*.

In general, higher confidence levels correspond to wider confidence intervals (so you can have greater confidence that the interval encompasses the true value), and lower confidence level intervals are narrower. As an example, a 90 percent CI for the same data is a smaller range (115–125 mg/dL) and the 99 percent CI is a larger range (112–128 mg/dL).

Although a 99 percent CI may be attractive, it can be hard to achieve in practice because an exponentially larger sample is needed (as described earlier in this section). Also, the wide range it provides can be relatively unhelpful. While dropping to a 90 percent CI would reduce the range and sample size needed, having only 90 percent confidence that the true value is in the range is also not very helpful. This may be why there seems to be an industry standard to use the 95 percent confidence level when calculating and reporting CIs.

The confidence level is sometimes abbreviated CL, just like the confidence limit, which can be confusing. Fortunately, the distinction is usually clear from the context in which CL appears. When it's not clear, we spell out what CL stands for.

FEEL CONFIDENT: DON'T LIVE ON AN ISLAND!

Imagine that you enroll a sample of participants from some defined population in a study and obtain a sample statistic. As an example, you calculate a mean blood glucose level from a sample of 50 adult diabetics representing the background population of all adult diabetics. Assume you calculate a 95 percent CI around this statistic, and then you assert that you are 95 percent confident that your CI contains the true population value. But what does that even mean? How can anyone be 95 percent confident? What does that feel like?

There is a popular simulation to illustrate the interpretation of CIs and help learners understand what it is like to be 95 percent confident. Imagine that you have a Microsoft Excel spreadsheet, and you make up an entire population of 100 adult diabetics (maybe they live on an island?). You make up a blood glucose measurement for each of them and type it into the spreadsheet. Then, when you take the average of this entire column, you get the true population parameter (in our simulation). Next, randomly choose a sample of 50 measurements from your population of 100, and calculate a sample mean and a 95 percent CI. Your sample mean will probably be different than the population parameter, but that's okay — that's just sampling error.

Here's where the simulation gets hard. You actually have to take 100 samples of 50. For each sample, you need to calculate the mean and 95 percent CI. You may find yourself making a list of the means and CIs from your 100 samples on a different tab in the spreadsheet. Once you are done with that part, go back and refresh your memory as to what the original population parameter really is. Get that number, then review all 100 CIs you calculated from all 100 samples of 50 you took from your imaginary population. Because you made 95 percent CIs, 95 out of your 100 CIs will contain the true population parameter (and 5 of them won't)! This simulation is a way of demonstrating a proof of the central limit theorem (CLT), and helps learners understand what it means to be 95 percent confident about their CI.

Taking sides with confidence intervals

As demonstrated in the simulation described in the sidebar "Feel Confident: Don't Live on an Island!", 95 percent CIs contain the true population value 95 percent of the time, and fail to contain the true value the other 5 percent of the time. Usually, 95 percent confidence limits are calculated to be balanced, so that the 5 percent failures are split evenly. This means that the true population parameter is actually less than the lower confidence limit 2.5 percent of the time, and it is actually greater than the upper confidence limit 2.5 percent of the time. This is called a two-sided, *balanced* CI.

In some situations, you may want *all* the failures to be on one side. In other words, you want a *one-sided* confidence limit. Cars that run on gasoline may have a declaration by their manufacturer that they go an average distance of at least 40 miles per gallon (mpg). If you were to test this by keeping track of distance traveled and gas usage on a sample of car trips, you may only be concerned if the average was below the lower confidence limit, but not care if it was above the upper confidence limit. This makes the boundary on one side infinite (which would really save you money on gas!). For example, from the results of your study, you could have an observed value of 45 mpg, with a one-sided confidence interval that goes from 42 mpg to plus infinity mpg!

TIP

In biostatistics, it is traditional to always use two-way CIs rather than one-way CIs, as these are seen as most conservative.

Calculating Confidence Intervals

Although an SE and a CI are different calculations intended to express different information, they are related in that the SE is used in the CI calculation. SEs and CIs are calculated using different formulas (depending on the type of sample statistic for which you are calculating the SE and CI). In the following sections, we describe methods of calculating SEs and CIs for commonly used sample statistics.

Before you begin: Formulas for confidence limits in large samples

Most of the methods we describe in the following sections are based on the assumption that your sample statistic has a sampling distribution that's approximately normal (Chapter 3 covers sampling distributions). There are strong theoretical reasons to assume a normal or nearly normal sampling distribution if you draw a large enough samples.

REMEMBER

For any normally distributed sample statistic, the lower and upper confidence limits can be calculated from the observed value of the statistic (V) and standard error (SE) of the statistic:

$$CL_L = V - k \times SE$$

$$CL_U = V - k \times SE$$

TIP

As you can see, CI calculations include a k x SE component, which is both added to and subtracted from the estimate to get the limits. This component is called the *margin of error* (ME).

Confidence limits computed this way are often referred to as *normal-based, asymptotic,* or *central-limit-theorem* (CLT) confidence limits. The value of k in the formulas depends on the desired confidence level and can be obtained from a table of critical values for the normal distribution. Table 10-1 lists the k values for some commonly used confidence levels.

TABLE 10-1

Multipliers for Normal-Based Confidence Intervals

Confidence Level	Tail Probability	k Value
50%	0.50	0.67
80%	0.20	1.28
90%	0.10	1.64
95%	0.05	1.96
98%	0.02	2.33
99%	0.01	2.58

TIP

For the most commonly used confidence level, 95 percent, k is 1.96, or approximately 2. This leads to the very simple approximation that 95 percent upper confidence limit is about two SEs above the value, and the lower confidence limit is about two SEs below the value.

The confidence interval around a mean

Suppose that you enroll a sample of 25 adult diabetics ($N = 25$) as participants in a study, and find that they have an average fasting blood glucose level of 130 mg/dL with a standard deviation (SD) of ±40 mg/dL. What is the 95 percent confidence interval around that 130 mg/dL estimated mean?

To calculate the confidence limits around a mean using the formulas in the preceding section, you first calculate the SE, which in this case is the standard error of the mean (SEM). The formula for the SEM is $SEM = SD / \sqrt{N}$, where SD is the SD of the sample values, and N is the number of values included in the calculation. For the fasting blood glucose study sample, where your SD was 40 mg/dL and your sample size was 25, the SEM is $SEM = 40 / \sqrt{25}$, which is equal to 40/5, or 8 mg/dL.

Using $k = 1.96$ for a 95 percent confidence level (from Table 10-1), the sample mean of 130 mg/dL, and the SD you just calculated of 8 mg/dL, you can compute the lower and upper confidence limits around the mean using these formulas:

$$CL_L = 130 - 1.96 \times 8 = 114.3$$

$$CL_U = 130 + 1.96 \times 8 = 145.7$$

On the basis of your calculations, you would report your result this way: mean glucose = 130 mg/dL (95 percent CI = 114 – 116 mg/dL).

REMEMBER

Please note that you should not report numbers to more decimal places than their precision warrants. In this example, the digits after the decimal point are practically meaningless, so the numbers are rounded off.

TIP

A version of the formula in the preceding section is designed to be utilized with smaller samples, and uses k values derived from a table of critical values of the Student t distribution. To calculate CIs this way, you need to know the number of degrees of freedom (df). For a mean value, the df is always equal to $N - 1$, so in our case, df = $25 - 1 = 24$. Using a Student t table (see Chapter 24), you can find that the Student-based k value for a 95 percent confidence level and 24 degrees of freedom is equal to 2.06, which is a little bit larger than the normal-based k value of 1.96. Using this k value instead of 1.96, you can calculate the 95 percent confidence limits as 113.52 mg/dL and 146.48 mg/dL, which happen to round off to the same whole numbers as the normal-based confidence limits. Generally, you don't have to use these more-complicated Student-based k values unless your N is quite small (say, less than 25).

The confidence interval around a proportion

If you were to conduct a study by enrolling and measuring a sample of 100 adult patients with diabetes, and you found that 70 of them had their diabetes under control, you'd estimate that 70 percent of the population of adult diabetics has their diabetes under control. What is the 95 percent CI around that 70 percent estimate?

There are multiple approximate formulas for CIs around an observed proportion, which are also called *binomial* CIs. Let's start by unpacking the simplest method for calculating binomial CIs, which is based on approximating the binomial distribution using a normal distribution (see Chapter 25). The N is the denominator of the proportion, and you should only use this method when N is large (meaning at least 50). You should also only use this method if the proportion estimate is not very close to 0 or 1. A good rule of thumb is the proportion estimate should be between 0.2 and 0.8.

Using this method, you first calculate the SE of the proportion using this formula: $SE = \sqrt{p(1-p)/N}$ where p stands for proportion. Next, you use the normal-based formulas in the earlier section "Before you begin: Formulas for confidence limits in large samples" to calculate the ME and the confidence limits.

Using the numbers from the sample of 100 adult diabetics (of whom 70 have their diabetes under control), you have $p = 0.7$ and $N = 100$. Using those numbers, the SE for the proportion is $\sqrt{0.7(1-0.7)/100}$ or 0.046. From Table 10-1, k is 1.96 for 95 percent confidence limits. So for the confidence limits, $CL_L = 0.7 - 1.96 \times 0.046$ and $CL_U = 0.7 + 1.96 \times 0.046$. If you calculate these out, you get a 95 percent CI of 0.61 to 0.79 (around the original estimate of 0.7). To express these fractions as percentages, you report your result this way: "The percentage of adult diabetics in the sample whose diabetes was under control was 70 percent (95 percent CI = 61 – 79 percent)."

The confidence interval around an event count or rate

Suppose that you learned that at a large hospital, there were 36 incidents of patients having a serious fall resulting in injury in the last three months. If that's the only incident report data you have to go on, then your best estimate of the monthly serious fall rate is simply the observed count (N), divided by the length of time (T) during which the N counts were observed: 36/3, or 12.0 serious falls per month. What is the 95 percent CI around that estimate?

There are many approximate formulas for the CIs around an observed event count or rate, which is also called a *Poisson CI*. The simplest method to calculate a Poisson CI is based on approximating the Poisson distribution by a normal distribution (see Chapter 24). It should be used only when N is large (at least 50). You first calculate the SE of the event rate using this formula: $SE = \sqrt{N/T}$. Next, you use the normal-based formulas in the earlier section "Before you begin: Formulas for confidence limits in large samples" to calculate the lower and upper confidence limits.

Using the numbers from hospital falls example, $N = 36$ and $T = 3$, so the SE for the event rate is $\sqrt{36}/3$, which is the same as the square root of 2, which is 1.41. According to Table 10-1, k is 1.96 for 95 percent CLs. So $CL_L = 12.0 - 1.96 \times 1.41$ and $CL_U = 12.0 + 1.96 \times 1.41$, which works out to 95 percent confidence limits of 9.24 and 14.76. You report your result this way: "The serious fall rate was 12.0 (95 percent CI = 9.24 – 14.76) per month."

To calculate the CI around the event count itself, you estimate the SE of the count N as $SE = \sqrt{N}$, then calculate the CI around the observed count using the formulas in the earlier section "Before you begin: Formulas for confidence limits in large samples." So the SE of the 36 observed serious falls in a three-month period is simply $\sqrt{36}$, which equals 6.0. So for the confidence limits, we have $CL_L = 36.0 - 1.96 \times 6.0$ and $CL_U = 36.0 + 1.96 \times 6.0$. In this case, the ME is 11.76, which works out to a 95 percent CI of 24.2 to 47.8 serious falls in the three-month period.

TIP

Many other approximate formulas for CIs around observed event counts and rates are available, most of which are more reliable when your N is small. These formulas are too complicated to attempt by hand, but fortunately, many statistical packages can do these calculations for you. Your best bet is to get the name of the formula, and then look in the documentation for the statistical software you're using to see if it supports a command for that particular CI formula.

Relating Confidence Intervals and Significance Testing

In Chapter 3, we introduce the concepts and terminology of significance testing, and in Chapters 11 through 14, we describe specific significance tests. If you read these chapters, you may have come to the correct conclusion that it is possible to assess statistical significance by using CIs. To do this, you first select a number that measures the amount of effect for which you are testing (known as the *effect size*). This effect size can be the difference between two means or the difference between two proportions. The effect size can also be a ratio, such as the ratio of two means, or other ratios that provide a comparison, such as an odds ratio, a relative risk ratio, or a hazard ratio (to name a few). The complete absence of any effect corresponds to a difference of 0, or a ratio of 1, so we call these the "no-effect" values.

REMEMBER

The following statements are always true:

>> If the 95 percent CI around the observed effect size *includes the no-effect value,* then the effect is *not* statistically significant. This means that if the 95 percent CI of a difference includes 0 or of a ratio includes 1, the difference is not large enough to be statistically significant at $\alpha = 0.05$, and we fail to reject the null.

>> If the 95 percent CI around the observed effect size *does not include the no-effect value,* then the effect *is* statistically significant. This means that if the 95 percent CI of a difference is entirely above or entirely below 0, or is entirely above or entirely below 1 with respect to a ratio, the difference is statistically significant at $\alpha = 0.05$, and we reject the null.

The same kind of correspondence is true for other confidence levels and significance levels. For example, a 90 percent confidence level corresponds to the $\alpha = 0.10$ significance level, and a 99 percent confidence level corresponds to the $\alpha = 0.01$ significance level, and so on.

So you have two different but related ways to estimate if an effect you see in your sample is a true effect. You can use significance tests, or else you can use CIs. Which one is better? Even though the two methods are consistent with one another, in biostatistics, we are encouraged for ethical reasons to report the CIs rather than the result of significant tests.

» The CI around the mean effect clearly shows you the observed effect size, as well as the size of the actual interval (indicating your level of uncertainty about the effect size estimate). It tells you not only whether the effect is statistically significant, but also can give you an intuitive sense of whether the effect is clinically important, also known as clinically significant.

» In contrast, the p value is the result of the complex interplay between the observed effect size, the sample size, and the size of random fluctuations. These are all boiled down into a single p value that doesn't tell you whether the effect was large or small, or whether it's clinically significant or negligible.

4

Comparing Groups

Chapter **11**

Comparing Average Values between Groups

omparing average values between groups of numbers is part of almost all biostatistical analyses, and over the years, statisticians have developed dozens of tests for this purpose. These tests include several different flavors of the Student t test, analyses of variance (ANOVA), and a dizzying collection of tests named after the men who popularized them, including Welch, Wilcoxon, Mann-Whitney, and Kruskal-Wallis, to name just a few. The multitude of tests is enough to make your head spin, which leaves many researchers with the uneasy feeling that they may be using the wrong statistical test on their data.

In this chapter, we guide you through the menagerie of statistical tests for comparing groups of numbers. We start by explaining why there are so many tests available, then guide you as to which ones are right for which situations. Next, we show you how to execute these tests using R software, and how to interpret the output. We focus on tests that are usually provided by modern statistical programs (like those discussed in Chapter 4, which also explains how to install and get started with R).

Grasping Why Different Situations Need Different Tests

You may wonder why there are so many tests for such a simple task as comparing averages. Well, "comparing averages" doesn't refer to a specific situation. It's a broad term that can apply to different situations where you are trying to compare averages. These situations can differ from each other on the basis of these and other factors, which are listed here in order of most to least common:

>> **Within or between:** You could be testing differences *within* groups or differences *between* groups.

>> **Number of time points:** You could be testing differences occurring at one point or over a number of time points.

>> **Number of groups:** You could be testing differences between two groups or between three or more groups.

>> **Distribution of outcome:** Your outcome measurement could follow the normal distribution or some other distribution (see Chapter 3).

>> **Variation:** You could be testing the differences in variation or spread across groups (see Chapter 3).

These different factors can occur in any and all combinations, so there are a lot of potential scenarios. In the following sections, we review situations you may frequently encounter when analyzing biological data, and advise you as to how to select the most appropriate testing approach given the situation.

Comparing the mean of a group of numbers to a hypothesized value

Sometimes you have a measurement from the literature (called a *historical control*) that provides a hypothesized value of your measurement, and you want to statistically compare the average of a group to this mean. This situation is common when you are comparing a value that was calculated based on statistical norms derived based on the population (such as the IQ test, where 100 has been scaled to be the population mean).

Typically, comparing a group mean to a historical control warrants using the *one-group Student t test* that we describe in the later section "Surveying Student t tests." For data that are not normally distributed, the *Wilcoxon Signed-Ranks (WSR) test* can be used instead, although it is not used often so we do not cover it in this chapter. (If you need a review on what *normally distributed* means, see Chapter 3.)

Comparing the mean of two groups of numbers

Comparing the mean of two groups of numbers is probably the most common situation encountered in biostatistics. You may be comparing mean levels of a protein that is a hypothesized disease biomarker between a group of patients known to have the disease and a group of healthy controls. Or, you may be comparing a measurement of drug efficacy between two groups of patients with the same condition who are taking two different drugs. Or, you may be comparing measurements of breast cancer treatment efficacy in women on one health insurance plan compared to those on another health insurance plan.

REMEMBER

Such comparisons are generally handled by the famous *unpaired* or *"independent sample" Student t test* (usually just called *the t test*) that we describe later in the section "Surveying Student t tests." Importantly, the t test is based on two assumptions about the distribution of the measurement value being tested in the two groups:

» **The values must be normally distributed** (called the *normality assumption*). For data that are not normally distributed, instead of the t-test, you can use the nonparametric *Wilcoxon Sum-of-Ranks test* (also called the *Mann-Whitney U test* and the *Mann-Whitney test*). We demonstrate the Wilcoxon Sum-of-Ranks test later in this chapter in the section "Running nonparametric tests."

» **The standard deviation (SD) of the values must be close for both groups** (called the *equal variance* assumption). As a reminder, the SD is the square root of the *variance*. To remember why accounting for variation is important in sampling, review Chapter 3. Also, Chapter 9 provides more information about the importance of SD. If the two groups you are comparing have very different SDs, you should not use a Student t test, because it may not give reliable results, especially if you are also comparing groups of different sizes. A rule of thumb is that one group's SD divided by another group's SD should not be more than 1.5 to quality for a Student t test. If you feel your data do not qualify, you can use an alternative called the *Welch test* (also called the *Welch t test*, or the *unequal-variance t test*). As you see later in this chapter under "Surveying Student t tests," because the Welch test accounts for both equal and unequal variance, it is the only one that is included in R statistical software.

Comparing the means of three or more groups of numbers

Comparing the means of three or more groups of numbers is an obvious extension of the two-group comparison in the preceding section. For example, you may have recorded some biological measurement, like a value indicating level of response to treatment among three diagnostic groups (such as mild, moderate, and severe periodontitis). A comparison of the means of three or more groups is handled by the *analysis of variance* (ANOVA), which we describe later in this chapter under "Assessing the ANOVA." When there is one grouping variable, like severity of periodontitis, you have a *one-way ANOVA*. If the grouping variable has three levels (like mild, moderate, and severe periodontitis), it's called a *one-way, three-level ANOVA*.

The null hypothesis of the one-way ANOVA is that all the groups have the same mean. The alternative hypothesis is that at least one group has a mean that is statistically significantly different from at least one of the other groups. The ANOVA produces a single p value, and if that p is less than your chosen criterion (typically $\alpha = 0.05$), you conclude that *at least* one of the means must be statistically significantly different from *at least* one of the other means. (For a refresher on hypothesis testing and p values, see Chapter 3.) But the problem with ANOVA is that if it is statistically significant, it doesn't tell you *which* groups have means that are statistically significantly different. If you have a statistically significant ANOVA, you have to follow-up with one or more so-called *post-hoc* tests (described later under "Assessing the ANOVA"), which test for differences between the means of each pair of groups in your ANOVA.

You can also use the ANOVA to compare just two groups. However, this *one-way, two-level ANOVA* produces exactly the same p value as the classic unpaired equal-variance Student t test.

Comparing means in data grouped on several different variables

The ANOVA is a very flexible method in that it can accommodate comparing means across several grouping variables at once. As an example, you could use an ANOVA for comparing treatment response among participants with different levels of the condition (such as mild, moderate, and severe periodontitis), who come from different clinics (such as Clinic A and Clinic B), and have undergone different treatment approaches (such as using mouthwash or not). An ANOVA involving three different grouping variables is called a *three-way ANOVA* (and compares at a more granular level).

REMEMBER

In ANOVA terminology, the term *way* refers to how many grouping variables are involved, and the term *level* refers to the number of different levels within any one grouping variable.

Like the t test, the ANOVA also assumes that the value you are comparing follows a normal distribution, and that the SDs of the groups you are comparing are similar. If your data are not normally distributed, you can use the nonparametric *Kruskal-Wallis test* instead of the one-way ANOVA, which we demonstrate later in the section "Running nonparametric tests."

Adjusting for a confounding variable when comparing means

Sometimes you are aware the variable you are comparing, such as reduction in blood pressure, is influenced by not only a treatment approach (such as drug A compared to drug B), but also by other confounding variables (such as age, whether the patient has diabetes, whether the patient smokes tobacco, and so on). These *confounders* are considered *nuisance variables* because they have a known impact on the outcome, and may be more prevalent in some groups than others. If a large proportion of the group on drug A were over age 65, and only a small proportion of those on drug B were over age 65, older age would have an influence on the outcome that would not be attributable to the drug. Such a situation would be *confounded by age*. (See Chapter 20 for a comprehensive review of confounding.)

When you are comparing means between groups, you are doing a *bivariate* comparison, meaning you are only involving two variables: the group variable and the outcome. Adjusting for confounding must be done through a *multivariate* analysis using regression.

Comparing means from sets of matched numbers

Often when biostatisticians consider comparing means between two or more groups, they are thinking of *independent* samples of data. When dealing with study participants, independent samples means that the data you are comparing come from different groups of participants who are not connected to each other statistically or literally. But in some scenarios, your intention is to compare means from *matched* data, meaning some sort of pairing exists in the data. Here are some common examples of matched data:

>> The values come from the same participants, but at two or more different times, such as before and after some kind of treatment, intervention, or event.

>> The values come from a crossover clinical trial, in which the same participant receives two or more treatments at two or more consecutive phases of the trial.

>> The values come from two or more different participants who have been paired, or matched, in some way as part of the study design. For example, in a study of participants who have Alzheimer's disease compared to healthy participants, investigators may choose to age-match each Alzheimer's patient to a healthy control when they recruit so both groups have the same age distribution.

Comparing means of matched pairs

If you have paired data, you *must* use a paired comparison. Paired comparisons are usually handled by the *paired student t test* that we describe later in this chapter under "Surveying Student t tests." If your data aren't normally distributed, you can use the nonparametric *Wilcoxon Signed-Ranks test* instead.

REMEMBER

The paired Student t test and the one-group Student t test are actually the same test. When you run a paired t test, the statistical software first calculates the difference between each pair of numbers. If comparing a post-treatment value to a pretreatment value, the software would start by subtracting one value from the other for each participant. Finally, the software would run a test to see if those mean differences were statistically significantly different from the hypothesized value of 0 using a one-group test.

Using Statistical Tests for Comparing Averages

Now that you have reviewed the different types of comparisons, you can continue to consider the basic concepts behind them as you dig more deeply. In this section, we discuss executing these tests in statistical software and interpreting the output. We do that with several tests, including Student t tests, the ANOVA, and nonparametric tests.

TIP

We opted not to clutter this chapter with pages of mathematical formulas for the following tests because based on our own experience, we believe you'll probably never have to do one of these tests by hand. If you really want to see the formulas, we recommend putting the name of the test in quotes in a search engine and looking on the Internet.

Surveying Student t tests

In this section, we present the general approach to conducting a Student t test. We walk through the computational steps common to the different kinds of t tests, including one-group, paired, and independent. As we do that, we explain the computational differences between the different test types. Finally, we demonstrate how to run the t tests using open source software R, and explain how to interpret the output (see Chapter 4 for more information about getting started with R).

Understanding the general approach to a t test

REMEMBER

As reviewed earlier, t tests are designed to compare two means only. If you measure the means of two groups, you see that they almost always come out to be different numbers. The Student t tests are intended to answer the question, *Is the observed difference in means larger than what you would expect from random fluctuations alone?* The different t tests take the same general approach to answer this question, using the following steps:

1. **Calculate the difference (*D*) between the mean values you are comparing.**

2. **Calculate the *precision* of the difference, which is the magnitude of the random fluctuations in that difference.**

   For the t test, calculate the standard error (SE) of that difference (see Chapter 10 for a refresher on SE).

3. **Calculate the *test statistic,* which in this case is *t.***

   The test statistic expresses the size of the D relative to the size of its SE. That is: $t = D / SE$.

4. **Calculate the degrees of freedom (*df*) of the *t* statistic.**

   df is a tricky concept, but is easy to calculate. For *t*, the *df* is the total number of observations minus the number of means you calculated from those observations.

5. **Use the *t* and *df* to calculate the p value.**

   The p value is the probability that random fluctuations alone could produce a t value at least as large as the value you just calculated based upon the Student t distribution.

The Student t statistic is always calculated using the general equation *D/SE*. Each specific type of t test we discussed earlier — including one-group, paired, unpaired, and Welch — calculates *D*, *SE,* and *df* slightly differently. These different calculations are summarized in Table 11-1.

TABLE 11-1 How t Tests Calculate Difference, Standard Error, and Degrees of Freedom

	One-Group	Paired	Unpaired t Equal Variance	Welch t Unequal Variance
D	Difference between mean of observations and a hypothesized value *(h)*	Mean of paired differences	Difference between means of the two groups	Difference between means of the two groups
SE	SE of the observations	SE of paired differences	SE of difference, based on a pooled estimate of SD within each group	SE of difference, from SE of each mean, by propagation of errors
df	Number of observations – 1	Number of pairs – 1	Total number of observations – 2	"Effective" df, based on the size and SD of the two groups

Executing a t test

REMEMBER

Statistical software packages contain commands that can execute (or run) t tests (see Chapter 4 for more about these packages). The examples presented here use R, and in this section, we explain the data structure required for running the various t tests in R. For demonstration, we use data from the National Health and Nutrition Examination Survey (NHANES) from 2017–2020 file (available at wwwn. cdc.gov/nchs/nhanes/continuousnhanes/default.aspx?Cycle=2017–2020).

>> **For the one-group t test,** you need the column of data containing the variable whose mean you want to compare to the hypothesized value (*H*), and you need to know *H*. R and other software enable you to specify a value for *H* and assumes 0 if you don't specify anything. In the NHANES data, the fasting glucose variable is *LBXGLU*, so the R code to test the mean fasting glucose against a maximum healthy level of 100 mg/dL in an R dataframe named *GLUCOSE* is *t.test(GLUCOSE$LBXGLU, mu = 100)*.

>> **For the paired t test,** you need two columns of data representing the pair of numbers you want to enter into the paired t test. For example, in NHANES, systolic blood pressure (SBP) was measured in the same participant twice (variables *BPXOSY1* and *BPXOSY2*). To compare these with a paired t test in an R dataframe named *BP*, the code is *t.test(BP$BPXOSY1, BP$BPXOSY2, paired = TRUE)*.

>> **For the independent t test,** you need to have one column coded as the grouping variable (preferable with a two-state flag coded as *0* and *1*), and another column with the value you want to test. We created a two-state flag in the NHANES data called *MARRIED* where *1 = married* and *0 = all other marital statuses*. To compare mean fasting glucose level between these two groups in a dataframe named *NHANES*, we used this code: *t.test(NHANES$LBXGLU ~ NHANES$MARRIED)*.

Interpreting the output from a t test

Listing 11-1 is the output from a one-sample t-test, where we tested the mean fasting glucose in the NHANES participants against the hypothesized mean of 100 mg/dL:

LISTING 11-1: **R Output from a One-Sample Student t Test**

```
> t.test(GLUCOSE$LBXGLU, mu = 100)

    One Sample t-test

data:    GLUCOSE$LBXGLU
t = 21.209, df = 4743, p-value < 2.2e-16
alternative hypothesis: true mean is not equal to 100
95 percent confidence interval:
   110.1485   112.2158
sample estimates:
mean of x
   111.1821
```

The R output starts by stating what test was run and what data were used, and then reports the t statistic (21.209), the df (4743), and the p value, which is written in scientific notation: $< 2.2e{-}16$. If you have trouble interpreting this notation, just remove the < and then copy and paste the rest of the number into a cell in Microsoft Excel. If you do that, you will see in the formula bar that the number resolves to 0.0000000000000022 — which is a very low p value! The shorthand used for this in biostatistics is $p < 0.0001$, meaning it is sufficiently small. Because of this small p value, we reject the null hypothesis and say that the mean glucose of NHANES participants is statistically significantly different from 100 mg/dL.

But in what direction? For that, it is necessary to read down further in the R output, under 95 percent confidence interval. It says the interval is 110.1485 mg/dL to 112.2158 mg/dL (if you need a refresher on confidence intervals, read Chapter 10). Because the entire interval is greater than 100 mg/dL, you can conclude that the NHANES mean is statistically significantly greater than 100 mg/dL.

Now, let's examine the output from the paired t test of SBP measured two times in the same participant, which is shown in Listing 11-2.

```
> t.test(BP$BPXOSY1, BP$BPXOSY2, paired = TRUE)


    Paired t-test

data:       BP$BPXOSY1 and BP$BPXOSY2
t = 4.3065, df = 10325, p-value = 1.674e-05
alternative hypothesis: true mean difference is not equal to 0
95 percent confidence interval:
   0.1444651   0.3858467
sample estimates:
mean difference
      0.2651559
```

Notice a difference between the output shown in Listings 11-1 and 11-2. In Listing 11-1, the third line of output says, "alternative hypothesis: true mean is not equal to 100." That is because we specified the null hypothesis of 100 when we coded the one-sample t test. Because we did a paired t test in Listing 11-2, this null hypothesis now concerns 0 because we are trying to see if there is a statistically significant difference between the first SBP reading and the second in the same individuals. Why should they be very different at all? In Listing 11-2, the p value is listed as 1.674e–05, which resolves to 0.00001674 (to be stated as p < 0.0001). We were surprised to see a statistically significant difference! The output says that the 95 percent confidence interval of the difference is 0.1444651 mmHg to 0.3858467 mmHg, so this small difference may be *statistically* significant while not being *clinically* significant.

Let's examine the output from our independent t test of mean fasting glucose values in NHANES participants who were married compared to participants with all other marital statuses. This output is shown in Listing 11-3.

```
> t.test(NHANES$LBXGLU &#x0007E; NHANES$MARRIED)


    Welch Two Sample t-test

data:       NHANES$LBXGLU BY NHANES$MARRIED
t = -4.595, df = 4731.2, p-value = 4.439e-06
alternative hypothesis: true difference in means between group $
95 percent confidence interval:
   -6.900665   -2.773287
sample estimates:
mean in group 0   mean in group 1
       108.8034          113.6404
```

Importantly, at the top of Listing 11-3, notice that it says "Welch Two Sample t-test." This is because R insists on using Welch's test instead of the Student t test for independent t tests because Welch's test accounts for unequal variance (as well as equal variance) between groups, as discussed earlier. In the output under the alternative hypothesis, notice that it says R is testing whether the true difference in means between group 0 and group 1 is not equal to 0 (remember, $1 = married$ and $0 = all\ other\ marital\ statuses$). R calculated a p value of 4.439e–06, which resolves to 0.000004439 — definitely p < 0.0001! The groups are definitely statistically significantly different when it comes to average fasting glucose.

But which group is higher? Well, for that, you can look at the last line of the output, where it says that the mean in group 0 (all marital statuses except married) is 108.8034 mg/dL, and the mean in group 1 (married) is 113.6404 mg/dL. So does getting married raise your fasting glucose? Before you try to answer that, please make sure you read up on confounding in Chapter 20!

But what if you just wanted to know if the variance in the fasting glucose measurement in the married group was equal or unequal to the other group, even though you were doing a Welch test that accommodates both? For that, you can do an F test. Because we are not sure which group's fasting glucose would be higher, we choose a two-sided F test and use this code: *var.test(LBXGLU ~ MARRIED, NHANES, alternative = "two.sided")*, which produces the output shown in Listing 11-4.

LISTING 11-4: **R Output from an F Test**

```
> var.test(LBXGLU ~ MARRIED, NHANES, alternative = "two.sided")

            F test to compare two variances

data: LBXGLU by MARRIED
F = 0.97066, num df = 2410, denom df = 2332, p-value = 0.4684
alternative hypothesis: true ratio of variances is not equal to$
95 percent confidence interval:
   0.8955321    1.0520382
sample estimates:
ratio of variances
         0.9706621
```

As shown in Listing 11-4, the p value on the F test is 0.4684. As a rule of thumb:

>> If p > 0.05, you would assume equal variances.

>> If p ≤ 0.05, you would assume unequal variances.

In this case, because the p value is greater than 0.05, equal variances can be assumed, and these data would qualify for the classic Student t test. As described earlier, R gets around this by always using the Welch's t test, which accommodates both unequal and equal variances.

Assessing the ANOVA

In this section, we present the basic concepts underlying the analysis of variance (ANOVA), which compares the means of three or more groups. We also describe some of the more popular post-hoc tests used to follow a statistically significant ANOVA. Finally, we show you how to run commands to execute an ANOVA and post-hoc tests in R, and interpret the output.

Grasping how the ANOVA works

As described earlier in "Surveying Student t tests," it is only possible to run a t test on two groups. This is why we demonstrated the t test comparing married NHANES participants (*M*) to all other marital statuses (*OTH*). We were testing the null hypothesis $M - OTH = 0$ because we were only allowed to compare two groups! So when comparing three groups, such as married (*M*), never married (*NM*), and all others (*OTH*), it's natural to think of pairing up the groups and running three t tests (meaning testing $M - NM$, then testing $M - OTH$, then testing $NM - OTH$). But running an exhaustive set of two-group t tests increases the likelihood of *Type I error*, which is where you get a statistically significant comparison that is just by chance (for a review, read Chapter 3). And this is just with three groups!

WARNING

The general rule is that *N* groups can be paired up in $N(N-1)/2$ different ways, so in a study with six groups, you'd have $6 \times 5/2$, or 15 two-group comparisons, which is way too many.

The term *one-way ANOVA* refers to an ANOVA with only one grouping variable in it. The grouping variable usually has three or more levels because if it has only two, most analysts just do a t test. In an ANOVA, you are testing how spread out the means of the various levels are from each other. It is not unusual for students to be asked to calculate an ANOVA manually in a statistics class, but we skip that here and just describe the result. One result derived from an ANOVA calculation is expressed in a test statistic called the *F ratio* (designated simply as *F*). The F is the ratio of how much variability there is *between* the groups relative to how much variability there is *within* the groups. If the null hypothesis is true, and no true difference exists between the groups (meaning the average fasting glucose in $M = NM = OTH$), then the F ratio should be close to 1. Also, F's sampling fluctuations should follow the *Fisher F distribution* (see Chapter 24), which is actually a family of distribution functions characterized by the following two numbers seen in the ANOVA calculation:

>> **The numerator degrees of freedom:** This number is often designated as df_N or df_1, which is one less than the number of groups.

>> **The denominator degrees of freedom:** This number is designated as df_D or df_2, which is the total number of observations minus the number of groups.

The p value can be calculated from the values of F, df_1, and df_2, and the software performs this calculation for you. If the p value from the ANOVA is statistically significant — less than 0.05 or your chosen α level — then you can conclude that the group means are not all equal and you can reject the null hypothesis. Technically, what that means is that at least one mean was so far away from another mean that it made the F test result come out far away from 1, causing the p value to be statistically significant.

Picking through post-hoc tests

Suppose that the ANOVA is not statistically significant (meaning F was larger than 0.05). It means that there is no point in doing any t tests, because all the means are close to each other. But if the ANOVA is statistically significant, we are left with the question: *Which group means are higher or lower than others?* Answering that question requires us to do *post-hoc tests*, which are t tests done after an ANOVA (*post hoc* is Latin for "after this").

Although using post-hoc tests can be helpful, controlling Type I error is not that easy in reality. There can be issues with the data that may make you not trust the results of your post-hoc tests, such having too many levels to the group you are testing in your ANOVA, or having one or more of the levels with very few participants (so the results are unstable). Still, if you have a statistically significant ANOVA, you should do post-hoc t tests, just so you know the answer to the question stated earlier.

REMEMBER

It's okay to do these post-hoc tests; you just have to take a *penalty*. A penalty is where you deliberately make something harder for yourself in statistics. In this case, we take a penalty by making it deliberately harder to conclude a p value on a t test is statistically significant. We do that by adjusting the α to be lower than 0.05. How much we adjust it depends on the post-hoc test we choose.

>> **The Bonferroni adjustment** uses this calculation to determine the new, lower alpha: α/N, where N is the number of groups. As you can tell, the Bonferroni adjustment is easy to do manually! In the case of our three marital groups (*M*, *NM*, and *OTH*), our adjusted Bonferroni α would be 0.05/3, which is 0.016. This means that for a post-hoc t test of average fasting glucose between two of the three marital groups, the p value would not be interpreted as significant unless the it was less than 0.016 (which is a tougher

criterion than only having to be less than 0.05). Even though the Bonferroni adjustment is easy to do by hand, because most analysts use statistical packages when doing these calculations, it is not used very often in practice.

>> **Tukey's HSD ("honestly" significant difference) test** adjusts α in a different way than Bonferroni. It is intended to be used when there are equally-sized groups in each level of the variable (also called *balanced* groups).

>> **The Tukey-Kramer test** is a generalization of the original Tukey's HSD test to designed to handle different-sized *(also called unbalanced)* groups. Since Tukey-Kramer also handles balanced groups, in R statistical software, only the Tukey-Kramer test is available, and not Tukey's HSD test (as demonstrated later in this chapter in the section "Executing and interpreting post-hoc t tests").

>> **Scheffe's test** compares all pairs of groups, but also lets you bundle certain groups together if doing so makes physical sense. For example, if you have two treatment groups and a control group (such as Drug A, Drug B, and Control), you may want to determine whether either drug is different from the control. In other words, you may want to test Drug A and Drug B as one group against the control group, in which case you use Scheffe's test. Scheffe's test is the safest to use if you are worried your analysis may be suffering from Type I error because it is the most conservative. On the other hand, it is less powerful than the other tests, meaning it will miss a real difference in your data more often than the other tests.

Running an ANOVA

Running a one-way ANOVA in R is similar to running an independent t test (see the earlier section "Executing a t test"). However, in this case, we save the results as an object, and then run R code on that object to get the output of our results.

Let's turn back to the NHANES data. First, we need to prepare our grouping variable, which is the three-level variable *MARITAL* (where *1 = married, 2 = never married,* and *3 = all over marital statuses*). Next, we identify our dependent variable, which is our fasting glucose variable called *LBXGLU*. Finally, we employ the *aov* command to run the ANOVA in R, and save the results in an object called *GLUCOSE_aov*. We use the following code: *GLUCOSE_aov <- aov(LBXGLU ~ as.factor(MARITAL), data = NHANES)*. (The reason we have to use the *as.factor* command on the *MARITAL* variable is to make R handle it as an ordinal variable in the calculation, not a numeric one.) Next, we can get our output by running a *summary* command on this object using this code: *summary(GLUCOSE_aov)*.

Interpreting the output of an ANOVA

We describe the R output here, but output from other statistical packages will have similar information. The output begins with the *variance table* (or simply the *ANOVA table*). You can tell it is a table because it looks like it has a column with no heading followed by columns with the following headings: *Df* (for df), *Sum Sq* (for the sum of squares), *Mean Sq* (mean square), *F value* (value of F statistic), and *Pr(>F)* (p value for the F test). You may recall that in order for an ANOVA test to be statistically significant at $\alpha = 0.05$, the p value on the F must be < 0.05. It is easy to identify that $F = 12.59$ on the output because it is labeled F value. But the p value on the F is labeled *Pr(>F)*, and that's not very obvious. As you saw before, the p value is in scientific notation, but resolves to 0.00000353, which is < 0.05, so it is statistically significant.

TIP

If you use R for this, you will notice that at the bottom of the output it says *Signif. codes: 0 '***' 0.001 '**' 0.01 '*' 0.05 '.' 0.1 ' ' 1*. This is R explaining its coding system for p values. It means that if a p value in output is followed by three asterisks, this is a code for < 0.001. Two asterisks is a code for $p < 0.01$, and one asterisk indicates $p < 0.05$. A period indicates $p < 0.1$, and no notation indicates the p value is greater than or equal to 0.1 — meaning by most standards, it is not statistically significant at all. Other statistical packages often use similar coding to make it easy for analysts to pick out statistically significant p values in the output.

WARNING

Several statistical packages that do ANOVAs offer one or more post-hoc tests as optional output, so programmers tend to request output for both ANOVAs and post-hoc tests, even before they know whether the ANOVA is statistically significant or not, which can be confusing. ANOVA output from other software can include a lot of extra information, such as a table of the mean, variance, standard deviation, and count of the observations in each group. It may also include a test for *homogeneity of variances,* which tests whether all groups have nearly the same SDs. In R, the ANOVA output is very lean, and you have to request information like this in separate commands.

Executing and interpreting post-hoc t tests

In the previous example, the ANOVA was statistically significant, so it qualifies for post-hoc pairwise t tests. Now that we are at this step, we need to select which adjustment to use. We already have an idea of what would happen if we used the Bonferroni adjustment. We'd have to run t tests like we did before, only this time we'd have to use the three-level *MARITAL* variable and run three t tests: One with *M* and *NM*, a second with *M* and *OTH*, and a third with *M* and *OTH*. For each p value we got, we would have to compare it to the adjusted Bonferroni α of 0.016 instead of 0.05. By evaluating each p value, you can determine which pairs of groups are statistically significantly different using the Bonferroni adjustment.

But Bonferroni is not commonly used in statistical software. In R, the most common post-hoc adjustments employed are Tukey-Kramer (using the *TukeyHSD* command) and Scheffe (using the *ScheffeTest* command from the package *Desc-Tools*). The reason why the Tukey HSD is not available in R is that the Tukey-Kramer can handle both balanced and unbalanced groups. In the case of marital statuses and fasting glucose levels in NHANES, the Tukey-Kramer is probably the most appropriate test because we do not need the special features of the Scheffe test. However, we explain the output anyway so that you can understand how to interpret it.

To run the Tukey-Kramer test in R, we use the following code: *TukeyHSD(GLUCOSE_aov, conf.level=.95)*. Notice that the code refers to the ANOVA object we made previously called GLUCOSE_aov. The Tukey-Kramer output begins by restating the test, and the contents of the ANOVA object *GLUCOSE_aov*.

Next is a table (also known as a *matrix*) with five columns. The first column does not have a heading, but indicates which levels of *MARITAL* are being compared in each row (for example, *2-1* means that *1 = M* is being compared to *2 = NM*). The column *diff* indicates the mean difference between the groups being compared, with *lwr* and *upr* referring to the lower and upper 95 percent confidence limits of this difference, respectively. (R is using the 95 percent confidence limits because we specified *conf.level = .95* in our code.) Finally, in the last column labeled *p adj* is the p value for each test. As you can see by the output, using the Tukey-Kramer test and $\alpha = 0.05$, M and NM are statistically significantly different (p = 0.0000102), and OTH and M are statistically significantly different (p = 0.0030753), but NM and OTH are not statistically significantly different (p = 0.1101964).

TIP

When doing a set of post-hoc tests in any software, the output will be formatted as a table, with each comparison listed on its own row, and information about the comparison listed in the columns.

In a real scenario, after completing your post-hoc test, you would stop here and interpret your findings. But because we want to explain the Scheffe test, we can take an opportunity compare what we find when we run that one, too. Let's start by loading the *DescTools* package using the R code *library(DescTools)* (Chapter 4 explains how to use packages in R). Next, let's try the Scheffe test by using the following code on our existing ANOVA object: *ScheffeTest(GLUCOSE_aov)*.

The Scheffe test output is arranged in a similar matrix, but also includes R's significance codes. This time, according to R's coding system, M and NM are statistically significantly different at p < 0.001, and M and OTH are statistically significantly different at p < 0.01. Although the actual numbers are slightly different, the interpretation is the same as what you saw using the Tukey-Kramer test.

TIP

Sometimes you may not know which post-hoc test to select for your ANOVA. If you have an advisor or you are on a research team, you should discuss which one is best. However, if you run the one you select and do not trust the results, it's not a bad idea to run the other ones and keep track of the results. The p values will always come out different, but if the interpretation changes — meaning different comparisons are statistically significant, depending upon what test you choose — you may want to rethink doing post-hoc tests. This means that the results you are getting are unstable.

Running nonparametric tests

As a reminder, the Wilcoxon Sum-of-Ranks test is the nonparametric alternative to the t test, which you can use if your data do not follow a normal distribution. Like with the t test, you can run a Wilcoxon Sum-of-Ranks test in R with options that gives you results if you are doing a paired t test. But to simply repeat the independent t test we did earlier comparing mean fasting glucose in married NHANES participants compared to all other marital statuses, you would run this code: *wilcox.test(NHANES$LBXGLU ~ NHANES$MARRIED)*.

The Kruskal-Wallis test is a nonparametric ANOVA alternative. Like the ANOVA, you can use the Kruskal-Wallis to test whether the mean fasting glucose is equal in the three-level marital status variable *MARITAL*. The R code for the Kruskal-Wallis test is different from the ANOVA code because it does not require you to produce an object for the summary statistics. The following code prints the results to the output: *kruskal.test(LBXGLU ~ MARITAL, data = NHANES)*.

Nonparametric tests don't compare group *means* or test for a nonzero *mean* difference. Rather, they compare group medians, or they deal with ranking the order of variables and analyze those ranks. Because it this, the output from R and other programs will likely focus on reporting the p value of the test.

WARNING

Only use a nonparametric test if you are absolutely sure your data do not qualify for a parametric test (meaning t test, ANOVA, and others that require a particular distribution). Parametric tests are more powerful. In the NHANES example, the data would qualify for a parametric test; we only showed you the code for non-parametric tests as an example.

Estimating the Sample Size You Need for Comparing Averages

There are several ways to estimate the sample size you need in order to be able to detect if there is a significant result on a t test or an ANOVA. (Check out Chapter 3 for a refresher on the concepts of power and sample size.)

Using formulas for manual calculation

Chapter 25 provides a set of formulas that let you estimate how many participants you need for several kinds of t tests and ANOVAs. As with all sample-size calculations, you need to be prepared to specify two parameters: the *effect size of importance,* which is the smallest between-group difference that's worth knowing about, and the amount of *random variability* in your data, expressed as the within-group SD. If you plug these values into the formulas in Chapter 25, you can calculate desired sample size.

Software and web pages

All the modern statistical programs covered in Chapter 4 provide power and sample-size calculations for most standard statistical tests. As described in Chapter 4, G*Power is menu-driven, and can be used for sample size calculations for many tests, including t tests and ANOVAs. If you are using G*Power, to estimate sample size for t tests, choose *t tests* from the test family drop-down menu, and for ANOVA, choose *F tests.* Then, from the *statistical test* drop-down menu, choose the test you plan to use and set *type of power analysis* to "A priori: Compute required sample size – given α, power, and effect size." Then enter the parameters and click *determine* to calculate the sample size.

TIP

In terms of web pages, the website https://statpages.info lists several dozen web pages that perform power and sample-size calculations for t tests and ANOVAs.

Chapter **12**

Comparing Proportions and Analyzing Cross-Tabulations

S uppose that you are studying pain relief in patients with chronic arthritis. Some are taking nonsteroidal anti-inflammatory drugs (NSAIDs), which are over-the-counter pain medications. But others are trying cannabidiol (CBD), a new potential natural treatment for arthritis pain. You enroll 100 chronic arthritis patients in your study and you find that 60 participants are using CBD, while the other 40 are using NSAIDs. You survey them to see if they get adequate pain relief. Then you record what each participant says (pain relief or no pain relief). Your data file has two *dichotomous* categorical variables: the treatment group (CBD or NSAIDs), and the outcome (pain relief or no pain relief).

You find that 10 of the 40 participants taking NSAIDs reported pain relief, which is 25 percent. But 33 of the 60 taking CBD reported pain relief, which is 55 percent. CBD appears to increase the percentage of participants experiencing pain relief by 30 percentage points. But can you be sure this isn't just a random sampling fluctuation?

Data from two potentially associated categorical variables is summarized as a *cross-tabulation*, which is also called a *cross-tab* or a *two-way table*. Because we are studying the association between two variables, this is a form of *bivariate analysis*. The rows of the cross-tab represent the different categories (or *levels*) of one variable, and the columns represent the different levels of the other variable. The cells of the table contain the count of the number of participants with the indicated levels for the row and column variables. If one variable can be thought of as the "cause" or "predictor" of the other, the cause variable becomes the rows, and the "outcome" or "effect" variable becomes the columns. If the cause and outcome variables are both dichotomous, meaning they have only two levels (like in this example), then the cross-tab has two rows and two columns. This structure contains four cells containing counts, and is referred to as a 2-by-2 (or 2×2) cross-tab, or a *fourfold table*. Cross-tabs are displayed with an extra row at the bottom and an extra column at the right to contain the sums of the cells in the rows and columns of the table. These sums are called *marginal totals*, or just *marginals*.

Comparing proportions based on a fourfold table is the simplest example of testing the association between two categorical variables. More generally, the variables can have any number of categories, so the cross-tab can be larger than 2×2, with multiple rows and many columns. But the basic question to be answered is always the same: *Is the spread of numbers across the columns so different from one row to the next that the numbers can't be explained away as random fluctuations?* Another way of asking the same question is: *Is being a member of a particular row associated with being a member of a particular column?*

In this chapter, we describe two tests you can use to answer this question: the Pearson chi-square test, and the Fisher Exact test. We also explain how to estimate power and sample sizes for the chi-square and Fisher Exact tests.

REMEMBER

Like with other statistical tests, you can run all the tests in this chapter from individual-level data in a database, where there is one record per participant. But the tests in this chapter can also be executed using data that has already been summarized in the form of a cross-tab:

>> Most statistical software is set up to work with *individual-level data.* In that case, your data file needs to have two columns for the association you want to test: one containing the categorical variable representing the treatment group (or whatever category is on the y-axis), and one containing the categorical variable representing the outcome. If you have the correct columns, all you have to do is tell the statistical software you are using which test or tests you want to run, and which variables to use in the test.

» Most statistical software is also set up so that you can do these tests using *summarized data* (rather than individual-level data), so long as you set an option in your programming when running the tests. In contrast, online calculators that execute these tests *expect* you to have already cross-tabulated the data. These calculators usually present a screen showing an empty table, and you enter the counts into the table's cells to run the calculation.

Examining Two Variables with the Pearson Chi-Square Test

The most commonly used statistical test of association between two categorical variables is called the *chi-square test of association* developed by Karl Pearson around the year 1900. It's called the chi-square test because it involves calculating a number called a *test statistic* that fluctuates in accordance with the chi-square distribution. Many other statistical tests also use the chi-square distribution, but the test of association is by far the most popular. In this book, whenever we refer to a chi-square test without specifying which one, we are referring to the Pearson chi-square test of association between two categorical variables. (Please note that some books use the notation X^2 or x^2 instead of saying the term *chi-square*.)

Understanding how the chi-square test works

You don't have to understand the equations behind the chi-square test if you have a computer to do them, which is optimal, though it is possible to calculate the test manually. This means you technically don't have to read this section. But we encourage you to do so anyway, because we think you'll have a better appreciation for the strengths and limitations of the test if you know its mathematical under-pinnings. Here, we walk you through conducting a chi-square test manually (which is possible to do in Microsoft Excel).

Calculating observed and expected counts

REMEMBER

All statistical significance tests start with a *null hypothesis* (H_0) that asserts that no real effect is present in the population, and any effect you think you see in your sample is due only to random fluctuations. (See Chapter 3 for more information.) The H_0 for the chi-square test asserts that there's no association between the levels of the row variable and the levels of the column variable, so you should expect the relative spread of cell counts across the columns to be the same for each row.

Figure 12-1 shows how this works out for the observed data taken from the example in this chapter's introduction. You can see from the marginal "Total" row that the overall rate of pain relief (for both groups combined) is 43/100, or 43 percent.

Observed Counts		Pain Relief	No Pain Relief	Total
Treatment	CBD:	33	27	60
	NSAIDs:	10	30	40
	Total:	43	57	100

© John Wiley & Sons, Inc.

Figure 12-1 presents the actual data you observed from your survey, where the observed counts are placed in each of the four cells. As part of the chi-square test statistic calculation, you now need to calculate an *expected* count for each cell. This is done by taking the product of the row and column marginals and dividing them by the total. So, to determine the expected count in the CBD/pain relief cell, you would multiply 43 (row marginal) by 60 (column marginal), then divide this by 100 (total) which comes out 25.8. Figure 12-2 presents the fourfold table with the expected counts in the cells.

Expected Counts if the Null Hypothesis Is True		Pain Relief	No Pain Relief	Total
Treatment	CBD:	25.8	34.2	60
	NSAIDs:	17.2	22.8	40
	Total:	43	57	100

© John Wiley & Sons, Inc.

The reason you need these expected counts is that they represent what would happen under the null hypothesis (meaning if the null hypothesis were true). If the null hypothesis were true:

>> In the CBD-treated group, you'd expect about 25.8 participants to experience pain relief (43 percent of 60), with the remaining 34.2 reporting no pain relief.

>> In the NSAIDs-treated group, you'd expect about 17.2 participants to feel pain relief (43 percent of 40) with the remaining 22.8 reporting no pain relief.

As you can see, this expected table assumes that you still have the overall pain relief rate of 43 percent, but that you also have the pain relief rates in each group equal to 43 percent. This is what would happen under the null hypothesis.

Now that you have observed and expected counts, you're no doubt curious as to how each cell in the observed table differs from its companion cell in the expected table. To get these numbers, you can subtract each expected count from the observed count in each cell to get a *difference table* (observed – expected), as shown in Figure 12-3.

FIGURE 12-3:
Differences
between
observed and
expected cell
counts if the null
hypothesis is
true.

Differences between Observed and Expected Counts		Outcome		
		Pain Relief	No Pain Relief	Total
Treatment	**CBD:**	+7.2	–7.2	0
	NSAIDs:	–7.2	+7.2	0
	Total:	0	0	0

© John Wiley & Sons, Inc.

As you review Figure 12-3, because you know the observed and expected tables in Figures 12-1 and 12-2 always have the same marginal totals by design, you should not be surprised to observe that the marginal totals in the difference table are all equal to zero. All four cells in the center of this difference table have the same absolute value (7.2), with a plus and a minus value in each row and each column.

REMEMBER

The pattern just described is always the case for 2×2 tables. For larger tables, the difference numbers aren't all the same, but they always sum up to zero for each row and each column.

The values in the difference table in Figure 12-3 show how far off from H_0 your observed data are. The question remains: Are those difference values larger than what may have arisen from random fluctuations alone if H_0 is really true? You need some kind of measurement unit by which to judge how unlikely those difference values are. Recall from Chapter 10 that the *standard error* (SE) expresses the general magnitude of random sampling, so looking at the SE as a type of measurement unit is a good way for judging the size of the differences you may expect to see from random fluctuations alone. It turns out that it is easy to approximate the SE of the differences because this is approximately equal to the square root of the expected counts. The rigorous proof behind this is too complicated for most mathophobes (as well as some normal people) to understand. Nevertheless, a simple informal explanation is based on the idea that random event occurrences typically follow the Poisson distribution for which the SE of the event count equals the square root of the expected count (as discussed in Chapter 10).

Summarizing and combining scaled differences

For the upper-left cell in the cross-tab (CBD–treated participants who experience pain relief), you see the following:

>> The observed count (Ob) is 33.

>> The expected count (Ex) is 25.8.

>> The difference (Diff) is $33 - 25.8$, or $+7.2$.

>> The SE of the difference is $\sqrt{25.8}$ or 5.08

You can "scale" the Ob-Ex difference (in terms of unit of SE) by dividing it by the SE measurement unit, getting the ratio $(\text{Diff} / \text{SE}) = +7.2 / 5.08$, or 1.42. This means that the difference between the *observed* number of CBD-treated participants who experience pain relief and the number you would have *expected* if the CBD had no effect on survival is about 1.42 times as large as you would have expected from random sampling fluctuations alone. You can do the same calculation for the other three cells and summarize these scaled differences. Figure 12-4 shows the differences between observed and expected cell counts, scaled according to the estimated standard errors of the differences.

FIGURE 12-4:
Differences between observed and expected cell counts.

Scaled Differences (Ob−Ex)/Sqrt(Ex)		Outcome	
		Pain Relief	No Pain Relief
Treatment	**CBD:**	1.42	−1.23
	NSAIDs:	−1.74	1.51

© John Wiley & Sons, Inc.

The next step is to combine these individual scaled differences into an overall measure of the difference between what you observed and what you would have expected if the CBD or NSAID use really did not impact pain relief differentially. You can't just add them up because the negative and positive differences would cancel each other out. You want all differences (positive and negative) to contribute to the overall measure of how far your observations are from what you expected under H_0.

Instead of summing the differences, statisticians prefer to sum the *squares* of differences, because the squares are always positive. This is exactly what's done in the chi-square test. Figure 12-5 shows the squared scaled differences, which are calculated from the observed and expected counts in Figures 12-1 and 12-2 using the formula $(\text{Ob} - \text{Ex})^2/\text{Ex}$ (rather than by squaring the rounded-off numbers in Figure 12-4, which would be less accurate).

Squared Scaled Differences $(\text{Ob} - \text{Ex})^2/\text{Ex}$		Outcome	
		Pain Relief	No Pain Relief
Treatment	CBD:	2.01	1.52
	NSAIDs:	3.01	2.27

© John Wiley & Sons, Inc.

You then add up these squared scaled differences: $2.01 + 1.52 + 3.01 + 2.27 = 8.81$ to get the chi-square test statistic. This sum is an excellent test statistic to measure the overall departure of your data from the null hypothesis:

REMEMBER

>> If the null hypothesis is true (use of CBD or NSAID does not impact pain relief status), this statistic should be quite small.

>> If one of the levels of treatment has a disproportionate association with the outcome (in either direction), it will affect the whole table, and the result will be a larger test statistic.

Determining the p value

Now that you calculated the test statistic, the only remaining task before interpretation is to determine the *p value*. The p value represents the probability that random fluctuations alone, in the absence of any true effect of CBD or NSAIDs on pain relief, could lead to a value of 8.81 or greater for this test statistic. (We introduce p values in Chapter 3.) Once again, the rigorous proof is very complicated, so we present an informal explanation:

When the expected cell counts are very large, the Poisson distribution becomes very close to a normal distribution (see Chapter 24 for more on the Poisson distribution). If the H_0 is true, each scaled difference should be an approximately normally distributed random variable with a mean of zero and a standard deviation of 1. The mean is zero because you subtract the expected value from the observed value, and the standard deviation is 1 because it is divided by the SE. The sum of the squares of one or more normally distributed random numbers is a number that follows the chi-square distribution (also covered in Chapter 24). So the test statistic from this test should follow the chi-square distribution. Now it is obvious why it is named the chi-square test! The next step is to obtain the p value for the test statistic. To do that manually, you would look up the test statistic (which is 8.81 in our case) in a chi-square table.

REMEMBER

In actuality, the chi-square distribution refers to a family of distributions. Which chi-square distribution you are using depends upon a number called the *degrees of freedom,* abbreviated d.f. or df or by the Greek lowercase letter *nu* (v) (in this book we use df). The df is a measure of the *probability of independence* between the value of the predictor (row) variable and value of the column (outcome) variable.

How would you calculate the df for a chi-square test? The answer is it depends on the number of rows in the cross-tab. For the 2×2 cross-tab (fourfold table) in this example, you added up the four values in Figure 12-5, so you may think that you should look up the 8.81 chi-square value with 4 df. But you'd be wrong. Note the italicized word *independence* in the preceding paragraph. And keep in mind that the differences $(Ob - Ex)$ in any row or column always add up to zero. The four terms making up the 8.81 total aren't independent of each other. It turns out that the chi-square test statistic for a fourfold table has only 1 df, not 4. In general, an N-by-M table, with N rows, M columns, and therefore $N \times M$ cells, has only $(N-1)(M-1)$ df because of the constraints on the row and column sums. In our case, N — which is the number of rows — is 2, so N-1 is 1. Also, M — which is the number of columns — is 2, so M-1 is 1 also (and 1 times 1 is 1). Don't feel bad if this wrinkle caught you by surprise — even Karl Pearson who invented the chi-square test got that part wrong!

So, if you were to manually look up the chi-square test statistic of 8.81 in a chi-square table, you would have to look under the distribution for 1 df to find out the p value. Alternatively, if you got this far and you wanted to use the statistical software R to look up the p value, you would use the following code: *pchisq(8.81, 1, lower.tail = FALSE)*. Either way, the p value for chi-square = 8.81, with 1 df, is 0.003. This means that there's only a 0.003 probability that random fluctuations could produce the effect seen, where CBD performs so differently than NSAIDs with respect to pain relief in chronic arthritis patients. A 0.003 probability is the same as 1 chance in 333 (because $1/0.003 = 333$), meaning very unlikely, but not impossible. So, if you set $\alpha = 0.05$, because $0.003 < 0.05$, your conclusion would be that in the chronic arthritis patients in our sample, whether the participant took CBD or NSAIDs was statistically significantly associated with whether or not they felt pain relief.

Putting it all together with some notation and formulas

TIP

The calculations of the Pearson chi-square test can be summarized concisely using the cell-naming conventions shown in Figure 12-6, along with the standard summation notation described in Chapter 2.

	Column 1	Column 2	Total
Row 1:	$Ob_{1,1}$	$Ob_{1,2}$	R_1
Row 2:	$Ob_{2,1}$	$Ob_{2,2}$	R_2
Total:	C_1	C_2	T

FIGURE 12-6: A general way of naming the cells of a cross-tab table.

Using these conventions, the basic formulas for the Pearson chi-square test are as follows:

- ❯❯ **Expected values:** $Ex_{i,j} = \dfrac{R_i \times C_j}{T}, \ i = 1, 2, \ldots N; \ j = 1, 2, \ldots M$

- ❯❯ **Chi-square statistic:** $\chi^2 = \displaystyle\sum_{i=1}^{N} \sum_{j=1}^{M} \dfrac{(Ob_{i,j} - Ex_{i,j})^2}{Ex_{i,j}}$

- ❯❯ **Degrees of freedom:** $\mathrm{df} = (N-1)(M-1)$

where i and j are array indices that indicate the row and column, respectively, of each cell.

Pointing out the pros and cons of the chi-square test

The Pearson chi-square test is very popular for several reasons:

- ❯❯ It's easy! The calculations are simple to do manually in Microsoft Excel (although this is not recommended because the risk of making a typing mistake is high). As described earlier, statistical software packages like the ones discussed in Chapter 4 can perform the chi-square test for both individual-level data as well as summarized cross-tabulated data. Also, several websites can perform the test, and the test has been implemented on smartphones and tablets.

>> It's flexible! The test works for tables with any number of rows and columns, and it easily handles cell counts of any magnitude. Statistical software can usually complete the calculations quickly, even on big data sets.

But the chi-square test has some shortcomings:

>> It's not an exact test. The p value it produces is only approximate, so using $p < 0.05$ as your criterion for statistical significance (meaning setting $\alpha = 0.05$) doesn't necessarily guarantee that your Type I error rate will be only 5 percent. Remember, your Type I error rate is the likelihood you will claim statistical significance on a difference that is not true (see Chapter 3 for an introduction to Type I errors). The level of accuracy of the statistical significance is high when all the cells in the table have large counts, but it becomes unreliable when one or more cell counts is very small (or zero). There are different recommendations as to the minimum counts you need per cell in order to confidently use the chi-square test. A rule of thumb that many analysts use is that you should have at least five observations in each cell of your table (or better yet, at least five *expected* counts in each cell).

>> It's not good at detecting trends. The chi-square test isn't good at detecting small but steady progressive trends across the successive categories of an *ordinal* variable (see Chapter 4 if you're not sure what *ordinal* is). It may give a significant result if the trend is strong enough, but it's not designed specifically to work with ordinal categorical data. In those cases, you should use a Mantel-Haenszel chi-square test for trend, which is outside the scope of this book.

Modifying the chi-square test: The Yates continuity correction

There is a little drama around the original Pearson chi-square of association test that needs to be mentioned here. Yates, who was a contemporary of Pearson, developed what is called the *Yates continuity correction*. Yates argued that in the special case of the fourfold table, adding this correction results in more reliable p values. The correction consists of subtracting 0.5 from the magnitude of the (Ob – Ex) difference before squaring it.

Let's apply the Yates continuity correction for your analysis of the sample data in the earlier section "Understanding how the chi-square test works." Take a look at Figure 12-3, which has the differences between the values in the observed and expected cells. The application of the Yates correction changes the 7.20 (or −7.20) difference in each cell to 6.70 (or −6.70). This lowers the chi-square value from

8.81 down to 7.63 and increases the p value from 0.0030 to 0.0057, which is still very significant — the chance of random fluctuations producing such an apparent effect in your sample is only about 1 in 175 (because $1/0.0057 = 175$).

TECHNICAL STUFF

Even though the Yates correction to the Pearson chi-square test is only applicable to the fourfold table (and not tables with more rows or columns), some statisticians feel the Yates correction is too strict. Nevertheless, it has been automatically built into statistical software like R, so if you run a Pearson chi-square using most commercial software, it automatically uses the Yates correction when analyzing a fourfold table (see Chapter 4 for a discussion of statistical software).

Focusing on the Fisher Exact Test

The Pearson chi-square test described earlier isn't the only way to analyze cross-tabulated data. Remember that one of the cons was that it is not an exact test? Famous but controversial statistician R. A. Fisher invented another test in the 1920s that gives the exact p value for tables that can handle very small cell counts (even cell counts of zero!). Not surprisingly, this test is called the *Fisher Exact* test (also sometimes referred to *Fisher's exact test*, or just *Fisher*).

Understanding how the Fisher Exact test works

Like with the chi-square, you don't have to know the details of the Fisher Exact test to use it. If you have a computer do the calculations for you (which we always recommend), you technically don't have to read this section. But we encourage you to read this section anyway so you'll have a better appreciation for the strengths and limitations of this test.

REMEMBER

This test is conceptually pretty simple. Instead of taking the product of the marginals and dividing it by the total for each cell as is done with the chi-square test statistic, Fisher exact test looks at every possible table that has the same marginal totals as your observed table. You calculate the exact probability (Pr) of getting each individual table using a formula that, for a fourfold table (using the notation for Figure 12-6), is

$$Pr = \frac{(R_1!)(R_2!)(C_1!)(C_2!)}{(Ob_{1,1}!)(Ob_{1,2}!)(Ob_{2,1}!)(Ob_{2,2}!)(T!)}$$

Those exclamation points indicate calculating the factorials of the cell counts (see Chapter 2). For the example in Figure 12-1, the observed table has a probability of

$$Pr = \frac{(60!)(40!)(43!)(57!)}{(33!)(27!)(10!)(30!)(100!)} = 0.00196$$

Other possible tables with the same marginal totals as the observed table have their own Pr values, which may be larger than, smaller than, or equal to the Pr value of the observed table. The Pr values for all possible tables with a specified set of marginal totals always add up to exactly 1.

The Fisher Exact test p value is obtained by adding up the Pr values for all tables that are at least as different from the H_0 as your observed table. For a fourfold table that means adding up all the Pr values that are less than (or equal to) the Pr value for your observed table.

For the example in Figure 12-1, the p value comes out to 0.00385, which means that there's only 1 chance in 260 (because $1/0.00385 = 260$) that random fluctuations could have produced such an apparent effect in your sample.

Noting the pros and cons of the Fisher Exact test

The big advantages of the Fisher Exact test are as follows:

>> It gives the exact p value.

>> It is exact for all tables, with large or small (or even zero) cell counts.

WARNING

Why do people still use the chi-square test, which is approximate and doesn't work for tables with small cell counts? Well, there are several problems with the Fisher Exact test:

>> The Fisher calculations are a *lot* more complicated, especially for tables larger than 2×2. Many statistical software packages either don't offer the Fisher Exact test or offer it only for fourfold tables. Even if they offer it, you may execute the test and find that it fails to finish the test, and you have to break into the program to stop the procedure. Also, some interactive web pages perform the Fisher Exact test for fourfold tables (including www.socscistatistics.com/tests/fisher/default2.aspx). Only the major statistical software packages (like SAS, SPSS, and R, described in Chapter 4) offer the Fisher Exact test for tables larger than 2×2 because the calculations are so intense. For this reason, the Fisher Exact test is only practical for small cell counts.

>> The calculations can become numerically unstable for large cell counts, even in a 2×2 table. The equations involve the factorials of the cell counts and marginal totals, and these can get very large — even for modest sample sizes — often exceeding the largest number that a computer program can handle. Many programs and web pages that offer the Fisher Exact test for fourfold tables fail with data from more than 100 subjects.

>> Another issue is — like the chi-square test — the Fisher Exact test is not for detecting gradual trends across ordinal categories.

Calculating Power and Sample Size for Chi-Square and Fisher Exact Tests

Note: The basic ideas of power and sample-size calculations are described in Chapter 3, and you should review that information before going further here.

Earlier in the section "Examining Two Variables with the Pearson Chi-Square Test," we used an example of an observational study design in which study participants were patients who chose which treatment they were using. In this section, we use an example from a clinical trial study design in which study participants are assigned to a treatment group. The point is that the tests in this section work on all types of study designs.

Let's calculate sample size together. Suppose that you're planning a study to test whether giving a certain dietary supplement to a pregnant woman reduces her chances of developing morning sickness during the first trimester of pregnancy, which is the first three months. This condition normally occurs in 80 percent of pregnant women, and if the supplement can reduce that incidence rate to only 60 percent, it would be considered a large enough reduction to be clinically significant. So, you plan to enroll a group of pregnant women who are early in their first trimester and randomize them to receive either the dietary supplement or a placebo that looks, smells, and tastes exactly like the supplement. You will randomly assign each participant to the either the supplement group or the placebo group in a process called *randomization*. The participants will not be told which group they are in, which is called *blinding*. (There is nothing unethical about this situation because all participants will agree before participating in the study that they would be willing to take the product associated with each randomized group, regardless of the one to which they are randomized.)

You'll have them take the product during their first trimester, and you'll survey them to record whether they experience morning sickness during that time (using explicit criteria for what constitutes morning sickness). Then you'll tabulate the results in a 2 × 2 cross-tab. The table will look similar to Figure 12-1, but instead will say "supplement" and "placebo" as the label on the two rows, and "did" and "did not" experience morning sickness as the headings on the two columns. And you'll test for a significant effect with a chi-square or Fisher Exact test. So, your sample size calculation question is: *How many subjects must you enroll to have at least an 80 percent chance of getting* $p < 0.05$ *on the test if the supplement truly can reduce the incidence from 80 percent to 60 percent?*

TIP

You have several ways to estimate the required sample size. The most general and most accurate way is to use power/sample-size software such as G*Power, which is described in detail in Chapter 4. Or you can use the online sample-size calculator at https://clincalc.com/stats/samplesize.aspx, which produces the same results.

TIP

You need to enroll additional subjects to allow for possible attrition during the study. If you expect *x* percent of the subjects to drop out, your enrollment should be:

Enrollment = 100 × Analyzable Number / (100 − *x*)

So, if you expect 15 percent of enrolled subjects to drop out and therefore be unanalyzable, you need to enroll 100 × 197/(100 − 15), or about 231 participants.

» Digging into sampling strategies for fourfold tables

» Using fourfold tables in different scenarios

Chapter **13**

Taking a Closer Look at Fourfold Tables

n Chapter 12, we show you how to compare proportions between two or more groups with a cross-tab table. In general, a cross-tab shows the relationship between two categorical variables. Each row of the table represents one particular category of one of the variables, and each column of the table represents one particular category of the other variable. The table can have two or more rows and two or more columns, depending on the number of different categories or levels present in each of the two variables. (To refresh your memory about categorical variables, read Chapter 8.)

Imagine that you are comparing the performance of three treatments (Drug A, Drug B, and Drug C) in patients who could have four possible outcomes: improved, stayed the same, got worse, or left the study due to side effects. In such a case, your treatment variable would have three levels so your cross-tab would have three rows, and your outcome variable would have four levels so your cross-tab would have four columns.

But this chapter only focuses on the special case that occurs when both categorical variables in the table have only two levels. Other words for two-level variables are *dichotomous* and *binary*. A few examples of dichotomous variables are hypertension status (hypertension or no hypertension), obesity status (obese or not obese), and pregnancy status (pregnant or not pregnant). The cross-tab of two dichotomous variables has two rows and two columns. Because a 2×2 cross-tab table has four cells, it's commonly called a *fourfold table*. Another name you may see for this table is a *contingency table.*

Chapter 12 includes a discussion of fourfold tables, and all that is included in Chapter 12 applies not only to fourfold tables but also to larger cross-tab tables. But because the fourfold table plays a pivotal role in public health with regard to certain calculations used commonly in epidemiology and biostatistics, it warrants a chapter all its own — this one! In this chapter, we describe several common research scenarios in which fourfold tables are used, which are: comparing proportions, testing for association, evaluating exposure and outcome associations, quantifying the performance of diagnostic tests, assessing the effectiveness of therapies, and measuring inter-rater and intra-rater reliability. In each scenario, we describe how to calculate several common measures called *indices* (singular: *index*), along with their confidence intervals. We also describe ways of sampling called *sampling strategies* (see Chapter 6 for more on sampling).

Focusing on the Fundamentals of Fourfold Tables

In contemplating statistical testing in a fourfold table, consider the process. As described in Chapter 12, you first formulate a null hypothesis (H_0) about the four-fold table, set the significance level (such as $\alpha = 0.05$), calculate a test statistic, find the corresponding p value, and interpret the result. With a fourfold table, one obvious test to use is the chi-square test (if necessary assumptions are met). The chi-square test evaluates whether membership in a particular row is statistically significantly associated with membership in a particular column. The *p value* on the chi-square test is the probability that random fluctuations alone, in the absence of any real effect in the population, could have produced an observed effect at least as large as what you saw in your sample. If the p value is less than α (which is 0.05 in your scenario), the effect is said to be *statistically significant,* and the null is rejected. Assessing significance using a chi-square test is the most common approach to testing a cross-tab of any size, including a fourfold table. But fourfold tables can serve as the basis for developing other metrics besides chi-square tests that can be useful in other ways, which are discussed in this chapter.

TIP

In the rest of this chapter, we describe many useful calculations that you can derive from the cell counts in a fourfold table. The statistical software that cross-tabulates your raw data can provide these indices depending upon the commands it has available (see Chapter 4 for a review of statistical software). Thankfully (and uncharacteristically), unlike in most chapters in this book, the formulas for many indices derived from fourfold tables are simple enough to do manually with a calculator (or using Microsoft Excel). All you need are the counts or frequencies of each of the four cells. For these indices, you can also use a web page for calculation, which is available here: `https://statpages.info/ctab2x2.html`. This chapter demonstrates how to calculate these indices in R (a free, open-source software described in Chapter 4).

Like any other value you calculate from a sample, an index calculated from a four-fold table is a *sample statistic,* which is an estimate of the corresponding *population parameter*. A good researcher always wants to quote the *precision* of that estimate. In Chapter 10, we describe how to calculate the standard error (SE) and confidence interval (CI) for sample statistics such as means and proportions. Likewise, in this chapter, we show you how to calculate the SE and CI for the various indices you can derive from a fourfold table.

Though an index itself may be easy to calculate manually, its SE or CI usually is not. Approximate formulas are available for some of the more common indices. These formulas are usually based on the fact that the random sampling fluctuations of an index (or its logarithm) are often nearly normally distributed if the sample size is large enough. We provide approximate formulas for SEs where they're available, and demonstrate how to calculate them in R when possible.

REMEMBER

For consistency, all the formulas in this chapter refer to the four cell counts of the fourfold table, and the row totals, column totals, and grand total, in the same standard way (see Figure 13-1). This convention is used in many online resources and textbooks.

	Column 1	Column 2	Total
Row 1	a	b	r1
Row 2	c	d	r2
Total	c1	c2	t

FIGURE 13-1: These designations for cell counts and totals are used throughout this chapter.

© John Wiley & Sons, Inc.

Choosing the Correct Sampling Strategy

In this section, we assume you are designing a cross-sectional study (see Chapter 7 for a review of study design terminology). Using such a design, though you could not assess cause-and-effect, you could evaluate the association between an exposure (hypothesized cause) and outcome. For example, you may hypothesize that being obese (exposure) causes a patient to develop hypertension (abbreviated HTN, outcome) over time. However, in a cross-sectional study, exposure and outcome are measured at the same time, so you can only look for associations. If your exposure and outcome are binary (such as obese: yes/no and HTN: yes/no), you can use a fourfold table for this evaluation. But you would have to develop a sampling strategy that would support your analytic plan.

TIP

The example given here is for the use of a fourfold table to interpret a cross-sectional study. If you have heard of a fourfold table being analyzed as part of a *cohort study* or *longitudinal study,* that is referring to a series of cross-sectional studies done over time to the same group or *cohort.* Each round of data collection is called a *wave,* and fourfold tables can be developed cross-sectionally (using data from one wave), or longitudinally (using data from two waves).

As described in Chapter 6, you could try simple random sampling (SRS), but this may not provide you with a balanced number of participants who are positive for the exposure compared to negative to the exposure. If you are worried about this, you could try stratified sampling on the exposure (such as requiring half the sample to be obese, and half the sample to not be obese). Although other sampling strategies described in Chapter 6 could be used, SRS and stratified sampling are the most common to use in cross-sectional study. Why is your sampling strategy so important? As you see in the rest of this chapter, some indices are meaningful only if the sampling is done accordingly so as to support a particular study design.

Producing Fourfold Tables in a Variety of Situations

Fourfold tables can arise from a number of different scenarios, including the following:

>> Comparing proportions between two groups (see Chapter 12)

>> Testing whether two binary variables are associated

>> Assessing associations between exposures and outcomes

>> Evaluating diagnostic procedures

>> Evaluating therapies

>> Evaluating inter-rater reliability

Note: These scenarios can also give rise to tables larger than 2×2, and fourfold tables can arise in other scenarios besides these.

Describing the association between two binary variables

Suppose you conduct a cross-sectional study by enrolling a random sample of 60 adults from the local population as participants in your study with the hypothesis that being obese is associated with having HTN. For the exposure, suppose you measure their height and weight, and use these values to calculate their body mass index (BMI). You then use their BMI to classify them as either obese or non-obese. For the outcome, you also measure their blood pressure in order to categorize them as having HTN or not having HTN. This is simple random sampling (SRS), as described in the earlier section "Choosing the Correct Sampling Strategy." You can summarize your data in a fourfold table (see Figure 13-2).

The table in Figure 13-2 indicates that more than half of the obese participants have HTN and more than half of the non-obese participants don't have HTN — so there appears to be a relationship between being a membership in a particular row and simultaneously being a member of a particular column. You can show this apparent association is statistically significant in this sample using either a Yates chi-square or a Fisher Exact test on this table (as we describe in Chapter 12). If you do these tests, your p values will be $p = 0.016$ and $p = 0.013$, respectively, and at $\alpha = 0.05$, you will be comfortable rejecting the null.

FIGURE 13-2: A fourfold table summarizing obesity and hypertension in a sample of 60 participants.

	Hypertension	No Hypertension	Total
Obese	14 (a)	7 (b)	21 (r1)
Not Obese	12 (c)	27 (d)	39 (r2)
Total	26 (c1)	34 (c2)	60 (t)

© John Wiley & Sons, Inc.

But when you present the results of this study, just saying that a statistically significant association exists between obesity status and HTN status isn't enough. You should also indicate how strong this relationship is and in what direction it goes. A simple solution to this is to present the test statistic and p value to represent how strong the relationship is, and to present the actual results as row or column percentages to indicate the direction. For the data in Figure 13-2, you could say that being obese was associated with having HTN, because 14/21 = 66 percent of obese participants also had HTN, while only 12/39 = 31 percent of non-obese participants had HTN.

Quantifying associations

How strongly is an exposure associated with an outcome? If you are considering this question with respect to exposures and outcomes that are continuous variables, you would try to answer it with a scatter plot and start looking for correlation and linear relationships, as discussed in Chapter 15. But in our case, with a fourfold table, you are essentially asking: how strongly are the two levels of the exposure represented in the rows associated with the two levels of the outcome represented in the columns? In the case of a cohort study — where the exposure is measured in participants without the outcome who are followed longitudinally to see if they get the outcome — you can ask if the exposure was associated with *risk* of the outcome or *protection* from the outcome. In a cohort design, you could ask, "How much does being obese increase the likelihood of getting HTN?" You can calculate two indices from the fourfold table that describe this increase, as you discover in the following sections.

Relative risk and the risk ratio

In a cohort study, you seek to quantify the amount of risk (or probability) for the outcome that is conferred by having the exposure. The risk of getting a negative outcome is estimated as the fraction of participants who experience the outcome during follow-up (because in a cohort design, all participants do not have the outcome when they enter the study). Another term for risk is *cumulative incidence rate* (CIR). You can calculate the CIR for the whole study, as well as separately for each stratum of the exposure (in our case, obese and nonobese). Using the notation in Figure 13-1, the CIR for participants with the exposure is $a/r1$. For the example from Figure 13-2, it's 14 / 21, which is 0.667 (66.7 percent). And for those without the exposure, the CIR is represented by $c/r2$. For this example, the CIR is calculated as 12 / 39, which is 0.308 (30.8 percent).

REMEMBER

The term *exposure* specifies a hypothesized cause of an outcome. If it is found that a certain exposure typically causes risk for an outcome, it is called a *risk factor,* and if it is found to confer protection, it is called a *protective factor.* Higher education has been found to be a protective factor against many negative outcomes (such as most injuries), and obesity has been found to be a risk factor for many negative outcomes (such as HTN and Type II diabetes).

The term *relative risk* refers to the amount of risk one group has relative to another. This chapter discusses different measures of relative risk that are to be used with different study designs. It is important to acknowledge here that technically, the term *risk* can only apply to cohort studies because you can only be at risk if you possess the exposure but not the outcome for some period of time in a study, and only cohort studies have this design feature. However, the other study designs — including cross-sectional and case-control — intend to estimate the relative risk you would get if you had done a cohort study, so they produce estimates of relative risk (see Chapter 7).

In a cohort study, the measure of relative risk used is called the *risk ratio* (also called cumulative incidence ratio). To calculate the risk ratio, first calculate the CIR in the exposed, calculate the CIR in the unexposed, then take a ratio of the CIR in the exposed to the CIR in the unexposed. This formula could be expressed as: $RR = (a/r1)/(c/r2)$.

For this example, as calculated earlier, the CIR for the exposed was 0.667, and the CIR for the unexposed was 0.308. Therefore, the risk-ratio calculation would be 0.667 / 0.308, which is 2.17. So, in this cohort study, obese participants were slightly more than twice as likely to be diagnosed as having HTN during follow-up than non-obese subjects.

REMEMBER

Calculating a risk ratio as a measure of relative risk is appropriate for a cohort study. However, there are restrictions when creating measures of relative risk for cross-sectional and case-control designs. In a cross-sectional study, you would not calculate a CIR in the exposed and the unexposed because the exposure and outcome are measured at the same time, so there's no time for any participants to experience any risk during the study. Instead, you would calculate the *prevalence* of the outcome in the exposed — which is $a/r1$ — and the prevalence of the outcome in the unexposed — which is $c/r2$ (read Chapter 14 to for a discussion of prevalence). Notice that even though we use different wording, these are the same formulas as for the CIR. Then, instead of a risk ratio, in a cross-sectional study you would use a *prevalence ratio,* which is calculated the same way as the risk ratio: $PR = (a/r1)/(c/r2)$.

WARNING

In a case-control study, for a measure of relative risk, you *must* use the odds ratio (discussed later in the section "Odds ratio"). You cannot use the risk ratio or prevalence ratio in a case-control study. The odds ratio can also be used as a measure of relative risk in a cross-sectional study, and can technically be used in a cohort study, although the preferred measure is the risk ratio.

Let's go back to discussing the risk ratio. You can calculate an approximate 95 percent confidence interval (CI) around the observed risk ratio using the following formulas, which assume that the logarithm of the risk ratio is normally distributed:

1. **Calculate the standard error (SE) of the log of risk ratio using the following formula:**

$$SE = \sqrt{b/(a \times r1) + d/(c \times r2)}$$

2. **Calculate Q with the following formula:** $Q = e^{1.96 \times SE}$ **where Q is simply a convenient intermediate quantity that will be used in the next part of the calculation, and e is the mathematical constant 2.718.**

3. **Find the lower and upper limits of the CI with the following formula:**

$$95\% \, CI = \left(\frac{RR}{Q} \right) to \, (RR \times Q)$$

For confidence levels other than 95 percent, replace the z-score of 1.96 in Step 2 with the corresponding z-score shown in Table 10-1 of Chapter 10. As an example, for 90 percent confidence levels, use 1.64, and for 99 percent confidence levels, use 2.58.

For the example in Figure 13-2, you calculate 95 percent CI around the observed risk ratio as follows:

1. $SE = \sqrt{7 / (14 \times 21) + 27 / (12 \times 39)}$, **which is 0.2855.**

2. $Q = e^{1.96 \times 0.2855}$, **which is 1.75.**

3. **The** $95\% \, CI = \left(\frac{2.17}{1.75} \right)$ **to** (2.17×1.75), **which is 1.24 to 3.80.**

Using this formula, the risk ratio would be expressed as 2.17, 95 percent CI 1.24 to 3.80.

You could also use R to calculate a risk ratio and 95 percent CI for the fourfold table in Figure 13-2 with the following steps:

1. **Create a matrix.**

   Create a matrix called *obese_HTN* with this code: *obese_HTN <- matrix(c(14,12,7,27),nrow = 2, ncol = 2)*.

2. **Load a library.**

   For many epidemiologic calculations, you can use the *epitools* package in R and use a command from this package to calculate the risk ratio and 95 percent CI. Load the *epitools* library with this command: *library(epitools)*.

3. **Run the command on the matrix.**

   In this case, run the *riskratio.wald* command on the *obese_HTN* matrix you created in Step 1: *riskratio.wald(obese_HTN)*.

The output is shown in Listing 13-1.

LISTING 13-1: **R output from risk ratio calculation on data from Figure 13-2**

```
> riskratio.wald(obese_HTN)
$data
              Outcome
Predictor     Disease1 Disease2 Total
    Exposed1  14            7        21
    Exposed2  12           27        39
    Total     26           34        60


$measure
              risk ratio with 95% C.I.
Predictor     estimate       lower          upper
    Exposed1  1.000000       NA             NA
    Exposed2  2.076923       1.09512        3.938939


$p.value
              two-sided
Predictor     midp.exact     fisher.exact   chi.square
    Exposed1  NA             NA             NA
    Exposed2  0.009518722    0.01318013     0.00744125


$correction
[1] FALSE

attr(,"method")
[1] "Unconditional MLE & normal approximation (Wald) CI"
>
```

Notice that the output is organized under the following headings: *$data*, *$measure*, *$p.value*, and *$correction*. Under the *$measure* section is a centered title that says *risk ratio with 95% C.I.* — which is more than a hint! Under that is a table with the following column headings: *Predictor, estimate, lower, and upper*. The estimate column has the risk ratio estimate (which you already calculated by hand and rounded off to 2.17). The lower and upper columns have the confidence limits, which R calculated as 1.09512 (round to 1.10) and 3.938939 (round to 3.94), respectively. You may notice that because R used a slightly different SE formula than our manual calculation, R's CI was slightly wider.

Odds ratio

The *odds* of an event occurring is the probability of it happening divided by the probability of it not happening. Assuming you use p to represent a probability, you could write the odds equation this way: $p/(1-p)$. In a fourfold table, you would represent the odds of the outcome in the exposed as a/b. You would also represent the odds of the outcome in the unexposed as c/d.

Let's apply this to the scenario depicted in Figure 13-2. This is a study of 60 individuals, where the exposure is obesity status (yes/no) and the outcome is HTN status (yes/no). Using the data from Figure 13-2, the odds of having the outcome for exposed participants would be calculated as a/b, which would be 14 / 7, which is 2.00. And the odds of having the outcome in the unexposed participants is c/d, which would be 12 / 27, which is 0.444.

Odds have no units. They are not expressed as percentages. See Chapter 3 for a more detailed discussion of odds.

TIP

When considering cross-sectional and cohort studies, the *odds ratio* (OR) represents the ratio of the odds of the outcome in the exposed to the odds of the outcome in the unexposed. In case-control studies, because of the sampling approach, the OR represents the ratio of the odds of exposure among those with the outcome to the odds of exposure among those without the outcome. But because any fourfold table has only one OR no matter how you calculate it, the actual value of the OR stays the same, but how it is described and interpreted depends upon the study design.

REMEMBER

Let's assume that Figure 13-2 presents data on a cross-sectional study, so we will look at the OR from that perspective. Because you calculate the odds in the exposed as a/b, and the odds in the unexposed as c/d, the odds ratio is calculated by dividing a/b by b/c like this: $OR = (a/b)/(c/d)$.

For this example, the OR is $(14/7)/(12/27)$, which is 2.00 / 0.444, which is 4.50. In this sample, assuming a cross-sectional study, participants who were positive for the exposure had 4.5 times the odds of also being positive for the outcome compared to participants who were negative for the exposure. In other words, obese participants had 4.5 times the odds of also having HTN compared to non-obese participants.

You can calculate an approximate 95 percent CI around the observed OR using the following formulas, which assume that the logarithm of the OR is normally distributed:

1. **Calculate the standard error of the log of the OR with the following formula:**

$$SE = \sqrt{1/a + 1/b + 1/c + 1/d}$$

2. **Calculate Q with the following formula: $Q = e^{1.96 \times SE}$, where Q is simply a convenient intermediate quantity that will be used in the next part of the calculation, and e is the mathematical constant 2.718.**

3. Find the limits of the confidence interval with the following formula:

$$95\% \text{ CI} = \left(\frac{OR}{Q} \right) \text{ to } (OR \times Q)$$

Like with the risk ratio CI, for confidence levels other than 95 percent, replace the z-score of 1.96 in Step 2 with the corresponding z-score shown in Table 10-1 of Chapter 10. As an example, for 90 percent confidence levels, use 1.64, and for 99 percent confidence levels, use 2.58.

For the example in Figure 13-2, you calculate 95 percent CI around the observed OR as follows:

1. $SE = \sqrt{1/14 + 1/7 + 1/12 + 1/27}$, which is 0.5785.

2. $Q = e^{1.96 \times 0.5785}$, which is 3.11.

3. $95\% \text{ CI} = \left(\frac{4.50}{3.11} \right)$ to (4.50×3.11), which is 1.45 to 14.0.

Using these calculations, the OR is estimated as 4.5, and the 95 percent CI as 1.45 to 14.0.

TECHNICAL
STUFF

To do this operation in R, you would follow the same steps as listed at the end of the previous section, except in Step 3, the command you'd run on the matrix is *oddsratio.wald()* using this code: *oddsratio.wald(obese_HTN)*. The output is laid out the same way as shown in Listing 13-1, with a *$measure* section titled *odds ratio with a 95% C.I.* In that section, it indicates that the lower and upper confidence limits are 1.448095 (rounded to 1.45) and 13.98389 (rounded to 13.98), respectively. This time, R's estimate of the 95 percent CI was close to the one you got with your manual calculation, but slightly narrower.

WARNING

A wide 95 percent CI is the sign of an unstable (and not very useful) estimate. Consider a 95 percent CI for an OR that goes from 1.45 to 14.0. If you are interpreting the results of a cohort study, you are saying that obesity could increase the odds of getting HTN by as little as 1.45, or as much as 14! Most researchers try to solve this problem by increasing their sample size to reduce the size of their SE, which will in turn reduce the width of the CI.

Evaluating diagnostic procedures

Many diagnostic procedures provide a positive or negative test result — such as a COVID-19 test. Ideally, this result should correspond to the true presence or absence of the medical condition for which the test was administered — meaning a positive COVID-19 test should mean you have COVID-19, and a negative test should mean you do not. The true presence or absence of a medical condition is best determined by some *gold standard* test that the medical community accepts as perfectly accurate in diagnosing the condition. For COVID-19, the polymerase chain reaction (PCR) test is considered a gold standard test because of its high level of accuracy. But gold standard diagnostic procedures (like PCR tests) can be time-consuming and expensive, and in the case of invasive procedures like biopsies, they may be very unpleasant for the patient. Therefore, quick, inexpensive, and relatively noninvasive *screening tests* are very valuable, even if they are not perfectly accurate. They just need to be accurate enough to help filter in the best candidates for a gold standard diagnostic test.

Most screening tests produce some *false positive* results, which is when the result of the test is positive, but the patient is actually negative for the condition. Screening tests also produce some *false negative* results, where the result is negative in patients where the condition is present. Because of this, it is important to know false positive rates, false negative rates, and other features of screening tests to consider their level of accuracy in your interpretation of their results.

You usually evaluate a new, experimental screening test for a particular medical condition by administering the new test to a group of participants. These participants include some who have the condition and some who do not. For all the participants in the study, their status with respect to the particular medical condition has been determined by the gold standard method, and you are seeing how well your new, experimental screening test compares. You can then cross-tabulate the new screening test results against the gold standard results representing the true condition in the participants. You would create a fourfold table in a framework as shown in Figure 13-3.

		True Status, by the Gold Standard		
		Condition Present	Condition Not Present	Total
Test Result	Positive	a = TP (True Positive)	b = FP (False Positive)	r1 = All Positive
	Negative	c = FN (False Negative)	d = TN (True Negative)	r2 = All Negative
	Total	c1 = All Present	c2 = All Not Present	t

FIGURE 13-3: This is how data are summarized when evaluating a proposed new diagnostic screening test.

© John Wiley & Sons, Inc.

Imagine that you are conducting a study at a primary care clinic. In the study, you administer a newly developed home pregnancy test to 100 women who come to a primary care appointment suspecting that they may be pregnant. This is convenience sampling from a population defined as "all women who think they may be pregnant," which is the population to whom a home pregnancy test would be marketed. At the appointment, all the participants would be given the gold standard pregnancy test, so by the end of the appointment, you would know their true pregnancy status according to the gold standard, as well as what your new home pregnancy test result said. Your results would next be cross-tabulated according to the framework shown in Figure 13-4.

FIGURE 13-4: Results from a study of a new experimental home pregnancy test.

		True Status		
		Pregnant	Not Pregnant	Total
Pregnancy Test Result	Positive	33 (a)	12 (b)	45 (r1)
	Negative	4 (c)	51 (d)	55 (r2)
	Total	37 (c1)	63 (c2)	100 (t)

© John Wiley & Sons, Inc.

The structure of the table in Figure 13-4 is important because if your results are arranged in that way, you can easily calculate at least five important characteristics of the experimental test (in our case, the home pregnancy test) from this table: accuracy, sensitivity, specificity, positive predictive value (PPV), and negative predictive value (NPV). We explain how in the following sections.

Overall accuracy

Overall accuracy measures how often a test result comes out the same as the gold standard result (meaning the test is correct). A perfectly accurate test never produces false positive or false negative results. In Figure 13-4, cells a and d represent correct test results, so the overall accuracy of the home pregnancy test is $(a+d)/t$. Using the data in Figure 13-4, accuracy $=(33+51)/100$, which is 0.84, or 84 percent.

Sensitivity and specificity

A perfectly *sensitive* test never produces a false negative result for an individual with the condition. Conversely, a perfectly *specific* test never produces a false positive result for an individual negative for the condition. The goal of developing a screening test is to balance the sensitivity against the specificity of the test based on the context of the condition, to optimize the accuracy and get the best of both worlds while minimizing both false positive and false negative results.

In a screening test with a sensitivity of 100 percent, the test result is always positive whenever the condition is truly present. In other words, the test will identify all individuals who truly have the condition. When a perfectly sensitive test comes out negative, you can be sure the person doesn't have the condition. You calculate *sensitivity* by dividing the number of true positive cases by the total number of cases where the condition was truly present: a/c_1 (that is, true positive/all present). Using the data in Figure 13-4, sensitivity = 33/37, which is 0.89. This means that the home test comes out positive in only 89 percent of truly pregnant women, and the other 11 percent were really pregnant, but had a false positive result in the test.

A perfectly *specific* test never produces a false positive result for an individual without the condition. In a test that has a specificity of 100 percent, whenever the condition is truly absent, the test always has a negative result. In other words, the test will identify all individuals who truly do not have the condition. When a perfectly specific test comes out positive, you can be sure the person has the condition. You calculate *specificity* by dividing the number of true negative cases by the total number of cases where the condition was truly absent: d/c_2 (that is, true negative/all not present). Using the data in Figure 13-4, specificity = 51/63, which is 0.81. This means that among the women who were not pregnant, the home test was negative only 81 percent of the time, and 11 percent of women who were truly negative tested as positive. (You can see why it is important to do studies like this before promoting the use of a particular screening test!)

But imagine you work in a lab that processes the results of screening tests, and you do not usually have access to the gold standard results. You may ask the question, "How likely is a particular screening test result to be correct, regardless of whether it is positive or negative?" When asking this about positive test results, you are asking about positive predictive value (PPV), and when asking about negative test results, you are asking about negative predictive value (NPV). These are covered in the following sections.

REMEMBER

Sensitivity and specificity are important characteristics of the test itself. Observe that the answers depend on the *prevalence* of the condition in the background population. If the study population were older women, then the prevalence of being pregnant would be lower, and that would impact the sensitivity and specificity. The prevalence will also impact the PPV and NPV, which we discuss in the next section. For these reasons, it is important to use natural sampling in such a study design.

Positive predictive value and negative predictive value

The *positive predictive value* (PPV, also called predictive value positive) is the fraction of all positive test results that are true positives. In the case of the pregnancy test scenario, the PPV would be the fraction of the time a positive screening test result means that the woman is truly pregnant. PPV is the likelihood that a positive test result is correct. You calculate PPV as $a/r1$. For the data in Figure 13-4, the PPV is $33/45$, which is 0.73. So, if the pregnancy test result is positive, there's a 73 percent chance that the woman is truly pregnant.

The *negative predictive value* (NPV, also called predictive value negative) is the fraction of all negative test results that are true negatives. In the case of the pregnancy test scenario, the NPV is the fraction of the time a negative screening test results means the woman is truly not pregnant. NPV is the likelihood a negative test result is correct. You calculate NPV as $d/r2$. For the data in Figure 13-4, the NPV is $51/55$, which is 0.93. So, if the pregnancy test result is negative, there's a 93 percent chance that the woman is truly not pregnant.

Investigating treatments

In conditions where there are no known treatments, one of the simplest ways to investigate a new treatment (such as a drug or surgical procedure) is to compare it to a placebo or sham condition using a clinical trial study design. Because many forms of dementia have no known treatment, it would be ethical to compare new treatments for dementia to placebo or a sham treatment in a clinical trial. In those cases, patients with the condition under study would be *randomized* (randomly assigned) to an active group (taking the real treatment) and a control group (that would receive the sham treatment), as randomization is a required feature of clinical trials. Because some of the participants in the control group may appear to improve, it is important that participants are blinded as to their group assignment, so that you can tell if outcomes are actually improved in the treatment compared to the control group.

Suppose you conduct a study where you enroll 200 patients with mild dementia symptoms, then randomize them so that 100 receive an experimental drug intended for mild dementia symptoms, and 100 receive a placebo. You have the participants take their assigned product for six weeks, then you record whether each participant felt that the product helped their dementia symptoms. You tabulate the results in a fourfold table, like Figure 13-5.

	Patient Was Helped	Patient Not Helped	Total
Real Treatment	70 (a)	30 (b)	100 (r1)
Placebo or Sham	50 (c)	50 (d)	100 (r2)
Total	120 (c1)	80 (c2)	200 (t)

FIGURE 13-5: Comparing a treatment to a placebo.

According to the data in Figure 13-5, 70 percent of participants taking the new drug report that it helped their dementia symptoms, which is quite impressive until you see that 50 percent of participants who received the placebo also reported improvement. When patients report therapeutic effect from a placebo, it's called the *placebo effect,* and it may come from a lot of different sources, including the patient's expectation of efficacy of the product. Nevertheless, if you conduct a Yates chi-square or Fisher Exact test on the data (as described in Chapter 12) at $\alpha = 0.05$, the results show treatment assignment was statistically significantly associated with whether or not the participant reported a treatment effect ($p = 0.006$ by either test).

Looking at inter- and intra-rater reliability

Many measurements in epidemiologic research are obtained by the subjective judgment of humans. Examples include the human interpretation of X-rays, CAT scans, ECG tracings, ultrasound images, biopsy specimens, and audio and video recordings of the behavior of study participants in various situations. Human researchers may generate quantitative measurements, such as determining the length of a bone on an ultrasound image. Human researchers may also generate classifications, such as determining the presence or absence of some atypical feature on an ECG tracing.

Humans who perform such determinations in studies are called *raters* because they are assigning *ratings,* which are values or classifiers that will be used in the study. For the measurements in your study, it is important to know how consistent such ratings are among different raters engaged in rating the same item. This is called *inter-rater reliability.* You will also be concerned with how reproducible the ratings are if one rater were to rate the same item multiple times. This is called *intra-rater reliability.*

When considering the consistency of a binary rating (like *yes* or *no*) for the same item between two raters, you can estimate *inter*-rater reliability by having each rater rate the same group of items. Imagine we had two raters rate the same 50 scans as yes or no in terms of whether each scan showed a tumor or not. We cross-tabbed the results and present them in Figure 13-6.

	Rated Yes by Rater 2	Rated No by Rater 2	Total
Rated Yes by Rater 1	22 (a)	5 (b)	27 (r1)
Rated No by Rater 1	7 (c)	16 (d)	23 (r2)
Total	29 (c1)	21 (c2)	50 (t)

© John Wiley & Sons, Inc.

FIGURE 13-6: Results of two raters reading the same set of 50 specimens and rating each specimen *yes* or *no*.

Looking at Figure 13-6, cell *a* contains a count of how many scans were rated *yes* — there is a tumor — by both Rater 1 and Rater 2. Cell *b* counts how many scans were rated *yes* by Rater 1 but *no* by Rater 2. Cell *c* counts how many scans were rated *no* by Rater 1 and *yes* by Rater 2, and cell *d* shows where Rater 1 and Rater 2 agreed and both rated the scan *no*. Cells *a* and *d* are considered *concordant* because both raters agreed, and *b* and *c* are *discordant* because both raters disagreed.

REMEMBER

Ideally, all the scans would be counted in concordant cells *a* or *d* of Figure 13-6, and discordant cells *b* and *c* would contain zeros. A measure of how close the data come to this ideal is called *Cohen's Kappa,* and is signified by the Greek lowercase kappa: κ. You calculate kappa as: $\kappa = 2(ad - bc) / (r1 \times c2 + r2 \times c1)$.

For the data in Figure 13-6, $\kappa = 2(22 \times 16 - 5 \times 7)/(27 \times 21 + 23 \times 29)$, which is 0.5138. How is this interpreted?

If the raters are in perfect agreement, then κ = 1. If you generate completely random ratings, you will see a κ = 0. You may think this means κ takes on a positive value between 0 and 1, but random sampling fluctuations can actually cause κ to be negative. This situation can be compared to a student taking a true/false test where the number of wrong answers is subtracted from the number of right answers as a penalty for guessing. When calculating κ, getting a score less than zero indicates the interesting combination of being both incorrect *and* unfortunate, and is penalized!

So, how do you interpret a κ of 0.5138? There's no universal agreement as to an acceptable value for κ. One common convention is that values of κ less than 0.4 are considered poor, those between 0.4 and 0.75 are acceptable, and those more than 0.75 are excellent. In this case, our raters may be performing acceptably.

For CIs forκ, you won't find an easy formula, but the fourfold table web page (`https://statpages.info/ctab2x2.html`) provides approximate CIs. For the preceding example, the 95 percent CI is 0.202 to 0.735. This means that for your two raters, their agreement was 0.514 (95 percent CI 0.202 to 0.735), which suggests that the agreement level was acceptable.

TIP

You can construct a similar table to Figure 13-6 for estimating *intra*-rater reliability. You would do this by having one rater rate the same groups of scans in two separate sessions. In this case, in the table in Figure 13-6, you'd replace the *by Rater* with *in Session* in the row and column labels.

Chapter **14**

Analyzing Incidence and Prevalence Rates in Epidemiologic Data

E*pidemiology* is the study of the causes of health and disease in human populations. It is sometimes defined as characterizing the *three Ds* — the *distribution* and *determinants* of human *disease* (although epidemiology technically also concerns more positive outcomes, such as human health and wellness). This chapter describes two concepts central to epidemiology: prevalence and incidence. Prevalence and incidence are also frequently encountered in other areas of human research as well. We describe how to calculate incidence rates and prevalence proportions. Then we concentrate on the analysis of incidence. (For an introduction to prevalence and to learn how to calculate prevalence ratios, see Chapter 13.) Later in this chapter, we describe how to calculate confidence intervals around incidence rates and rate ratios, and how to compare incidence rates between two populations.

Understanding Incidence and Prevalence

Incidence and prevalence are two related but distinct concepts. In the following sections, we define each of these concepts and provide examples. After that, we describe the relationship between incidence and prevalence.

Prevalence: The fraction of a population with a particular condition

REMEMBER

The *prevalence* of a condition in a population is the proportion of the population that has that condition at any given moment. It's calculated by creating a fraction with a numerator and a denominator. The denominator is the total population eligible to have the condition. The numerator is the number of individuals from the population who have the condition at a given time. If you divide this numerator by this denominator, you will calculate the prevalence of the condition in that population.

Prevalence can be expressed as a decimal fraction, a percentage, or a rate *per so many* (usually per 1,000, per 10,000, or per 100,000). For example, a 2021 survey found that 11.6 percent of the U.S. adult population has Type II diabetes. But a rarer outcome — such as a monthly hospitalization rate for those suffering from influenza — may be expressed as 31.7 per 100,000. The prevalence is expressed as the result of a calculation from this fraction, but stated as a rate so that it is easy to envision. It would be hard to envision that 0.0317 percent of influenza sufferers were hospitalized in one month. On the other hand, it is much easier to envision almost 32 people from a town with a population of 100,000 being hospitalized in one month — provided you also envision that everyone in the town had influenza.

Because prevalence is a proportion, it's analyzed in exactly the same way as any other proportion. The standard error (SE) of a prevalence ratio can be estimated by the formula in Chapter 13. Confidence intervals (CIs) for a prevalence estimate can be obtained from exact methods based on the binomial distribution or from formulas based on the normal approximation to the binomial distribution. Also, prevalence can be compared between two or more populations using the chi-square or Fisher Exact test. For this reason, the remainder of this chapter focuses on how to analyze incidence rates.

Incidence: Counting new cases

REMEMBER

The *incidence* of a condition is the rate at which new cases of that condition appear in a population. Incidence is generally expressed as an *incidence rate* (R), which — like prevalence — is a fraction. The numerator for incidence is defined as the number of observed events (N) in a particular time period. (Consider an *event* to mean that a member of the population goes from not having the condition to having the condition.) Take note that while incidence expresses the number of *new* cases of the condition in the numerator, in contrast, prevalence includes *all* cases — both new and existing — in the numerator. The denominator for incidence is defined as the number of individuals in the population who could have had the event multiplied by the interval of time being used. This is also called *time exposed* or *exposure (E)*. So, the equation for incidence is the number of observed events divided by the exposure, which is (E): $R = N/E$.

Exposure is measured in units of person-time, such as person-days or person-years. Incidence rates are expressed as the number of cases per unit of person-time. The unit of person-time is used so that the incidence rate can at least be the size of a whole number so it is easier to interpret and compare.

TIP

The incidence rate should be estimated by counting events over a narrow enough interval of time so that the number of observed events is a small fraction of the total population studied. One year is narrow enough for calculating incidence of Type II diabetes in adults because 0.02 percent of the adult population develops diabetes in a year. However, one year isn't narrow enough to be useful when considering the incidence of an acute condition like influenza. In influenza and other infectious diseases, the intervals of interest would be in terms of daily, weekly, and monthly trends. It's not very helpful to know that 30 percent of the population came down with influenza in a one-year period.

Consider City XYZ, which has a population of 300,000 adults. None of them has been diagnosed with Type II diabetes. Suppose that in 2023, 30 adults from City XYZ were newly diagnosed with Type II diabetes. The incidence of adult Type II diabetes in City XYZ would be calculated with a numerator of 30 cases and a denominator of 300,000 adults in one year. Using the incidence formula, this works out to 0.0001 new cases per person-year. As described before, in epidemiology, rates are reconfigured to have at least whole numbers so that they are easier to interpret and envision. For this example, you could express City XYZ's 2023 adult Type II diabetes incidence rate as 1 new case per 10,000 person-years, or as 10 new cases per 100,000 person-years.

Now imagine another city — City ABC — has a population of 80,0000 adults, and like with City XYZ, none of them had ever been diagnosed with Type II diabetes. Now, assume that in 2023, 24 adults from City ABC were newly diagnosed with Type II diabetes. City ABC's 2023 incidence rate would be calculated as 24 cases in 80,000 individuals in one year, which works out to 24/80,000 or 0.0003 new cases per person-year. To make the estimate comparable to City XYZ's estimate, let's express City ABC's estimate as 30 new cases per 100,000 person-years. So, the 2023 adult Type II diabetes incidence rate in City ABC — which is 30 new cases per 100,000 person-years — is three times as large as the 2023 adult Type II diabetes incidence rate for City XYZ, which is 10 new cases for 100,000 person-years. (Looks like City ABC's public health department needs to get advice from City XYZ!)

Understanding how incidence and prevalence are related

From the definitions and examples in the preceding sections, you see that incidence and prevalence are two related but distinct concepts. The incidence rate tells you how fast new cases of some condition arise in a population, and prevalence tells you what fraction of the population has that condition at any moment.

You may expect that conditions with higher incidence rates would have higher prevalence than conditions with lower incidence rates. This is true with common chronic conditions, such as hypertension. But if a condition is acute — including infectious diseases, such as influenza and COVID-19 — the duration of the condition may be short. In such a scenario, a high incidence rate may not be paired with a high prevalence. Relatively rare chronic diseases of long duration — such as dementia — have low yearly incidence rates, but as human health improves and humans live longer on average, the prevalence of dementia increases.

Analyzing Incidence Rates

The preceding sections show you how to calculate incidence rates and express them in larger units that are easier to envision. But, as we emphasize in Chapter 10, whenever you report an estimate you've calculated, you should also indicate the level of precision of that estimate. How precise are those incident rates? And how can you tell when the difference between two incidence rates is statistically significant? The next sections show you how to calculate standard errors (SEs) and confidence intervals (CIs) for incidence rates, and how to compare incidence rates between two populations.

Expressing the precision of an incidence rate

The precision of an incidence rate (R) is expressed using a confidence interval (CI). The SE of R typically is not reported, because the event rate usually isn't normally distributed. The SE is computed only as part of the CI calculation.

Random fluctuations in R are attributed entirely to fluctuations in the event count (N). We are assuming the exposure (described earlier in this chapter as the person-time in the denominator, abbreviated as E) is known exactly — or at least, much more precisely than N. Therefore, the CI for the event rate is based on the CI for N. Here's how you calculate the CI for R:

1. **Calculate the confidence interval (CI) for *N*.**

   Chapter 11 provides approximate SE and CI formulas based on the normal approximation to the Poisson distribution (see Chapter 24). These approximations are reasonable when N is large — meaning $N \geq 50$ events:

   $$95\% \text{ CI} = N - 1.96\sqrt{N} \quad \text{to} \quad N + 1.96\sqrt{N}$$

2. **Divide the lower and upper confidence limits for *N* by the exposure (*E*).**

   The answer is the CI for the incidence rate R.

Earlier in the chapter, we describe City ABC, which had a population of 80,000 adults without a diagnosis of Type II diabetes. In 2023, 24 new diabetes cases were identified in adults in City ABC, so the event count (N) is 24, and the exposure (E) is 80,000 person-years (because we are counting 80,000 persons for one year). Even though 24 is not that large, let's use this example to demonstrate calculating a CI for R. The incidence rate (R) is N/E, which is 24 per 80,000 person-years, or 30 per 100,000 person-years. How precise is this incidence rate?

To answer this, first, you should find the confidence limits for N. Using the approximate formula, the 95 percent CI around the event count of 24 is $24 - 1.96\sqrt{24}$ to $24 + 1.96\sqrt{24}$, or 14.4 to 33.6 events. Next, you divide the lower and upper confidence limits of N by the exposure using these formulas: 14.4/80,000 = 0.00018 for the lower limit, and 33.6/80,000 = 0.00042 for the upper limit. Finally, you can express these limits as 18.0 to 42.0 events per 100,00 person-years — the CI for the incidence rate. Your interpretation would be that City ABC's 2023 incidence rate for Type II diabetes in adults was 30.0 (95 percent CI 18.0 to 42.0) per 100,000 person-years.

Comparing incidences with the rate ratio

REMEMBER

When comparing incidence rates between two populations, you should calculate a *rate ratio* (RR) by dividing one incidence rate by the other. So for two groups with event counts N_1 and N_2, exposures E_1 and E_2, and incidence rates R_1 and R_2, respectively, you calculate the RR for Group 2 relative to Group 1 as a reference, like this:

$$RR = \frac{R_2}{R_1} = \frac{N_2/E_2}{N_1/E_1}$$

Let's revisit the example of 2023 incidence of Type II diabetes in adults in City XYZ compared to City ABC. For City XYZ, you have $N_1 = 30$ and $E_1 = 300,000$. For City ABC, you have $N_1 = 24$ and $E_2 = 80,000$. The RR for City ABC relative to City XYZ is $RR = (24/80,000)/(30/300,000)$, or 3.0, indicating that City ABC has three times the adult Type II diabetes incidence in 2023 compared to City XYZ. You could calculate the difference ($R_2 - R_1$) between two incidence rates if you wanted to, but in epidemiology, RRs are used much more often than rate differences.

Calculating confidence intervals for a rate ratio

Whenever you report an RR you've calculated, you should also indicate how precise it is. The exact calculation of a CI around RR is quite difficult, but if your observed event counts are large enough (meaning ≥ 10), then the following approximate formula for the 95 percent CI around an RR works reasonably well: 95% CI $= RR/Q$ to $RR \times Q$ where $Q = e^{1.96\sqrt{1/N_1 + 1/N_2}}$.

For other confidence levels, you can replace the 1.96 in the Q formula with the appropriate critical z value for the normal distribution.

So, for the 2023 adult Type II diabetes example, you would set $N_1 = 30$, $N_2 = 24$, and $RR = 3.0$. The equation would be $Q = e^{1.96\sqrt{1/24 + 1/30}}$, so the 95 percent lower and upper confidence limits would be $3.0/1.71$ and 3.0×1.71, meaning the CI of the RR would be from 1.75 to 5.13. You would interpret this by saying that that 2023 RR for adult Type II diabetes incidence is 3.0 times the rate in City ABC compared to City XYZ (95 percent CI 1.75 to 5.13).

Comparing two event rates

The examples in this chapter have compared incidence (or event) rates of adult Type II diabetes in 2023 between City XYZ and City ABC. These two event rates are represented as R_1 for City XYZ, and R_2 for City ABC. They are based on City XYZ having an N_1 of 30 events and City ABC having an N_2 of 24 events, and on exposures E_1 and E_2 for City XYZ and City ABC, respectively. The difference in event rates between City XYZ and City ABC can be tested for significance by calculating the 95 percent CI around the RR, and observing whether that CI includes the value of 1.0. Because the RR is a ratio, having 1.0 included in the CI indicates that City XYZ's and City ABC's rates could be identical. If the 95 percent CI around the

RR includes 1, the RR isn't statistically significantly different from 1, so the two rates aren't significantly different from each other (assuming $\alpha = 0.05$). But if the 95 percent CI is either entirely above or entirely below 1.0, the RR is statistically significantly different from 1, so the two rates are significantly different from each other (assuming $\alpha = 0.05$).

For the City ABC and City XYZ adult Type II diabetes 2023 rate comparison, the observed RR was 3.0, with a 95 percent confidence interval of 1.75 to 5.13. This CI does not include 1.0 — in fact, it is entirely above 1.0. So, the RR is significantly greater than 1, and you would conclude that City ABC has a statistically significantly higher adult Type II diabetes incidence rate than City XYZ (assuming $\alpha = 0.05$).

Comparing two event counts with identical exposure

If — and only if — the two exposures (E_1 and E_2) are identical, there's an *extremely* simple rule for testing whether two event counts (N_1 and N_2) are significantly different from each other at the level of $\alpha = 0.05$: If $\frac{(N_1 - N_2)^2}{N_1 + N_2} > 4$, then the Ns are statistically significantly different (at $\alpha = 0.05$).

REMEMBER

To interpret the formula into words, if the square of the difference is more than four times the sum, then the event counts are statistically significantly different at $\alpha = 0.05$. The value of 4 in this rule approximates 3.84, the chi-square value corresponding to $p = 0.05$.

Imagine you learned that in City XYZ, there were 30 fatal car accidents in 2022. In the following year, 2023, you learned City XYZ had 40 fatal car accidents. You may wonder: *Is driving in City XYZ getting more dangerous every year? Or was the observed increase from 2022 to 2023 due to random fluctuations?* Using the simple rule, you can calculate $(30 - 40)^2 / (30 + 40) = 100/70 = 1.4$, which is less than 4. Having 30 events — which in this case are fatal car accidents — isn't statistically significantly different from having 40 events in the same time period. As you see from the result, the increase of 10 in one year is likely statistical noise. But had the number of events increased more dramatically — say from 30 to 50 events — the increase would have been statistically significant. This is because $(30 - 50)^2 / (30 + 50) = 400/80 = 5.0$, which is greater than 4.

Estimating the Required Sample Size

As in all sample-size calculations, you need to specify the desired statistical power and the α level of the test. Let's set power to 80 percent and α to 0.05, as these are common settings. When comparing event rates (R_1 and R_2) between two groups with R_1 as the reference group, you must also specify:

>> The expected rate in the reference group (R_1)

>> The effect size of importance, expressed as the rate ratio $RR = R_2/R_1$

>> The expected ratio of exposure in the two groups (E_2/E_1)

For example, suppose that you're designing a study to test whether rotavirus gastroenteritis has a higher incidence in City XYZ compared to City ABC. You'll enroll an equal number City XYZ and City ABC residents, and follow them for one year to see whether they get rotavirus. Suppose that the one-year incidence of rotavirus in City XYZ is 1 case per 100 person-years (an incidence rate of 0.01 case per patient-year, or 1 percent per year). You want to have an 80 percent likelihood of getting a statistically significant result assuming $p = 0.05$ (you want to set power at 80 percent and $\alpha = 0.05$). When comparing the incidence rates, you are only concerned if they differ by more than 25 percent, which translates to a RR of 1.25. This means you expect to see $0.01 \times 1.25 = 0.0125$ cases per patient-year in City ABC.

If you want to use G*Power to do your power calculation (see Chapter 4), under Test family, choose *z tests* for population-level tests. Under Statistical test, choose *Proportions: Difference between two independent proportions* because the two rates are independent. Under Type of power analysis, choose *A priori: Compute required sample size − given α, power and effect size*, and under the Input Parameters section, choose *two tails* so you can test if one is higher or lower than the other. Set Proportion p1 to 0.01 (to represent City XYZ's incidence rate), Proportion p2 to 0.0125 (to represent City ABC's expected incidence rate), α err prob (α) to 0.05, and Power (1-β err prob) (power) to 0.8 for 80 percent, and keep a balanced Allocation ration N2/N1 of 1. After clicking Calculate, you'll see you need at least 27,937 person-years of observation in each group, meaning observing 57,000 participants over a one-year study. The shockingly large target sample size illustrates a challenge when studying incidence rates of rare illnesses.

5

Looking for Relationships with Correlation and Regression

Understand *correlation*, which is the strength and direction of the relationship between two variables, and *regression*, which is a set of techniques for describing the relationship between two variables.

Get a handle on straight-line regression, which is the simplest kind of regression.

Do *multiple regression* analysis, which is regression when there's more than one predictor variable.

Find out about other useful kinds of regression you encounter in biological research, such as Poisson regression and nonlinear regression.

Chapter **15**

Introducing Correlation and Regression

orrelation, regression, curve-fitting, model-building — these terms all describe a set of general statistical techniques that deal with the relation-ships among variables. Introductory statistics courses usually present only the simplest form of correlation and regression, equivalent to fitting a straight line to a set of data. But in the real world, correlations and regressions are seldom that simple — statistical problems may involve more than two variables, and the relationship among them can be quite complicated.

REMEMBER

The words *correlation* and *regression* are often used interchangeably, but they refer to two different concepts:

>> **Correlation** refers to the strength and direction of the relationship between two variables, or among a group of variables.

>> **Regression** refers to a set of techniques for describing how the values of a variable or a group of variables may cause, predict, or be associated with the values of another variable.

You can study correlation and regression for many years and not master all of it. In this chapter, we cover the kinds of correlation and regression most often encountered in biological research and explain the differences between them. We also explain some terminology used throughout Parts 5 and 6.

Correlation: Estimating How Strongly Two Variables Are Associated

Correlation refers to the extent to which two variables are related. In the following sections, we describe the *Pearson correlation coefficient* and discuss ways to analyze correlation coefficients.

Lining up the Pearson correlation coefficient

REMEMBER

The Pearson correlation coefficient is represented by the symbol r and measures the extent to which two variables (X and Y) tend to lie along a straight line when graphed. If the variables have no relationship, r will be 0, and the points will be scattered across the graph. If the relationship is *perfect* the points will lie exactly along a straight line, and r will either be:

>> **+1:** If the variables have a *direct* or *positive* relationship, meaning when one goes up, the other goes up, or

>> **−1:** If the variables have an *inverse* or *negative* relationship, meaning when one goes up, the other goes down

Correlation coefficients can be positive (indicating upward-sloping data) or negative (indicating downward-sloping data). Figure 15-1 shows what several different values of r look like.

Note: The Pearson correlation coefficient measures the extent to which the points lie along a *straight* line. If your data follow a curved line, the r value may be low or zero, as shown in Figure 15-2. All three graphs in Figure 15-2 have the same amount of random scatter in the points, but they have quite different r values. Pearson r is based on a straight-line relationship and is too small (or even zero) if the relationship is nonlinear. So, you shouldn't interpret $r = 0$ as evidence of lack of association or independence between two variables. It could indicate only the lack of a *straight-line* relationship between the two variables.

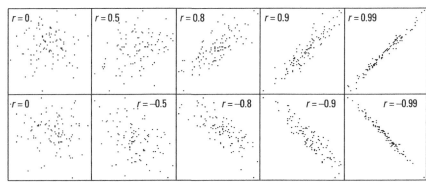

FIGURE 15-1:
100 data points, with varying degrees of correlation.

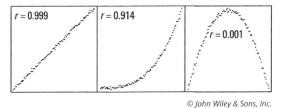

FIGURE 15-2:
Pearson r is based on a straight-line relationship.

Analyzing correlation coefficients

In the following sections, we show the common kinds of statistical analyses that you can perform on correlation coefficients.

Testing whether r is statistically significantly different from zero

Before beginning your calculations for correlation coefficients, remember that the data used in a correlation — the "ingredients" to a correlation — are the values of two variables referring to the same experimental unit. An example would be measurements of height (X) and weight (Y) in a sample of individuals. Because your raw data (the X and Y values) always have random fluctuations due to either sampling error or measurement imprecision, a calculated correlation coefficient is also subject to random fluctuations.

Even when X and Y are completely independent, your calculated r value is almost never exactly zero. One way to test for a statistically significant association between X and Y is to test whether r is statistically *significantly* different from zero by calculating a p value from the r value (see Chapter 3 for a refresher on p values).

The correlation coefficient has a strange sampling distribution, so it is not useful for statistical testing. Instead, the quantity t can be calculated from the observed correlation coefficient r, based on N observations, by the formula $t = r/\sqrt{(1-r^2)/(N-2)}$. Because t fluctuates in accordance with the Student t distribution with $N - 2$ degrees of freedom (df), it is useful for statistical testing (see Chapter 11 for more about t).

For example, if $r = 0.500$ for a sample of 12 participants, then $t = 0.5/\sqrt{(1-0.5^2)/(12-2)}$, which works out to $t = 1.8257$, with 10 degrees of freedom. You can use the online calculator at https://statpages.info/pdfs.html and calculate the p by entering the t and df values. You can also do this in R by using the code:

```
2 * pt(q = 1.8257, df = 10, lower.tail = FALSE).
```

Either way, you get p $= 0.098$, which is greater than 0.05. At $\alpha = 0.05$, the r value of 0.500 is not statistically significantly different from zero (see Chapter 12 for more about α).

How precise is an r value?

You can calculate confidence limits around an observed r value using a somewhat roundabout process. The quantity z, calculated by the *Fisher z transformation* $z = \frac{1}{2}\log[(1+r)/(1-r)]$, is approximately normally distributed with a standard deviation of $1/\sqrt{N-3}$. Therefore, using the formulas for normal-based confidence intervals (see Chapter 10), you can calculate the lower and upper 95 percent confidence limits around z: $z_{\text{Lower}} = z - 1.96/\sqrt{N-3}$ and $Z_{\text{Upper}} = z + 1.96/\sqrt{N-3}$. You can turn these into the corresponding confidence limits around r by the reverse of the z transformation: $r = (e^{2x} - 1)/(e^{2z} + 1)$ for $z = z_{\text{Lower}}$ and $z = z_{\text{Upper}}$.

Here are the steps for calculating 95 percent confidence limits around an observed r value of 0.05 for a sample of 12 participants (N = 12):

1. **Calculate the Fisher *z* transformation of the observed *r* value:**

   $$z = \frac{1}{2}\log((1+0.5)/(1-0.5)) = 0.549$$

2. **Calculate the lower and upper 95 percent confidence limits for *z*:**

   $$z_{\text{Lower}} = 0.549 - 1.96/\sqrt{12-3} = -0.104$$
   $$z_{\text{Upper}} = 0.549 + 1.96/\sqrt{12-3} = +1.203$$

3. **Calculate the lower and upper 95 percent confidence limits for *r*:**

$$r_{\text{Lower}} = (e^{2 \times (-0.104)} - 1)/(e^{2 \times (-0.104)} + 1) = -0.104$$
$$r_{\text{Upper}} = (e^{2 \times 1.203} - 1)/(e^{2 \times 1.203} + 1) = 0.835$$

Notice that the 95 percent confidence interval goes from –0.104 to +0.835, a range that includes the value zero. This means that the true *r* value could indeed be zero, which is consistent with the non-significant p value of 0.098 that you obtained from the significance test of *r* in the preceding section.

Determining whether two r values are statistically significantly different

Suppose that you have two correlation coefficients and you want to test whether they are statistically significantly different. It doesn't matter whether the two *r* values are based on the same variables or are from the same group of participants. Imagine that a significance test for comparing two correlation coefficient values (which we will call r_1 and r_2) that were obtained from N_1 and N_2 participants, respectively. You can utilize the Fisher *z* transformation to get z_1 and z_2. The difference $(z_1 - z_2)$ has a standard error (SE) of $SE_{z_2 - z_1} = \sqrt{1/(N_1 - 3) + 1/(N_2 - 3)}$. You obtain the test statistic for the comparison by dividing the difference by its SE. You can convert this to a p value by referring to a table (or web page) of the normal distribution.

For example, if you want to compare an r_1 value of 0.4 based on an N_1 of 100 participants with an r_2 value of 0.6 based on an N_2 of 150 participants, you perform the following steps:

1. **Calculate the Fisher *z* transformation of each observed *r* value:**

$$z_1 = \frac{1}{2} \log[(1 + 0.4)/(1 - 0.4)] = 0.424$$
$$z_2 = \frac{1}{2} \log[(1 + 0.6)/(1 - 0.6)] = 0.693$$

2. **Calculate the $(z_2 - z_1)$ difference:**

$$0.693 - 0.424 = 0.269$$

3. **Calculate the SE of the $(z_2 - z_1)$ difference:**

$$SE_{z_2 - z_1} = \sqrt{1/(100 - 3) + 1/(150 - 3)} = 0.131$$

4. **Calculate the test statistic:**

$$0.269/0.131 = 2.05$$

5. **Look up 2.05 in a normal distribution table or web page such as** `https://statpages.info/pdfs.html` **(or edit and run the R code provided earlier in "Testing whether r is statistically significantly different from zero"), and observe that the p value is 0.039 for a two-sided test.**

A two-sided test is used when you're interested in knowing whether either *r* is larger than the other. The p value of 0.039 is less than 0.05, meaning that the two correlation coefficients are statistically significantly different from each other at $\alpha = 0.05$.

Determining the required sample size for a correlation test

REMEMBER

If you are planning to conduct a study where the outcome is a correlation between two variables designated *X* and *Y*, you need to be sure to enroll a large enough sample so that if the correlation is indeed statistically significant, you have enough sample for *r* to show it. As described in Chapter 11 with the t test and the ANOVA, the sample size can be estimated through one big equation, where you plug the estimated effect size along with the α and power you select into an equation, and calculate the sample size (see Chapter 3 for the scoop on effect size and selecting α and power).

For a sample-size calculation for a correlation coefficient, you need to plug in the following *design parameters* of the study into the equation:

>> **The desired α *level* of the test:** The p value that's considered significant when you're testing the correlation coefficient (usually 0.05).

>> **The desired *power* of the test:** The probability of rejecting the null hypothesis if the alternative hypothesis is true (usually set to 0.8 or 80 percent).

>> **The *effect size* of importance:** The smallest *r* value that is considered practically important, or *clinically significant*. If the true *r* is less than this value, then you don't care whether the test comes out significant, but if *r* is greater than this value, you want to get a significant result.

REMEMBER

It may be challenging to select an effect size, and context matters. One approach would be to start by referring to Figure 15-1 to select a potential effect size, then do a sample-size calculation and see the result. If the result requires more samples than you could ever enroll, then try making the effect size a little larger and redoing the calculation until you get a more reasonable answer.

TIP

You can use software like G*Power (see Chapter 4) to perform the sample-size calculation. If you use G*Power:

1. Under Test Family, choose *t-tests*.

2. Under Statistical Test, choose *Correlation: Point Biserial model*.

3. Under Type of Power Analysis, choose *A Priori: Compute required sample size – given α, power, and effect size*.

4. Under Tail(s), because either r could be greater, choose two.

5. Under Effect Size, which is the expected difference between r_1 and r_2, enter the effect size you expect.

6. Under α err prob, enter **0.05**.

7. Under Power (1-β err prob), enter **0.08**.

8. Click Calculate.

The answer will appear under *Total sample size*. As an example, if you enter these parameters and an effect size of 0.02, the total sample size will be 191.

Regression: Discovering the Equation that Connects the Variables

As described earlier, correlation assesses the relationship between two continuous numeric variables (as compared to categorical variables, as described in Chapter 8). This relationship can also be evaluated with *regression* analysis to provide more information about how these two variables are related. But perhaps more importantly, regression is not limited to continuous variables, nor is it limited to only two variables. Regression is about developing a formula that explains how all the variables in the regression are related. In the following sections, we explain the purpose of regression analysis, identify some terms and notation typically used, and describe common types of regression.

Understanding the purpose of regression analysis

You may wonder how fitting a formula to a set of data can be useful. There are actually many uses. With regression, you can

>> **Test for a significant association or relationship between two or more variables.** The process is similar to correlation, but is more generalized to produce a unique equation or formula relating to the variables.

>> **Get a compact representation of your data.** A well-fitting regression model succinctly summarizes the relationships between the variables in your data.

>> **Make precise predictions, or prognoses.** With a properly fitted survival function (see Chapter 23), you can generate a customized survival curve for a newly diagnosed cancer patient based on that patient's age, gender, weight, disease stage, tumor grade, and other factors to predict how long they will live. A bit morbid, perhaps, but you could certainly do it.

>> **Do mathematical manipulations easily and accurately on a fitted function that may be difficult or inaccurate to do graphically on the raw data.** These include making estimates within the range of the measured values (called *interpolation*) as well as outside the measured values (called *extrapolation*, and considered risky). You may also want to *smooth* the data, which is described in Chapter 19.

>> **Obtain numerical values for the parameters that appear in the regression model formula.** Chapter 19 explains how to make a regression model based on a theoretical rather than known statistical distribution (described in Chapter 3). Such a model is used to develop estimates like the ED_{50} of a drug, which is the dose that produces one-half the maximum effect.

Talking about terminology and mathematical notation

REMEMBER

A *regression model* is a formula that describes how one variable, the *dependent variable*, depends on one or more other variables, and on one or more *parameters*. (While it is technically possible to have more than one dependent variable in a model, a discussion of this type of regression is outside the scope of this book.) The dependent variable is also called the *outcome*, and the other variables are called *independent variables* or *predictors*. *Parameters* refer to the other terms that appear in the formula that make the function come as close as possible to the observed data which are determined by the statistical software you are using.

TIP

If you have only one independent variable, it's often designated by X, and the dependent variable is designated by Y. If you have more than one independent variable, variables are usually designated by letters toward the end of the alphabet (W, X, Y, Z). Parameters are often designated by letters toward the beginning of the alphabet *(a, b, c, d)*. There's no consistent rule regarding uppercase versus lower-case letters.

Sometimes a collection of predictor variables is designated by a subscripted variable (X_1, X_2 and so on) and the corresponding coefficients by another subscripted variable (b_1, b_2, and so on).

In mathematical texts, you may see a regression model with three predictors written in one of several ways, such as

» $Z = a + bX + cY + dV$ (different letters for each variable and parameter)

» $Y = b_0 + b_1X_1 + b_2X_2$ (using a general subscript-variable notation)

TIP

In practical work, using the actual names of the variables from your data and using meaningful terms for parameters is easiest to understand and least error-prone. For example, consider the equation for the first-order elimination of an injected drug from the blood, $Conc = Conc_0 \times e^{-k_e \times Time}$. This form, with its short but meaningful names for the two variables, *Conc* (blood concentration) and *Time* (time after injection), and the two parameters, $Conc_0$ (concentration at Time $= 0$) and k_e (elimination rate constant), would probably be more meaningful to a reader than $Y = a \times e^{-b \times X}$.

Classifying different kinds of regression

You can classify regression on the basis of

» How many predictors or independent variables appear in the model

» The type of data of the outcome variable

» What mathematical form to which the data appear to conform

There are different terms for different types of regression. In this book, we refer to regression models with one predictor in the model as *simple regression,* or *univariate regression*. We refer to regression models with multiple predictors as *multivariate regression*.

In the next section, we explain how the type of outcome variable determines which regression to select, and after that, we explain how the mathematical form of the data influences the type of regression you choose.

Examining the outcome variable's type of data

Here are the different regressions we cover in this book by type of outcome variable:

>> **Ordinary regression** (also called *linear* regression) is used when the outcome is a continuous variable whose random fluctuations are governed by the normal distribution (see Chapters 16 and 17).

>> **Logistic regression** is used when the outcome variable is a two-level or dichotomous variable whose fluctuations are governed by the binomial distribution (see Chapter 18).

>> **Poisson regression** is used when the outcome variable is the number of occurrences of a sporadic event whose fluctuations are governed by the Poisson distribution (see Chapter 19).

>> **Survival regression** when the outcome is a *time to event,* often called a *survival time*. Part 6 covers the entire topic of survival analysis, and Chapter 23 focuses on regression.

Figuring out what kind of function is being fitted

Another way to classify different types of regression analysis is according to whether the mathematical formula for the model is linear or nonlinear in the parameters.

In a *linear* function, you multiply each predictor variable by a parameter and then add these products to give the predicted value. You can also have one more parameter that isn't multiplied by anything — it's called the *constant term* or the *intercept*. Here are some linear functions:

>> $Y = a + bX$

>> $Y = a + bX + cX^2 + dX^3$

>> $Y = a + bX + cLog(W) + dX/Cos(Z)$

In these examples, Y is the dependent variable or the outcome, and X, W, and Z are the independent variables or predictors. Also, a, b, c, and d are parameters.

The predictor variables can appear in a formula in nonlinear form, like squared or cubed, inside functions like Log and Sin, and multiplied by each other. But as long as the coefficients appear only in a linear way, the function is still considered *linear in the parameters.* By that, we mean each coefficient is multiplied by a term involving predictor variables, with the terms added together in a linear equation.

A *nonlinear* function is anything that's not a linear function. For example:

$$Y = a/\left(b + e^{-c \times X}\right)$$

is nonlinear in the parameters, because the parameter b is in the denominator of a fraction, and the parameter c is in an exponent. The parameter a appears in a linear form, but if *any* of the parameters appear in a nonlinear way, the function is said to be nonlinear in the parameters. Nonlinear regressions are covered in Chapter 19.

Chapter **16**

Getting Straight Talk on Straight-Line Regression

hapter 15 refers to regression analyses in a general way. This chapter focuses on the simplest type of regression analysis: *straight-line regression*. You can visualize it as *fitting* a straight line to the points in a scatter plot from a set of data involving just two variables. Those two variables are generally referred to as *X* and *Y*. The *X* variable is formally called the *independent variable* (or the *predictor* or *cause*). The *Y* variable is called the *dependent variable* (or the *out-come* or *effect*).

Knowing When to Use Straight-Line Regression

TIP

You may see straight-line regression referred to in books and articles by several different names, including *linear regression, simple linear regression, linear univariate regression,* and *linear bivariate regression.* This abundance of references can be confusing, so we always use the term *straight-line regression.*

Straight-line regression is appropriate when *all* of these things are true:

>> You're interested in the relationship between two — and only two — numerical variables. At least one of them must be a continuous variable that serves as the dependent variable (*Y*).

>> You've made a scatter plot of the two variables and the data points seem to lie, more or less, along a straight line (as shown in Figures 16-1a and 16-1b). You shouldn't try to fit a straight line to data that appears to lie along a curved line (as shown in Figures 16-1c and 16-1d).

>> The data points appear to scatter randomly around the straight line over the entire range of the chart, with no extreme outliers (as shown in Figures 16-1a and 16-1b).

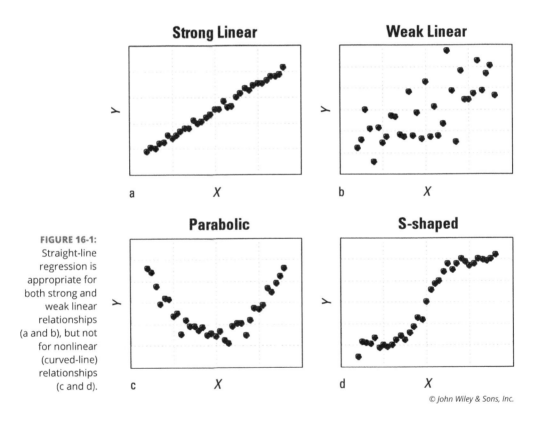

FIGURE 16-1: Straight-line regression is appropriate for both strong and weak linear relationships (a and b), but not for nonlinear (curved-line) relationships (c and d).

© *John Wiley & Sons, Inc.*

You should proceed with straight-line regression when one or more of the following are true:

>> You want to test whether there's a statistically significant association between the X and Y variables.

>> You want to know the value of the slope and/or intercept (also referred to as the Y *intercept*) of a line fitted through the X and Y data points.

>> You want to be able to predict the value of Y if you know the value of X.

Understanding the Basics of Straight-Line Regression

The formula of a straight line can be written like this: $Y = a + bX$. This formula breaks down this way:

>> Y is the dependent variable (or outcome).

>> X is the independent variable (or predictor).

>> a is the intercept, which is the value of Y when $X = 0$.

>> b is the slope, which is the amount Y changes when X increases by 1.

In straight-line regression, our goal is to develop the best-fitting line for our data. Using least-squares as a guide, the best-fitting line through a set of data is the one that minimizes the sum of the squares (SSQ) of the *residuals*. Residuals are the vertical distances of each point from the fitted line, as shown in Figure 16-2.

Good Fit   **Bad Fit**

FIGURE 16-2:
On average, a good-fitting line has smaller residuals than a bad-fitting line.

© *John Wiley & Sons, Inc.*

For curves, finding the best-fitting curve is a very complicated mathematical problem. What's nice about the straight-line regression is that it's so simple that you can calculate the least-squares parameters from explicit formulas. If you're interested (or if your professor insists that you're interested), we present a general outline of how those formulas are derived.

Think of a set of data containing X_i and Y_i, in which i is an index that identifies each observation in the set, as described in Chapter 2. From those data, SSQ can be calculated like this:

$$SSQ = \sum_i (a + bX_i - Y_i)^2$$

If you're good at first-semester calculus, you can find the values of a and b that minimize SSQ by setting the partial derivatives of SSQ with respect to a and b equal to 0. If you stink at calculus, trust that this leads to these two simultaneous equations:

$$a(N) + b(\Sigma Y) = (\Sigma Y)$$

$$a(\Sigma X) + b(\Sigma X^2) = (\Sigma XY)$$

where N is the number of observed data points.

These equations can be solved for a and b:

$$a = \frac{(\Sigma Y)(\Sigma X^2) - (\Sigma X)((\Sigma XY)}{(N)((\Sigma X^2) - (\Sigma X)^2}$$

$$b = \frac{(\Sigma XY) - (a)(\Sigma X)}{(\Sigma X^2)}$$

See Chapter 2 if you don't feel comfortable reading the mathematical notations or expressions in this section.

TIP

Running a Straight-Line Regression

Even if it is possible, it is not a good idea to calculate regressions manually or with a calculator. You'll go crazy trying to evaluate all those summations and other calculations, and you'll almost certainly make a mistake somewhere in your calculations.

WARNING

Fortunately, most statistical packages can perform a straight-line regression. Microsoft Excel has built-in functions for calculating the slope and intercept of the least-squares straight line. You can also find straight-line regression web pages (several are listed at https://statpages.info). If you use R, you can explore using the *lm()* command. (See Chapter 4 for an introduction to statistical software.) In the following sections, we list the basic steps for running a straight-line regression, complete with an example.

Taking a few basic steps

The exact steps you take to run a straight-line regression depend on what software you're using, but here's the general approach:

1. **Structure your data into the proper form.**

   Usually, the data consist of two columns of numbers, one representing the independent variable and the other representing the dependent variable.

2. **Tell the software which variable is the independent variable and which one is the dependent variable.**

   Depending on the software, you may type in the variable names, or pick them from a menu or list in your file.

3. **If the software offers output options, tell it that you want it to output these results:**

   - Graphs of observed and calculated values

   - Summaries and graphs of the residuals

   - Regression table

   - Goodness-of-fit measures

4. **Execute the regression in the software (tell it to run the regression).**

   Then go look for the output. You should see the output you requested in Step 3.

Walking through an example

To see how to run a straight-line regression and interpret the output, we use the following example throughout the rest of this chapter.

Consider how blood pressure (BP) is related to body weight. It may be reasonable to suspect that people who weigh more have higher BP. If you test this hypothesis on people and find that there really is an association between weight and BP, you may want to quantify that relationship. Maybe you want to say that every extra kilogram of weight tends to be associated with a certain amount of increased BP. Even though you are testing an association, the reality is that you believe that as people weigh more, it causes their BP to go up — not the other way around. So, you would characterize weight as the independent variable (*X*), and BP as the dependent variable (*Y*). The following sections take you through the steps of gathering data, creating a scatter plot, and interpreting the results.

Gathering the data

Suppose that you recruit a sample of 20 adults from a particular clinical population to participate in your study (see Chapter 6 for more on sampling). You weigh them and measure their systolic BP (SBP) as a measure of their BP. Table 16-1 shows a sample of weight and SBP data from 20 participants. Weight is recorded in kilograms (kg), and SBP is recorded in the strange-sounding units of *millimeters of mercury* (mmHg).

TABLE 16-1

Weight and Blood Pressure Data

Participant Study ID	Body Weight (kg)	SBP (mmHg)
1	74.4	109
2	85.1	114
3	78.3	94
4	77.2	109
5	63.8	104
6	77.9	132
7	78.9	127
8	60.9	98
9	75.6	126
10	74.5	126
11	82.2	116
12	99.8	121
13	78.0	111

Participant Study ID	Body Weight (kg)	SBP (mmHg)
14	71.8	116
15	90.2	115
16	105.4	133
17	100.4	128
18	80.9	128
19	81.8	105
20	109.0	127

Creating a scatter plot

It's not easy to identify patterns and trends between weight and SBP by looking at a table like Table 16-1. You get a much clearer picture of how the data are related if you make a scatter plot. You would place weight, the independent variable, on the X axis, and SBP, the dependent variable, on the Y axis, as shown in Figure 16-3.

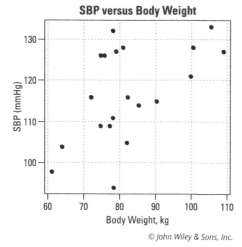

FIGURE 16-3:
Scatter plot of SBP versus body weight.

© John Wiley & Sons, Inc.

Examining the results

In Figure 16-3, you can see the following pattern:

>> **Low-weight participants have lower SBP,** which is represented by the points near the lower-left part of the graph.

>> **Higher-weight participants have higher SBP,** which is represented by the points near the upper-right part of the graph.

You can also tell that there aren't any higher-weight participants with a very low SBP, because the lower-right part of the graph is rather empty. But this relationship isn't completely convincing, because several participants in the lower weight range of 70 to 80 kg have SBPs over 125 mmHg.

REMEMBER

A correlation analysis (described in Chapter 15) will tell you how strong this type of association is, as well as its direction (which is positive in this case). The results of a correlation analysis help you decide whether or not the association is likely due to random fluctuations. Assuming it is not, proceeding to a regression analysis provides you with a mathematical formula that numerically expresses the relationship between the two variables (which are weight and SBP in this example).

Interpreting the Output of Straight-Line Regression

In the following sections, we walk you through the printed and graphical output of a typical straight-line regression run. Its looks will vary depending on your software. The output in this chapter was generated using R (see Chapter 4 to get started with R). But regardless of the software you use, you should be able to program the regression so the following elements appear on your output:

>> A statement of what you asked the program to do (the code you ran for the regression)

>> A summary of the residuals, including graphs that display the residuals and help you assess whether they're normally distributed

>> The regression table (providing the results of the regression model)

>> Measures of goodness-of-fit of the line to the data

Seeing what you told the program to do

In the example data set, the SBP variable is named *BPs*, and the weight variable is named *wgt*. In Figure 16-4, the first two lines produced by the statistical software reprint the code you ran. The code says that you wanted to fit a linear formula where the software estimates the parameters to the equation *SBP = weight* based on your observed SBP and weight values. The code used was *lm(formula = BPs ~ Wgt)*.

```
Call:
lm (formula = BPs ~ Wgt)

Residuals:
    Min      IQ    Median      3Q       Max
 -20.999  -4.720   -3.403    6.528    17.196

Coefficients:
              Estimate Std. Error t value Pr (>|t|)
(Intercept)    76.8602    14.6552   5.245 5.49e-05 ***
Wgt             0.4871     0.1760   2.767   0.0127 *
---
Signif. codes:        0 `***' 0.001 `**' 0.01 `*' 0.05 ` . ' 0.1 ` ' 1

Residual standard error: 9.838 on 18 degrees of freedom
Multiple R-squared: 0.2984,        Adjusted R-squared:   0.2594
F-statistic: 7.656 on 1 and 18 DF, p-value: 0.01271
```

FIGURE 16-4: Sample straight-line regression output from R.

The actual equation of the straight line is not *SBP = weight*, but more accurately *SBP = a + b × weight*, with the *a* (intercept) and *b* (slope) parameters having been left out of the model. This is a reminder that although the goal is to evaluate the *SBP = weight* model conceptually, in reality, this relationship will be numerically different with each data set we use.

Evaluating residuals

REMEMBER

The *residual* for a point is the vertical distance of that point from the fitted line. It's calculated as $Residual = Y - (a + b \times X)$, where *a* and *b* are the intercept and slope of the fitted straight line, respectively.

Most regression software outputs several measures of how the data points scatter above and below the fitted line, which provides an idea of the size of the residuals (see "Summary statistics for the residuals" for how to interpret these measures). The residuals for the sample data are shown in Figure 16-5.

FIGURE 16-5: Scattergram of SBP versus weight, with the fitted straight line and the residuals of each point from the line.

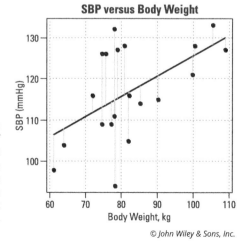

© John Wiley & Sons, Inc.

Summary statistics for the residuals

If you read about summarizing data in Chapter 9, you know that the distribution of values from a numerical variable are reported using summary statistics, such as mean, standard deviation, median, minimum, maximum, and quartiles. Summary statistics for residuals are what you should expect to find in the *residuals* section of your software's output. Here's what you see in Figure 16-4 at the top under *Residuals*:

>> **The minimum and maximum values:** These are labeled as *Min* and *Max*, respectively, and represent the two largest residuals, or the two points that lie farthest away from the least-squares line in either direction. The minimum is negative, indicating it is below the line, while the positive maximum is above the line. The minimum is almost 21 mmHg below the line, while the maximum lies about 17 mmHg above the line.

>> **The first and third quartiles:** These are labeled *IQ* and *3Q* on the output. Looking under IQ, which is the first quartile, you can tell that about 25 percent of the data points (which would be 5 out of 20) lie more than 4.7 mmHg below the fitted line. For the third quartile results, you see that another 25 percent lie more than 6.5 mmHg above the fitted line. The remaining 50 percent of the points lie within those two quartiles.

>> **The median:** Labeled *Median* on the output, a median of –3.4 tells you that half of the residuals, which is 10 of the 20 data points, are less than –3.4, and half are greater than –3.4. The negative sign means the median lies below the fitted line.

Note: The mean isn't included in these summary statistics because the mean of the residuals is always exactly 0 for any kind of regression that includes an intercept term.

REMEMBER

The *residual standard error,* often called the *root-mean-square (RMS) error* in regression output, is a measure of how tightly or loosely the points scatter above or below the fitted line. You can think of it as the *standard deviation (SD)* of the residuals, although it's computed in a slightly different way from the usual SD of a set of numbers. RMS uses $N - 2$ instead of $N - 1$ in the denominator of the SD formula. At the bottom of Figure 16-4, *Residual standard error* is expressed as 9.838 mmHg. You can think of it as another summary statistic for residuals

Graphs of the residuals

Most regression programs will produce different graphs of the residuals if requested in code. You can use these graphs to assess whether the data meet the criteria for executing a least-squares straight-line regression. Figure 16-6 shows two of the more common types of residual graphs. The one on the left is called a *residuals versus fitted* graph, and the one on the right is called *a normal Q-Q* graph.

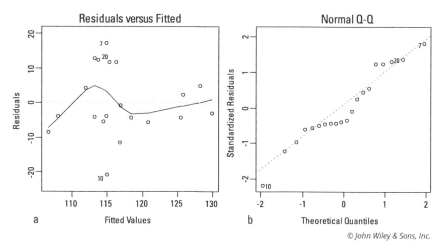

© John Wiley & Sons, Inc.

FIGURE 16-6:
The *residuals versus fitted* (a) and *normal* (b) *Q-Q* graphs help you determine whether your data meets the requirements for straight-line regression.

As stated at the beginning of this section, you calculate the residual for each point by subtracting the predicted *Y* from the observed *Y*. As shown in Figure 16-6, a *residuals versus fitted* graph displays the values of the residuals plotted along the *Y* axis and the predicted *Y* values from the fitted straight line plotted along the *X* axis. A *normal Q-Q* graph shows the *standardized residuals*, which are the residuals divided by the RMS value, along the *Y* axis, and theoretical quantiles along the *X* axis. *Theoretical quantiles* are what you'd expect the standardized residuals to be if they were exactly normally distributed.

REMEMBER

Together, the two graphs shown in Figure 16-6 provide insight into whether your data conforms to the requirements for straight-line regression:

>> Your data must lie above and below the line *randomly* across the whole range of data.

>> The average amount of scatter must be *fairly constant* across the whole range of data.

>> The residuals should be approximately normally distributed.

You need years of experience examining residual plots before you can interpret them confidently, so don't feel discouraged if you can't tell whether your data complies with the requirements for straight-line regression from these graphs. Here's how we interpret them, allowing for other biostatisticians to disagree:

>> We read the residuals versus fitted chart in Figure 16-6 to show the points lying equally above and below the fitted line, because this appears true whether you're looking at the left, middle, or right part of the graph.

>> Figure 18-6 shows most of the residuals lie within ±10 mmHg of the line, but several larger residuals appear to be where the SBP is around 115 mmHg. We think this is a little suspicious. If you see a pattern like this, you should examine your raw data to see whether there are unusual values associated with these particular participants.

>> If the residuals are normally distributed, then in the normal Q-Q chart in Figure 16-6, the points should lie close to the dotted diagonal line, and shouldn't display any overall curved shape. Our opinion is that the points follow the dotted line pretty well, so we're not concerned about lack of normality in the residuals.

Making your way through the regression table

REMEMBER

When doing regression, it is common to focus on the table of regression coefficients. It's likely where you look first when interpreting your results, and where you concentrate most of your attention. When you run a straight-line regression, statistical programs typically produce a table of regression coefficients that looks much like the one in Figure 16-4 under the heading *Coefficients*.

For straight-line regression, the coefficients table has two rows that correspond with the two parameters of the straight line:

>> **The intercept row:** This row is labeled *(Intercept)* in Figure 16-4, but can be labeled *Intercept* or *Constant* in other software.

>> **The slope row:** This row is usually labeled with the name of the independent variable in your data, so in Figure 16-4, it is named *Wgt*. It may be labeled *Slope* in some programs.

The table has several different columns, depending on the software. In Figure 16-4, the columns are *Estimate, Std. Error, t value, and Pr (>|t|)*. How to interpret the results from these columns is discussed in the next section.

The values of the coefficients (the intercept and the slope)

TIP

The first column of the table of regression coefficients usually shows the values of the slope and intercept of the fitted straight line (labeled *Estimate* in Figure 16-4). Other column headings include *Coefficient* or the single letter *B* or *C* (in uppercase or lowercase), depending on the software.

Looking at the rows in Figure 16-4, the intercept (labeled *(Intercept)*) is the predicted value of *Y* when *X* is equal to 0, and is expressed in the same units of measurement as the *Y* variable. The slope (labeled *Wgt*) is the amount the predicted value of *Y* changes when *X* increases by exactly one unit of measurement, and is expressed in units equal to the units of *Y* divided by the units of *X*.

In the example shown in Figure 16-4, the estimated value of the intercept is 76.8602 mmHg, and the estimated value of the slope is 0.4871 mmHg/kg.

>> The intercept value of 76.9 mmHg means that a person who weighs 0 kg is predicted to have a SBP of about 77 mmHg. But nobody weighs 0 kg! The intercept in this example (and in many straight-line relationships in biology) has no physiological meaning at all, because 0 kg is completely outside the range of possible human weights.

>> The slope value of 0.4871 mmHg/kg *does* have a real-world meaning. It means that every additional 1 kg of weight is associated with a 0.4871 mmHg increase in SBP. If we multiply both estimates by 10, we could say that every additional 10 kg of body weight is associated with almost a 5 mmHg SBP increase.

The standard errors of the coefficients

The second column in the regression table often contains the standard errors of the estimated parameters. In Figure 16-4, it is labeled *Std. Error*, but it could be stated as *SE* or use a similar term. We use SE to mean standard error for the rest of this chapter.

REMEMBER

Because data from your sample always have random fluctuations, any estimate you calculate from your data will be subject to random fluctuations, whether it is a simple summary statistic or a regression coefficient. The SE of your estimate tells you how precisely you were able to estimate the parameter from your data, which is very important if you plan to use the value of the slope (or the intercept) in a subsequent calculation.

Keep these facts in mind about SE:

>> **SEs always have the same units as the coefficients themselves.** In the example shown in Figure 16-4, the SE of the intercept has units of mmHg, and the SE of the slope has units of mmHg/kg.

>> **Round off the estimated values.** It is not helpful to report unnecessary digits. In this example, the SE of the intercept is about 14.7, so you can say that the estimate of the intercept in this regression is about 77 $\pm$ 15 mmHg. In the same way, you can say that the estimated slope is 0.49 $\pm$ 0.18 mmHg/kg.

When reporting regression coefficients in professional publications, you may state the SE like this: "The predicted increase in systolic blood pressure with weight (±1 SE) was 0.49 ± 0.18 mmHg/kg."

If you know the value of the SE, you can easily calculate a *confidence interval* (CI) around the estimate (see Chapter 10 for more information on CIs). These expressions provide a very good approximation of the 95 percent confidence limits (abbreviated CL), which mark the low and high ends of the CI around a regression coefficient:

$$Lower\ 95\%\ CL\ =\ Coefficient\ -\ 2 \times SE$$

$$Upper\ 95\%\ CL\ =\ Coefficient\ +\ 2 \times SE$$

More informally, these are written as $95\%\ CI = \text{coefficient} \pm 2 \times SE$.

So, the 95 percent CI around the slope in our example is calculated as $0.49 \pm 2 \times 0.176$, which works out to 0.49 ± 0.35, with the final confidence limits of 0.14 to 0.84 mmHg. If you submit a manuscript for publication, you may express the precision of the results in terms of CIs instead of SEs, like this: "The predicted increase in SBP as a function of body weight was 0.49 mmHg/kg ($95\%\ CI : 0.14 - 0.84$)."

The Student t value

In most output, there is a column in the regression table that shows the ratio of the coefficient divided by its SE. This column is labeled *t value* in Figure 16-4, but it can be labeled *t* or other names. This column is not very useful. You can think of this column as an intermediate quantity in the calculation of what you're really interested in, which is the p value for the coefficient.

The p value

A column in the regression tables (usually the last one) contains the p value, which indicates whether the regression coefficient is statistically significantly different from 0. In Figure 16-4, it is labeled $Pr(>|t|)$, but it can be called a variety of other names, including *p value*, *p*, and *Signif*.

In Figure 16-4, the p value for the intercept is shown as $5.49e - 05$, which is equal to 0.0000549 (see the description of scientific notation in Chapter 2). Assuming we set α at 0.05, the p value is much less than 0.05, so the intercept is statistically significantly different from zero. But recall that in this example (and usually in straight-line regression), the intercept doesn't have any real-world importance. It's equals the estimated SBP for a person who weighs 0 kg, which is nonsensical, so you probably don't care whether it's statistically significantly different from zero or not.

But the p value for the slope is very important. Assuming $\alpha = 0.05$, if it's less than 0.05, it means that the slope of the fitted straight line is statistically significantly different from zero. This means that the X and Y variables are statistically significantly associated with each other. A p value greater than 0.05 would indicate that the true slope could equal zero, and there would be no conclusive evidence for a statistically significant association between X and Y. In Figure 18-4, the p value for the slope is 0.0127, which means that the slope is statistically significantly different from zero. This tells you that in your model, body weight is statistically significantly associated with SBP.

TIP

If you want to test for a significant *correlation* between two variables at $\alpha = 05$, you can look at the p value for the slope of the least-squares straight line. If it's less than 0.05, then the X and Y variables are also statistically significantly correlated. The p value for the significance of the slope in a straight-line regression is always exactly the same as the p value for the correlation test of whether r is statistically significantly different from zero, as described in Chapter 15.

Wrapping up with measures of goodness-of-fit

The last few lines of output in Figure 16-4 contain several indicators of how well the straight line represents the data. The following sections describe this part of the output.

The correlation coefficient

Most straight-line regression programs provide the classic Pearson r correlation coefficient between X and Y (see Chapter 15 for details). But the program may provide you the correlation coefficient in a roundabout way by outputting r^2 rather than r itself. In Figure 16-4, at the bottom under *Multiple R-squared*, the r^2 is listed as 0.2984. If you want Pearson r, just use Microsoft Excel or a calculator to take square root of 0.2984 to get 0.546.

REMEMBER

The r^2 is always positive, because square of any number is always positive. But the correlation coefficient can be positive or negative, depending on whether the fitted line slopes upward or downward. If the fitted line slopes downward, make your r value negative.

Why did the program give you r^2 instead of r in the first place? It's because r^2 is a useful estimate called the *coefficient of determination*. It tells you what percent of the total variability in the Y variable can be explained by the fitted line.

>> An r^2 value of 1 means that the points lie exactly on the fitted line, with no scatter at all.

>> An r^2 value of 0 means that your data points are all over the place, with no tendency at all for the X and Y variables to be associated.

>> An r^2 value of 0.3 (as in this example) means that 30 percent of the variance in the dependent variable is explainable by the independent variable in this straight-line model.

Note: Figure 18-4 also lists the *Adjusted R-squared* at the bottom right. We talk about the adjusted r^2 value in Chapter 17 when we explain multiple regression, so for now, you can just ignore it.

The F statistic

The last line of the sample output in Figure 17-4 presents the F statistic and associated p value (under *F-statistic*). These estimates address this question: Is the straight-line model any good at all? In other words, how much better is the straight-line model, which contains an intercept and a predictor variable, at predicting the outcome compared to the *null model?*

REMEMBER

The *null model* is a model that contains only a single parameter representing a constant term with no predictor variables at all. In this case, the null model would only include the intercept.

Under $\alpha = 0.05$, if the p value associated with the F statistic is less than 0.05, then adding the predictor variable to the model makes it statistically significantly better at predicting SBP than the null model.

For this example, the p value of the F statistic is 0.013, which is statistically significant. It means using weight as a predictor of SBP is statistically significantly better than just guessing that everyone in the data set has the mean SBP (which is how the null model is compared).

Scientific fortune-telling with the prediction formula

As we describe in Chapter 15, one reason to do regression in biostatistics is to develop a prediction formula that allows you to make an educated guess about value of a dependent variable if you know the values of the independent variables. You are essentially developing a *predictive model.*

TIP

Some statistics programs show the actual equation of the best-fitting straight line. If yours doesn't, don't worry. Just substitute the coefficients of the intercept and slope for a and b in the straight-line equation: $Y = a + bX$.

With the output shown in Figure 16-4, where the intercept (*a*) is 76.9 and the slope (*b*) is 0.487, you can write the equation of the fitted straight line like this: SBP = 76.9 + 0.487 Weight.

Then you can use this equation to predict someone's SBP if you know their weight. So, if a person weighs 100 kilograms, you can estimate that that person's SBP will be around 76.9 + 100 × 0.487, which is 76.9 + 48.7, or about 125.6 mmHg. Your prediction probably won't be exactly on the nose, but it should be better than not using a predictive model and just guessing.

How far off will your prediction be? The residual SE provides a unit of measurement to answer this question. As we explain in the earlier section "Summary statistics for the residuals," the residual SE indicates how much the individual points tend to scatter above and below the fitted line. For the SBP example, this number is ± 9.8, so you can expect your prediction to be within about ± 10 mmHg most of the time.

Recognizing What Can Go Wrong with Straight-Line Regression

Fitting a straight line to a set of data is a relatively simple task, but you still have to be careful. A computer program does whatever you tell it to, even if it's something you shouldn't do.

WARNING

Those new to straight-line regression may slip up in the following ways:

>> **Fitting a straight line to curved data:** Examining the pattern of residuals in the residuals versus fitted chart in Figure 16-5 can let you know if you have this problem.

>> **Ignoring outliers in the data:** Outliers — especially those in the corners of a scatterplot like the one in Figure 16-3 — can mess up all the classical statistical analyses, and regression is no exception. One or two data points that are way off the main trend of the points will drag the fitted line away from the other points. That's because the strength with which each point tugs at the fitted line is proportionate to the square of its distance from the line, and outliers have a lot of distance, so they have a strong influence.

REMEMBER

Always look at a scatter plot of your data to make sure outliers aren't present. Examine the residuals to ensure they are distributed normally above and below the fitted line.

Calculating the Sample Size You Need

To estimate how many data points you need for a regression analysis, you need to first ask yourself why you're doing the regression in the first place.

>> **Do you want to show that the two variables are statistically significantly associated?** If so, you want to calculate the sample size required to achieve a certain statistical *power* for the significance test (see Chapter 3 for an introduction to statistical power).

>> **Do you want to estimate the value of the slope (or intercept) to within a certain margin of error?** If so, you want to calculate the sample size required to achieve a certain *precision* in your estimate.

Testing the statistical significance of a slope is exactly equivalent to testing the statistical significance of a correlation coefficient, so the sample-size calculations are also the same for the two types of tests. If you haven't already, check out Chapter 15, which contains guidance and formulas to estimate how many participants you need to test for any specified degree of correlation.

If you're using regression to estimate the value of a regression coefficient — for example, the slope of the straight line — then the sample-size calculations become more complicated. The precision of the slope depends on several factors:

>> **The number of data points:** More data points give you greater precision. SEs vary inversely with the square root of the sample size. Alternatively, the required sample size varies inversely with the square of the desired SE. So, if you quadruple the sample size, you cut the SE in half. This is a very important and generally applicable principle.

>> **Tightness of the fit of the observed points to the line:** The closer the data points hug the line, the more precisely you can estimate the regression coefficients. The effect is directly proportional, in that twice as much *Y*-scatter of the points produces twice as large a SE in the coefficients.

>> **How the data points are distributed across the range of the *X* variable:** This effect is hard to quantify, but in general, having the data points spread out evenly over the entire range of *X* produces more precision than having most of them clustered near the middle of the range.

Given these factors, how do you strategically design a study and gather data for a linear regression where you're mainly interested in estimating a regression coefficient to within a certain precision? One practical approach is to first conduct a study that is small and underpowered, called a *pilot study,* to estimate the SE of the regression coefficient. Imagine you enroll 20 participants and measure them, then create a regression model. If you're really lucky, the SE may be as small as you wanted, or even smaller, so you know if you conduct a larger study, you will have enough sample.

TIP

But the SE from a pilot study usually isn't small enough (unless you're a lot luckier that we've ever been). That's when you can reach for the square-root law as a remedy! Follow these steps to calculate the total sample size you need to get the precision you want:

1. **Divide the SE that you *got* from your pilot study by the SE you *want* your full study to achieve.**

2. **Take the square of this ratio.**

3. **Multiply the square of the ratio by the sample size of your pilot study.**

Imagine that you want to estimate the slope to a precision or SE of ±5. If a pilot study of 20 participants gives you a SE of ±8.4 units, then the ratio is 8.4 / 5, which is 1.68. Squaring this ratio gives you 2.82, which tells you that to get an SE of 5, you need 2.82 × 20, or about 56 participants. And because we assume you took our advice, we'll assume you've already recruited the first 20 participants for your pilot study. Now, you only have to recruit only another 36 participants to have a total of 56.

REMEMBER

Admittedly, this estimation is only approximate. But it does give you at least a ballpark idea of how big your sample size needs to be to achieve the desired precision.

Chapter **17**

More of a Good Thing: Multiple Regression

hapter 15 introduces the general concepts of *correlation* and *regression*, two related techniques for detecting and characterizing the relationship between two or more variables. Chapter 16 describes the simplest kind of regression — fitting a straight line to a set of data consisting of one independent variable (the *predictor*) and one dependent variable (the *outcome*). The formula relating the predictor to the outcome, known as the *model*, is of the form $Y = a + bX$, where Y is the outcome, X is the predictor, and a and b are *parameters* (also called regression coefficients). This kind of regression is usually the only one you encounter in an introductory statistics course, because it is a relatively simple way to do a regression. It's good for beginners to learn!

This chapter extends simple straight-line regression to more than one predictor — to what's called the *ordinary multiple linear regression* model, or more simply, *multiple regression*.

Understanding the Basics of Multiple Regression

In Chapter 16, we outline the derivation of the formulas for determining the parameters of a straight line so that the line — defined by an intercept at the Y axis and a slope — comes as close as possible to all the data points (imagine a scatter plot). The term *as close as possible* is operationalized as a *least-squares line*, meaning we are looking for the line where the sum of the squares (SSQ) of vertical distances of each point from to the line is the smallest. SSQ for a fitted line is smallest for the least-squares line than for any other line you could possibly draw.

The same idea can be extended to multiple regression models containing more than one predictor (which estimates more than two parameters). For two predictor variables, you're fitting a *plane*, which is a flat sheet. Imagine fitting a set of points to this plane in three dimensions (meaning you'd be adding a Z axis to your X and Y). Now, extend your imagination. For more than two predictors, in regression, you're fitting a *hyperplane* to points in four-or-more-dimensional space. Hyperplanes in multidimensional space may sound mind-blowing, but luckily for us, the actual formulas are simple algebraic extensions of the straight-line formulas.

In the following sections, we define some basic terms related to multiple regression, and explain when you should use it.

Defining a few important terms

REMEMBER

Multiple regression is formally known as the *ordinary multiple linear regression model*. What a mouthful! Here's what the terms mean:

>> **Ordinary:** The outcome variable is a continuous numerical variable whose random fluctuations are normally distributed (see Chapter 24 for more about normal distributions).

>> **Multiple:** The model has more than two predictor variables.

>> **Linear:** Each predictor variable is multiplied by a parameter, and these products are added together to estimate the predicted value of the outcome variable. You can also have one more parameter thrown in that isn't multiplied by anything — it's called the *constant term* or the *Intercept*. The following are examples of linear functions used in regression:

- $Y = a + bX$ (This is the straight-line model from Chapter 16, where X is the predictor variable, Y is the outcome, and a and b are parameters.)

- $Y = a + bX + cX^2 + dX^3$ (In this multiple regression model, variables can be squared or cubed. But as long as they're multiplied by a coefficient — which is a slope from the model — and the products are added together, the function is still considered linear in the parameters.)

- $Y = a + bX + cZ + dXZ$ (This multiple regression model is special because of the XZ term, which can be written as $X * Z$, and is called an *interaction*. It is where you multiple two predictors together to create a new interaction term in the model.)

In textbooks and published articles, you may see regression models written in various ways:

>> A collection of predictor variables may be designated by a subscripted variable and the corresponding coefficients by another subscripted variable, like this: $Y = b_0 + b_1X_1 + b_2X_2$.

>> In practical research work, the variables are often given meaningful names, like *Age, Gender, Height, Weight, Glucose,* and so on.

>> Linear models may be represented in a shorthand notation that shows only the variables, and not the parameters, like this: $Y = X + Z + X * Z$ instead of $Y = a + bX + cZ + dX * Z$ or $Y = 0 + X + Z + X * Z$ to specify that the model has no intercept. And sometimes you'll see a "~" instead of the "=". If you do, read the "~" as "is a function of," or "is predicted by."

Being aware of how the calculations work

Fitting a linear multiple regression model essentially involves creating a set of simultaneous equations, one for each parameter in the model. The equations involve the parameters from the model and the sums of various products of the dependent and independent variables. This is also true of the simultaneous equations for the straight-line regression in Chapter 16, which involve estimating the slope and intercept of the straight line and the sums of X, Y, X^2, and XY. Your statistical software solves these simultaneous equations to obtain the parameter values, just as is done in straight-line regression, except now, there are more equations to solve. In multiple as in straight-line regression, you can also get the information you need to estimate the standard errors (SEs) of the parameters.

Executing a Multiple Regression Analysis in Software

Before executing your multiple regression analysis, you may need to do some prep work on the variables you intend to include in your model. In the following sections, we explain how to handle the categorical variables you plan to include. We show you how to examine these variables through making several charts before you run your analysis. If you need guidance on what variables to consider for your models, read Chapter 20.

Preparing categorical variables

The predictors in a multiple regression model can be either numerical or categorical (Chapter 8 discusses the different types of data). In a categorical variable, each category is called a *level*. If a variable, like *Setting*, can have only two levels, like *Inpatient* or *Outpatient*, then it's called a *dichotomous* or a *binary* categorical variable. If it can have more than two levels, it is called a *multilevel* variable.

Figuring out the best way to introduce categorical predictors into a multiple regression model is always challenging. You have to set up your data the right way, or you'll get results that are either wrong, or difficult to interpret properly. Following are two important factors to consider.

Having enough participants in each level of each categorical variable

Before using a categorical variable in a multiple regression model, you should tabulate how many participants (or rows) are included in each level. If you have any sparse levels — row frequencies in the single digits — you will want to consider collapsing them into others. Usually, the more evenly distributed the number of rows are across all the levels, and the fewer levels there are, the more precise and reliable the results. If a level doesn't contain enough rows, the program may ignore that level, halt with a warning message, produce incorrect results, or crash. Worse, if it produces results, they will be impossible to interpret.

Imagine that you create a one-way frequency table of a Primary Diagnosis variable from a sample of study participant data. Your results are: Hypertension: 73, Diabetes: 35, Cancer: 1, and Other: 10. To deal with the sparse Cancer variable, you may want to create another variable in which Cancer is collapsed together with Other (which would then have 11 rows). Another approach is to create a binary variable with yes/no levels, such as: Hypertension: 73 and No Hypertension: 46. But binary variables don't take into account the other levels. You could also make a binary Diabetes variable, where 35 were coded as *yes* and the rest were *no*, and so on for Cancer and Other.

Similarly, if your model has two categorical variables with an *interaction term* (like Setting + Primary Diagnosis + Setting * Primary Diagnosis), you should prepare a two-way cross-tabulation of the two variables first (in our example, Setting by Primary Diagnosis). You will observe that you are limited by having to ensure that you have enough rows in each cell of the table to run your analysis. See Chapter 12 for details about cross-tabulations.

Choosing the reference level wisely

For each categorical variable in a multiple regression model, the program considers one of the categories to be the *reference level* and evaluates how each of the other levels affects the outcome, relative to that reference level. Statistical software lets you specify the reference level for a categorical variable, but you can also let the software choose it for you. The problem is that the software uses some arbitrary algorithm to make that choice (such as whatever level sorts alphabetically as first), and usually chooses one you don't want. Therefore, it is better if you instruct the software on the reference level to use for all categorical variables. For specific advice on choosing an appropriate reference level, read the next section, "Recoding categorical variables as numerical."

Recoding categorical variables as numerical

Data may be stored as character variables — meaning the variable for primary diagnosis (*PrimaryDx*) may be contain character data, such as *Hypertension, Diabetes, Cancer,* and *Other.* Because it is difficult for statistical programs to work with character data, these variables are usually recoded with a numerical code before being used in a regression. This means a new variable is created, and is coded as 1 for hypertension, 2 for diabetes, 3 for cancer, and so on.

TIP

It is best to code binary variables as 0 for not having the attribute or state, and 1 for having the attribute or state. So a binary variable named *Cancer* should be coded as *Cancer = 1* if the participant has cancer, and *Cancer = 0* if they do not.

For categorical variables with more than two levels, it's more complicated. Even if you recode the categorical variable from containing characters to a numeric code, this code cannot be used in regression unless we want to model the category as an ordinal variable. Imagine a variable coded as 1 = graduated high school, 2 = graduated college, and 3 = obtained post-graduate degree. If this variable was entered as a predictor in regression, it assumes equal steps going from code 1 to code 2, and from code 2 to code 3. Anyone who has applied to college or gone to graduate school knows these steps are not equal! To solve this problem, you could select one level for the reference group (let's choose 3), and then create two binary *indicator variables* for the other two levels — meaning one for 1 = graduated high school and 2 = graduated college. Here's another example of coding multilevel categorical variables as a set of indicator variables, where each level is assigned its own binary variable that is coded 1 if the level applies to the row, and 0 if it does not (see Table 17-1).

TABLE 17-1   **Coding a Multilevel Category into a Set of Binary Indicator Variables**

StudyID	PrimaryDx	HTN	Diab	Cancer	OtherDx
1	Hypertension	1	0	0	0
2	Diabetes	0	1	0	0
3	Cancer	0	0	1	0
4	Other	0	0	0	1
5	Diabetes	0	1	0	0

Table 17-1 shows theoretical coding for a data set containing the variables *StudyID* (for participant ID) and *PrimaryDx* (for participant primary diagnosis). As shown in Table 17-1, you take each level and make an indicator variable for it: Hypertension is *HTN*, diabetes is *Diab,* cancer is *Cancer,* and other is *OtherDx.* Instead of including the variable *PrimaryDx* in the model, you'd include the indicator variables for all levels of *PrimaryDx except* the reference level. So, if the reference level you selected for *PrimaryDx* was hypertension, you'd include *Diab, Cancer,* and *OtherDx* in the regression, but would *not* include *HTN.* To contrast this to the education example, in the set of variables in Table 17-1, participants can have a 1 for one or more indicator variables or just be in the reference group. However, with the education example, they can only be coded at one level, or be in the reference group.

REMEMBER

Don't forget to leave the reference-level indicator variable out of the regression, or your model will break!

Creating scatter charts before you jump into multiple regression analysis

One common mistake researchers make is immediately running a regression or another advanced statistical analysis before thoroughly examining their data. As soon as your data are available in electronic format, you should run error-checks, and generate summaries and histograms for each variable you plan to use in your regression. You need to assess the way the values of the variables are distributed as we describe in Chapter 11. And if you plan to analyze your data using multiple regression, you need special preparation. Namely, you should chart the relationship between each predictor variable and the outcome variable, and also the relationships *between the predictor variables themselves.*

Imagine that you are interested in whether the outcome of systolic blood pressure (SBP) can be predicted by age, body weight, or both. Table 17-2 shows a small data file with variables that could address this research question that we use throughout the remainder of this chapter. It contains the age, weight, and SBP of 16 study participants from a clinical population.

TABLE 17-2 **Sample Age, Weight, and Systolic Blood Pressure Data for a Multiple Regression Analysis**

Participant ID	Age (years)	Weight (kg)	SBP (mmHg)
1	60	58	117
2	61	90	120
3	74	96	145
4	57	72	129
5	63	62	132
6	68	79	130
7	66	69	110
8	77	96	163
9	63	96	136
10	54	54	115
11	63	67	118
12	76	99	132
13	60	74	111
14	61	73	112
15	65	85	147
16	79	80	138

Looking at Table 17-2, let's assume that your variable names are *StudyID* for Participant ID, *Age* for age, *Weight* for weight, and *SBP* for SBP. Imagine that you're planning to run a regression model with this formula (using the shorthand notation described in the earlier section "Defining a few important terms"): SBP ~ Age + Weight. In this case, you should first prepare several scatter charts: one of *SBP* (outcome) versus *Age* (predictor), one of *SBP* versus *Weight* (another outcome versus predictor), and one of *Age* versus *Weight* (both predictors). For regression models involving many predictors, there can be a lot of scatter charts! Fortunately, many statistics programs can automatically prepare a set of small *thumbnail* scatter charts for all possible pairings among a set of variables, arranged in a matrix as shown in Figure 17-1.

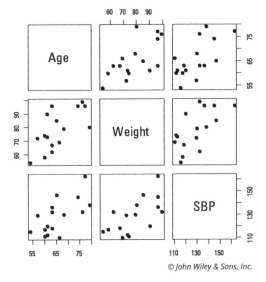

FIGURE 17-1:
A scatter chart matrix for a set of variables prior to multiple regression.

These charts can give you insight into which variables are associated with each other, how strongly they're associated, and their direction of association. They also show whether your data have outliers. The scatter charts in Figure 17-1 indicate that there are no extreme outliers in the data. Each scatter chart also shows some degree of positive correlation (as described in Chapter 15). In fact, if you refer to Figure 17-1, you may guess that the charts in Figure 17-1 correspond to correlation coefficients between 0.5 and 0.8. In addition to the scatter charts, you can also have your software calculate correlation coefficients (r values) between each pair of variables. For this example, here are the results: $r = 0.654$ for *Age* versus *Weight*, $r = 0.661$ for *Age* versus *SBP*, and $r = 0.646$ for *Weight* versus *SBP*.

Taking a few steps with your software

The exact steps you take to run a multiple regression depend on your software, but here's the general approach:

1. **Assemble your data into a file with one row per participant and one column for each variable you want in the model.**

2. **Tell the software which variable is the outcome and which are the predictors.**

3. **Specify whatever optional output you want from the software, which could include graphs, summaries of the *residuals* (observed minus predicted outcome values), and other useful results.**

4. **Execute the regression (run or submit the code).**

   Now, you should retrieve the output, and look for the optional output you requested.

Interpreting the Output of a Multiple Regression Analysis

The output from a multiple regression run is formatted like the output from the straight-line regression described in Chapter 16.

Examining typical multiple regression output

Figure 17-2 shows the output from a multiple regression analysis on the data in Table 17-2, using R statistical software as described in Chapter 4. Other statistical software produces similar output, but the results are arranged and formatted differently.

Here we describe the components of the output in Figure 17-2:

>> **Code:** The first line starting with *Call:* reflects back the code run to execute the regression, which contains the linear model using variable names: SBP ~ Age + Weight.

```
Call: lm(formula = SBP ~ Age + Weight )

Residuals:
     Min      1Q   Median      3Q      Max
 -15.3596  -9.6585   0.0242   6.7305  17.8369

Coefficients:
            Estimate Std. Error t value Pr(>|t|)
(Intercept)  42.7498    25.7325   1.661    0.121
Age           0.8446     0.5163   1.636    0.126
Weight        0.3894     0.2659   1.464    0.167

Residual standard error: 11.23 on 13 degrees of freedom
Multiple R-squared: 0.5171,     Adjusted R-squared: 0.4428
F-statistic: 6.959 on 2 and 13 DF,   p-value: 0.008817
```

FIGURE 17-2: Output from multiple regression using the data from Table 17-2.

>> **Residual information:** As a reminder, the residuals are the observed outcome values minus predicted values coming from the model. Under *Residuals*, the minimum, first quartile, median, third quartile and maximum are listed (under the headings *Min, IQ, Median, 3Q*, and *Max*, respectively). The maximum and minimum indicate that one observed SBP value was 17.8 mmHg greater than predicted by the model, and one was 15.4 mmHg smaller than predicted.

>> **Regression or coefficients table:** This is presented under *Coefficients:*, and includes a row for each parameter in the model. It also includes columns for the following:

● **Estimate:** The estimated *value* of the parameter, which tells you how much the outcome variable changes when the corresponding variable increases by exactly 1.0 unit, *holding all the other variables constant.* For example, the model predicts that if all participants have the same weight, every additional year of age is associated with an increase in SBP of 0.84 mmHg.

● **Standard error:** The standard error (SE) is the precision of the estimate, and is in the column labeled *Std. Error*. The SE for the *Age* coefficient is ± 0.52 mmHg per year, indicating the level of uncertainty around the 0.84 mmHg estimate.

● **t value:** The t value (which is labeled *t value*) is the value of the parameter divided by its SE. For *Age*, the t value is $0.8446 / 0.5163$, or 1.636.

● **p value:** The p value is designated *Pr(>|t|)* in this output. The p value indicates whether the parameter is statistically significantly different from zero at your chosen α level (let's assume 0.05). If $p < 0.05$, then the predictor variable is statistically significantly associated with the outcome after controlling for the effects of all the other predictors in the model. In this example, neither the *Age* coefficient (p = 0.126) nor the *Weight* coefficient (p = 0.167) is statistically significantly different from zero.

» **Model fit statistics:** These are calculations that describe how well the model fits your data overall.

- **Residual standard error**: In this example, the *Residual standard error:* (bottom of output) indicates that the observed-minus-predicted residuals have a standard deviation of 11.23 mmHg.

- **Multiple r^2:** This refers to the square of an overall correlation coefficient for the multivariate fit of the model, and is listed under *Multiple R-squared*.

- **F statistic:** The F statistic and associated p value (on the last line of the output) indicate whether the model predicts the outcome statistically significantly better than a *null model*. A *null model* contains only the intercept term and no predictor variables at all. The very low p value (0.0088) indicates that age and weight together predict SBP statistically significantly better than the null model.

Checking out optional output to request

Depending on your software, you may also be able to request several other useful calculations from the regression to be included:

» **Predicted values** for the dependent variable for each participant. This can be output either as a listing, or as a new variable placed into your data file.

» **Residuals** (observed minus predicted value) for each participant. Again, this can be output either as a listing, or as a new variable placed into your data file.

Deciding whether your data are suitable for regression analysis

REMEMBER

Before drawing conclusions from any statistical analysis, you need to make sure that your data fulfill assumptions on which that analysis was based. Two assumptions of ordinary linear regression include the following:

» The amount of variability in the residuals is fairly constant, and not dependent on the value of the dependent variable.

» The residuals are approximately normally distributed.

Figure 17-3 shows two graphs you can optionally request that help you determine or *diagnose* whether these assumptions are met, so they are called *diagnostic graphs* (or *plots*).

» Figure 17-3a provides an indication of *variability* of the residuals. To interpret this plot, visually evaluate whether the points seem to scatter evenly above and below the line, and whether the amount of scatter seems to be the same across the left, middle, and right parts of the graph. That seems to be the case in this figure.

» Figure 17-3b provides an indication of the *normality* of the residuals. To interpret this plot, visually evaluate whether the points appear to lie along the dotted line or are noticeably following a curve. In this figure, the points are consistent with a straight line except in the very lower-left part of the graph.

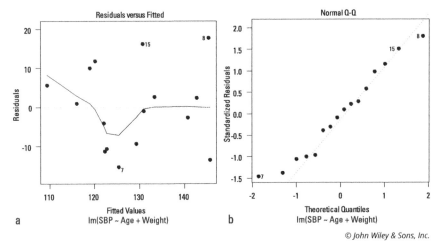

FIGURE 17-3: Diagnostic graphs from a regression.

© John Wiley & Sons, Inc.

Determining how well the model fits the data

Several calculations in standard regression output indicate how closely the model fits your data:

» The residual SE is the average scatter of the observed points from the fitted model. You want them to be close to the line. As shown in Figure 17-2, the residual SE is about ± 11 mmHg.

>> The multiple $r2$ value represents the amount of variability in the dependent variable explained by the model, so you want it to be high. As shown in Figure 17-2, it is 0.52 in this example, indicating a moderately good fit.

>> A statistically significant F statistic indicates that the model predicts the outcome significantly better than the null model. As shown in Figure 17-2, the p value on the F statistic is 0.009, which is statistically significant at $\alpha = 0.05$.

Figure 17-4 shows another way to judge how well the model predicts the outcome. It's a graph of observed and predicted values of the outcome variable, with a superimposed *identity line* (Observed = Predicted). Your program may offer this *observed versus predicted* graph, or you can generate it from the observed and predicted values of the dependent variable. For a perfect prediction model, the points would lie exactly on the identity line. The correlation coefficient of these points is the multiple r value for the regression.

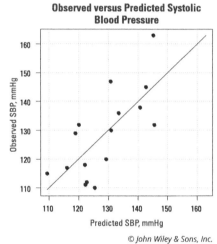

FIGURE 17-4: Observed versus predicted outcomes for the model SBP ~ Age + Weight, for the data in Table 17-2.

© John Wiley & Sons, Inc.

Watching Out for Special Situations that Arise in Multiple Regression

Here we describe two topics that come up in multiple regression: interactions (both synergistic and anti-synergistic), and collinearity. Both relate to how the simultaneous behavior of two predictors can influence an outcome.

Synergy and anti-synergy

Sometimes, two predictor variables exert a *synergistic effect* on an outcome. That is, if both predictors were to be associated with an increase in the outcome by one unit, the outcome would change by *more* than the sum of the two increases, which is what you'd expect from changing each value individually by one unit. You can test for synergy between two predictors with respect to an outcome by fitting a model that contains an *interaction term*, which is the product of those two variables. In this equation, we predict SBP using Age and Weight, and include an interaction term for Age and Weight:

$$SBP = Age + Weight + Age * Weight$$

If the estimate of the slope for the interaction term has a statistically significant p value, then the null hypothesis of *no interaction* is rejected, and the two variables are interpreted to have a significant interaction. If the sign on the interaction term is positive, it is a *synergistic* interaction, and if it is negative, it is called an *anti-synergistic* or *antagonistic* interaction.

WARNING

Introducing interaction terms into a fitted model and interpreting their significance — both clinically and statistically — must be done contextually. Interaction terms may not be appropriate for certain models, and may be required in others.

Collinearity and the mystery of the disappearing significance

When developing multiple regression models, you are usually considering more predictors than just two as we used in our example. You develop *iterative* models, meaning models with the same outcome variable, but different groups of predictors. You also use some sort of strategy in choosing the order in which you introduce the predictors into the iterative models, which is described in Chapter 20. So imagine that you used our example data set and — in one iteration — ran a model to predict *SBP* with *Age* and other predictors in it, and the coefficient for *Age* was statistically significant. Now, imagine you added *Weight* to that model, and in the new model, *Age* was no longer statistically significant! You've just been visited by the *collinearity* fairy.

In the example from Table 17-2, there's a statistically significant positive correlation between each predictor and the outcome. We figured this out when running the correlations for Figure 17-1, but you could check our work by using the data in Figure 17-2 in a straight-line regression, as described in Chapter 16. In contrast, the multiple regression output in Figure 17-2 shows that neither *Age* nor *Weight* are statistically significant in the model, meaning neither has regression coefficients that are statistically significantly different from zero! Why are they associated with the outcome in correlation but not multiple regression analysis?

The answer is collinearity. In the regression world, the term *collinearity* (also called *multicollinearity*) refers to a strong correlation between two or more of the predictor variables. If you run a correlation between *Age* and *Weight* (the two predictors), you'll find that they're statistically significantly correlated with each other. It is this situation that destroys your statistically significant p value seen on some predictors in iterative models when doing multiple regression.

The problem with collinearity is that you cannot tell which of the two predictor variables is actually influencing the outcome more, because they are fighting over explaining the variability in the dependent variable. Although models with collinearity are valid, they are hard to interpret if you are looking for cause-and-effect relationships, meaning you are doing *causal inference*. Chapter 20 provides philosophical guidance on dealing with collinearity in modeling.

Calculating How Many Participants You Need

REMEMBER

Studies should target enrolling a large enough sample size to ensure that you get a statistically significant result for your primary research hypothesis in the case that the effect you're testing in that hypothesis is large enough to be of clinical importance. So if the main hypothesis of your study is going to be tested by a multiple regression analysis, you should theoretically do a calculation to determine the sample size you need to support that analysis.

Unfortunately, that is not possible in practice, because the equations would be too complicated. Instead, considerations are aimed more toward being able to gather enough data to support a planned regression model. Imagine that you plan to gather data about a categorical variable where you believe only 5 percent of the participants will fall in a particular level. If you are concerned about including that level in your regression analysis, you would want to greatly increase your estimate for target sample size. Although regression models tend to *converge* in software if they include at least 100 rows, that may not be true depending upon the number and distribution of the values in the predictor variables and the outcome. It is best to use experience from similar studies to help you develop a target sample size and analytic plan for a multiple regression analysis.

Chapter **18**

A Yes-or-No Proposition: Logistic Regression

You can use logistic regression to analyze the relationship between one or more predictor variables (the X variables) and a categorical outcome variable (the Y variable). Typical categorical outcomes include the following two-level variables (which are also called *binary* or *dichotomous*):

» Lived or died by a certain date

» Did or didn't get diagnosed with Type II diabetes

» Responded or didn't respond to a treatment

» Did or did not choose a particular health insurance plan

In this chapter, we explain logistic regression. We describe the circumstances under which to use it, the important related concepts, how to execute it with software, and how to interpret the output. We also point out the pitfalls with logistic regression and show you how to determine the sample sizes you need to execute such a model.

Using Logistic Regression

Following are typical uses of logistic regression analysis:

>> To test whether one or more predictors and an outcome are statistically significantly associated. For example, to test whether age and/or obesity status are associated with increased likelihood to be diagnosed with Type II diabetes.

>> To overcome the limitations of the 2x2 cross-tab method (described in Chapter 12), which can analyze only one predictor at a time (and the predictor has to be binary). With logistic regression, you can analyze multiple predictor variables at a time. Each predictor can be a numeric variable or a categorical variable having two or more levels.

>> To quantify the *extent* or *magnitude* of an association between a particular predictor and an outcome that have been established to have an association. In other words, you are seeking to quantify the amount by which a specific predictor influences the chance of getting the outcome. As an example, you could quantify the amount obesity plays a role in the likelihood of a person being diagnosed with Type II diabetes.

>> To develop a formula to predict the probability of getting an outcome based on the values of the predictor variables. For example, you may want to predict the probability that a person will be diagnosed with Type II diabetes based on the person's age, gender, obesity status, exercise status, and medical history.

>> To make *yes* or *no* predictions about the outcome that take into account the consequences of false-positive and false-negative predictions. For example, you can generate a tentative cancer diagnosis from a set of observations and lab results using a formula that balances the different consequences of a false-positive versus a false-negative diagnosis.

>> To see how one predictor influences the outcome after adjusting for the influence of other variables. One example is to see how the number of minutes of exercise per day influences the chance of having a heart attack after controlling for the for the effects of age, gender, lipid levels, and other patient characteristics that could influence the outcome.

>> To determine the value of a predictor that produces a certain probability of getting the outcome. For example, you could determine the dose of a drug that produces a favorable clinical response in 80 percent of the patients treated with it, which is called the ED_{80}, or *80 percent effective dose*.

Understanding the Basics of Logistic Regression

In this section, we explain the concepts underlying logistic regression using an example from a fictitious animal study involving data on mortality due to radiation exposure. This example illustrates why straight-line regression wouldn't work and why you have to use logistic regression instead.

Gathering and graphing your data

As in the other chapters in Part 5, we present a real-world problem here. This example examines the lethality of exposure to gamma-ray radiation when given in acute, large doses. It is already known that gamma-ray radiation is deadly in large-enough doses, so this animal study is focused only at the short-term lethality of acute large doses. Table 18-1 presents data on 30 animals in two columns.

TABLE 18-1   **Radiation Dose and Survival Data for 30 Animals, Sorted Ascending by Dose Level**

Dose in REMs	Outcome (*0 = Lived; 1 = Died*)	Dose in REMS	Outcome (*0 = Lived; 1 = Died*)
0	0	433	0
10	0	457	1
31	0	559	1
82	0	560	1
92	0	604	1
107	0	632	0
142	0	686	1
173	0	691	1
175	0	702	1
232	0	705	1
266	0	774	1
299	0	853	1
303	1	879	1
326	0	915	1
404	1	977	1

In Table 18-1, *dose* is the radiation exposure expressed in units called *Roentgen Equivalent Man (REM)*. Because Table 18-1 is sorted ascending by dose, by looking at the *Dose* and *Outcome* columns, you can get a rough sense of how survival depends on dose. At low levels of radiation, almost all animals live, and at high doses, almost all animals die.

How can you analyze these data with logistic regression? First, make a scatter plot (see Chapter 16) with the predictor — the dose — on the *X* axis, and the outcome of death on the *Y* axis, as shown in Figure 18-1a.

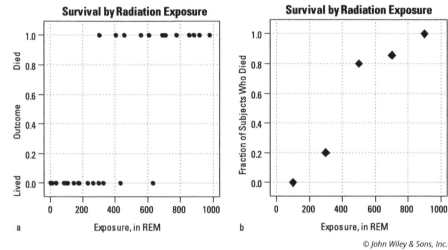

FIGURE 18-1: Dose versus mortality from Table 18-1: each individual's data (a) and grouped (b).

© John Wiley & Sons, Inc.

In Figure 18-1a, because the outcome variable is binary, the points are restricted to two horizontal lines, making the graph difficult to interpret. You can get a better picture of the dose-lethality relationship by grouping the doses into intervals. In Figure 18-1b, we grouped the intervals into 200 REM classes (see Chapter 9), and plotted the fraction of individuals in each interval who died. Clearly, Figure 18-1b shows the chance of dying increases with increasing dose.

Fitting a function with an S shape to your data

WARNING

Don't try to fit a straight line if you have a binary outcome variable because the relationship is almost certainly not a straight line. For one thing, the fraction of individuals who are positive for the outcome can never be smaller than 0 nor larger than 1. In contrast, a straight line, a parabola, or any polynomial distribution would very happily violate those limits at extreme doses, which is obviously illogical.

If you have a binary outcome, you need to fit a function that has an S shape. The formula calculating Y must be an expression involving X that — by design — can never produce a Y value outside of the range from 0 to 1, no matter how large or small X may become.

REMEMBER

Of the many mathematical expressions that produce S-shaped graphs, the *logistic* function is ideally suited to this kind of data. In its simplest form, the logistic function is written like this: $Y = 1/\left(1 + e^{-X}\right)$, where e is the mathematical constant 2.718, known as a natural logarithm (see Chapter 2). We will use e to represent this number for the rest of the chapter. Figure 18-2a shows the shape of the logistic function.

The logistic function shown in Figure 18-2 can be made more versatile for representing observed data by being *generalized*. The logistic function is generalized by adding two adjustable parameters named a and b like this: $Y = 1/\left(1 + e^{-(a+bX)}\right)$.

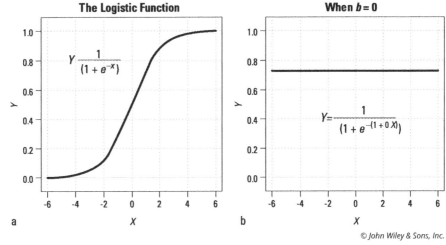

FIGURE 18-2:
The first graph (a) shows the shape of the logistic function. The second graph (b) shows that when b is 0, the logistic function becomes a horizontal straight line.

© John Wiley & Sons, Inc.

Notice that the $a + bX$ part looks just like the formula for a straight line (see Chapter 16). It's the rest of the logistic function that bends the straight line into its characteristic S shape. The middle of the S (where $Y = 0.5$) always occurs when $X = -b/a$. The steepness of the curve in the middle region is determined by b, as follows:

>> **If *b* is positive,** the logistic function is an upward-sloping S-shaped curve, like the one shown in Figure 18-2a.

>> **If _b_ is 0,** the logistic function is a horizontal straight line whose _Y_ value is equal to $1/(1 + e^a)$, as shown in Figure 18-2b.

>> **If _b_ is negative,** the curve is flipped upside down, as shown in Figure 18-3a. Notice that this is a mirror image of Figure 18-2a.

>> **If _b_ is a very large number, either positive or negative,** the logistic curve becomes so steep that it looks like what mathematicians call a _step function,_ as shown in Figure 18-3b.

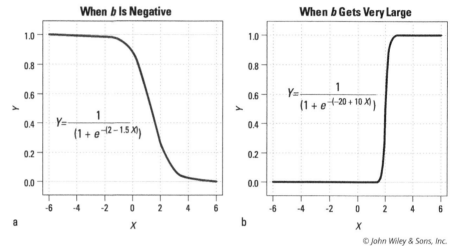

FIGURE 18-3: The first graph (a) shows that when b is negative, the logistic function slopes downward. The second graph (b) shows that when b is very large, the logistic function becomes a "step function."

© John Wiley & Sons, Inc.

WARNING

Because the logistic curve approaches the limits 0.0 and 1.0 for extreme values of the predictor(s), you should not use logistic regression in situations where the fraction of individuals positive for the outcome does not approach these two limits. Logistic regression is appropriate for the radiation example because none of the individuals died at a radiation exposure of zero REMs, and all of the individuals died at doses of 686 REMs and higher. If we imagine a study of patients with a disease where the outcome is a cure, if taking a drug in very high doses would not always cause a 100 percent cure, and the disease could resolve on its own without any drug, the data would not be appropriate. This is because some patients with high doses would still have an outcome value of 0, and some patients at zero dose would have an outcome value of 1.

REMEMBER

Logistic regression fits the logistic model to your data by finding the values of _a_ and _b_ that make the logistic curve come as close as possible to all your plotted points. With this fitted model, you can then predict the probability of the outcome. See the later section "Predicting probabilities with the fitted logistic formula" for more details.

GETTING INTO THE NITTY-GRITTY OF LOGISTIC REGRESSION

You don't need to know all the theoretical and computation details for logistic regression because the software will do them for you. However, you should have a general idea of what it is doing behind the scenes. The calculations are much more complicated than those for ordinary straight-line or multivariate least-squares regression. In fact, it's impossible to write down a set of formulas that give the logistic regression coefficients in terms of the observed X and Y values. The only way to obtain them is through a complex iterative procedure that would not be practical to do manually.

Logistic regression determines the values of the regression coefficients that are most consistent with the observed data using what's called the *maximum likelihood* criterion. The likelihood of any statistical model is the probability (based on the model) of obtaining the values you observed in your data. There's a likelihood value for each row in the data set, and a total likelihood (L) for the entire data set. The likelihood value for each data point is the predicted probability of getting the observed outcome result. For individuals who died (refer to Table 18-1), the likelihood is the probability of dying (Y) predicted by the logistic formula. For individuals who survived, the likelihood is the predicted probability of not dying, which is $(1 - Y)$. The total likelihood (L) for the whole set of individuals is the product of all the calculated likelihoods for each individual.

To find the values of the coefficients that maximize L, it is most practical to find the values that minimize the quantity *2 multiplied by the natural logarithm of L*, which also called the *–2 log likelihood* and abbreviated *–2LL*. Statisticians also call *–2LL* the *deviance*. The closer the curve designated by the regression formula comes to the observed points, the smaller this deviance value will be. The actual value of the deviance for a logistic regression model doesn't mean much by itself. It's the difference in deviance between two models you might be comparing that is important.

Once deviance is calculated, the final step is to identify the values of the coefficients that will minimize the deviance of the observed Y values from the fitted logistic curve. This may sound challenging, but statistical programs employ elegant and efficient ways to minimize such a complicated function involving several variables, and uses these methods to obtain the coefficients.

Handling multiple predictors in your logistic model

The data in Table 18-1 have only one predictor variable, but you may have several predictors of a binary outcome. If the data in Table 18-1 were about humans, you would assume the chance of dying from radiation exposure may depend not only on the radiation dose received, but also on age, gender, weight, general health, radiation wavelength, and the amount of time over which the person was exposed to radiation. In Chapter 17, we describe how the straight-line regression model can be generalized to handle multiple predictors. You can generalize the logistic formula to handle multiple predictors in the same way.

Suppose that the outcome variable Y is dependent on three predictors called X, V, and W. Then the multivariate logistic model looks like this:

$$Y = 1 / \left(1 + e^{-(a + bX + CV + dW)}\right)$$

Logistic regression finds the best-fitting values of the parameters a, b, c, and d given your data. That way, for any particular set of values for X, V, and W, you can use the equation to predict Y, which is the probability of being positive for the outcome.

Running a Logistic Regression Model with Software

REMEMBER

The theory behind logistic regression is difficult to grasp, and the calculations are complicated (see the sidebar "Getting into the nitty-gritty of logistic regression" for details). The good news is that most statistical software (as described in Chapter 4) can run a logistic regression model, and it is similar to running a straight-line or multiple linear regression model (see Chapters 16 and 17). Here are the steps:

1. **Make sure your data set has a column for the outcome variable that is coded as 1 where the individual is positive for the outcome, and 0 when they are negative.**

   If you do not have an outcome column coded this way, use the data management commands in your software to generate a new variable coded as 0 for those who do not have the outcome, and 1 for those who have the outcome, as shown in Table 18-1.

2. **Make sure your data set has a column for each predictor variable, and that these columns are coded the way you want them to be entered them into the model.**

The predictors can be quantitative, such as age or weight. They can also be categorical, like gender or treatment group. You will need to make decisions about how to recode these variables to enter them into the regression model. See Chapter 17, where we describe how to set up categorical predictor variables.

3. **Tell your software which variables are the predictors and which is the outcome.**

   Depending on the software, you may do this by typing the variable names, or by selecting the variables from a menu or list.

4. **Request the optional output from the software if available which may include:**

   - A summary of information about the variables, goodness-of-fit measures, and a graph of the fitted logistic curve

   - A table of regression coefficients, including odds ratios (ORs) and their 95 percent confidence intervals (CIs)

   - Predicted probabilities of getting the outcome for each individual, and a classification table of observed outcomes versus predicted outcomes

   - Measures of prediction accuracy, which include overall accuracy, sensitivity, and specificity, as well as a Receiver Operator Characteristics (ROC) curve

5. **Execute the model in the software.**

   Obtain the output you requested, and interpret the resulting model.

Interpreting the Output of Logistic Regression

Figure 18-4 shows two kinds of statistical software output from a logistic regression model produced from the data in Table 18-1. The output presented is not from a particular command in a particular software. Instead, typical output for the different items is presented to enable us to cover many different potential scenarios.

FIGURE 18-4:
Typical output
from a logistic
regression model.
The output on the
left (a) shows
statistical results
output for the
model, and the
output on the
right (b)
shows predicted
probabilities for
each individual
that can be
output as a
data set.

```
Outcome: Died; Predictors: Dose

Descriptives:
15 cases Died=0; 15 cases Died=1.

Deviance  (= -2 Log Likelihood) :
  Null Model:  41.589
  Final Model:  15.747
  Chi Square=  25.842;  df=1;  p<0.0001

Hosmer-Lemeshow Goodness of Fit Test:
  Chi Square=  4.161;  df=8;  p<0.842

Cox/Snell  R-square= 0.577
Nagelkerke  R-square= 0.770
AIC= 19.747

Coefficients and Standard Errors...
Variable        Coeff.      StdErr  p-value
Intercept      -4.8276      1.7521    0.0038
Dose     0.0115      0.0040    0.0038

Odds Ratios and 95% Confidence Intervals:
Variable       O.R.     Low      High
Dose     1.0115       1.0037       1.0194

Fitted Logistic Formula:
Prob (Death) =
  1 / (1 + Exp ( - (-4.828 + 0.01146 * Dose) ) )
```

Dose	Died	Pr Death	Predict
0	0	0.0079	0
10	0	0.0089	0
31	0	0.0113	0
82	0	0.0201	0
92	0	0.0225	0
107	0	0.0266	0
142	0	0.0391	0
173	0	0.0549	0
175	0	0.0561	0
232	0	1.1025	0
266	0	0.1443	0
299	0	0.1976	0
303	1	0.2049	0
326	0	0.2512	0
404	1	0.4505	0
433	0	0.5334	1
457	1	0.6008	1
559	1	0.8289	1
560	1	0.8305	1
604	1	0.8902	1
632	0	0.9179	1
686	1	0.9540	1
691	1	0.9565	1
702	1	0.9614	1
705	1	0.9627	1
774	1	0.9827	1
853	1	0.9929	1
879	1	0.9947	1
915	1	0.9965	1
977	1	0.9983	1

a. Statistical Output

b. Predicted Probabilities Output

© John Wiley & Sons, Inc.

Seeing summary information about the variables

At the top of Figure 18-4a, you can see information about the variables under *Descriptives*. It can include means and standard deviations of predictors that are numerical variables, and a count of how many individuals did or did not have the outcome event. In Figure 18-4a, you can see that 15 of the 30 individuals lived and 15 died.

Assessing the adequacy of the model

In Figure 18-4a, the middle section starting with *Deviance* and ending with *AIC* provides model fit information. These are measures that indicate how well the fitted function represents the data, which is called *goodness-of-fit*. Some have test statistics and an associated p value (see Chapter 3 for a refresher on p values), while others produce metrics. Although there are different model fit statistics, you will find that they usually agree on how well a model fits the data.

You may see the following model fit measures, depending on your software:

>> **A p value associated with the decrease in deviance between the null model and the final model:** This information is shown in Figure 18-4a under *Deviance*. Under $\alpha = 0.05$, if this p value < 0.05, it indicates that adding the predictor variables to the null model statistically significantly improves its ability to predict the outcome. In Figure 18-4a, p < 0.0001, which means that adding radiation dose to the model makes it statistically significantly better at predicting an individual animal's chance of dying than the null model. However, it's not very hard for a model with any predictors to be better than the null model, so this is not a very sensitive model fit statistic.

>> **A p value from the Hosmer-Lemeshow (H-L) test:** In Figure 18-4a, this is listed under *Hosmer-Lemeshow Goodness of Fit Test*. The null hypothesis for this test is your data are consistent with the logistic function's *S* shape, so if p < 0.05, your data do not qualify for logistic regression. The focus of the test is to see if the *S* is getting distorted at very high or very low levels of the predictor (as shown in Figure 18-4b). In Figure 18-4a, the H-L p value is 0.842, which means that the data are consistent with the shape of a logistic curve.

>> **One or more pseudo–r^2 values:** *Pseudo–r^2 values* indicate how much of the total variability in the outcome is explainable by the fitted model. They are analogous to how r^2 is interpreted in ordinary least-squares regression, as described in Chapter 17. In Figure 18-4a, two such values are provided under the labels *Cox/Snell R-square* and *Nagelkerke R-square*. The Cox/Snell r^2 is 0.577, and the Nagelkerke r^2 is 0.770, both of which indicate that a majority of the variability in the outcome is explainable by the logistic model.

TIP

>> **Akaike's Information Criterion (AIC):** AIC is a measure of the final model deviance adjusted for how many predictor variables are in the model. Like deviance, the smaller the AIC, the better the fit. The AIC is not very useful on its own, and is instead used for choosing between different models. When all the predictors in one model are *nested* — or included — in another model with more predictors, the AIC is helpful for comparing these models to see if it is worth adding the extra predictors.

Checking out the table of regression coefficients

REMEMBER

Your intention when developing a logistic regression model is to obtain estimates from the table of coefficients, which looks much like the coefficients table from ordinary straight-line or multivariate least-squares regression (see Chapters 16 and 17). In Figure 18-4a, they are listed under *Coefficients and Standard Errors*. Observe:

>> Every predictor variable appears on a separate row.

>> There's one row for the constant term labeled *Intercept*.

>> The first column usually lists the regression coefficients (under *Coeff.* in Figure 18-4a).

>> The second column usually lists the standard error (SE) of each coefficient (under *StdErr* in Figure 18-4a).

>> A p-value column indicates whether the coefficient is statistically significantly different from 0. This column may be labeled *Sig* or *Signif* or Pr(> |z|), but in Figure 18-4a, it is labeled *p-value*.

For each predictor variable, the output should also provide the odds ratio (OR) and its 95 percent confidence interval. These are usually presented in a separate table as they are in Figure 18-4a under *Odds Ratios and 95% Confidence Intervals*.

Predicting probabilities with the fitted logistic formula

TIP

The output may include the fitted logistic formula. At the bottom of Figure 18-4a, the formula is shown as:

$$\text{Prob(Death)} = 1/(1 + \text{Exp}(-(-4.828 + 0.01146 * \text{Dose})))$$

You can write out the formula manually by inserting the value of the regression coefficients from the regression table into the logistic formula. The final model produced by the logistic regression program from the data in Table 18-1 and the resulting logistic curve are shown in Figure 18-5.

Once you have the fitted logistic formula, you can predict the probability of having the outcome if you know the value of the predictor variable. For example, if an individual is exposed to 500 REM of radiation, the probability of the outcome is given by this formula: $\text{Probability of Death} = 1/\left(1 + e^{-(-4.828 + 0.01146 \times 500)}\right)$, which equals 0.71. An individual exposed to 500 REM of radiation has a predicted probability of 0.71 — or a 71 percent chance — of dying shortly thereafter. The predicted probabilities for each individual are shown in the data listed in Figure 18-4b. You can also calculate some points of special significance on a logistic curve, as you find out in the following sections.

WARNING

Be careful with your algebra when evaluating these formulas! The a coefficient in a logistic regression is often a negative number, and subtracting a negative number is like adding its absolute value.

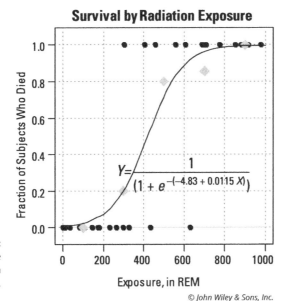

Survival by Radiation Exposure

$$Y = \frac{1}{\left(1 + e^{-(-4.83 + 0.0115\,X)}\right)}$$

(y-axis) Fraction of Subjects Who Died

1.0
0.8
0.6
0.4
0.2
0.0

(x-axis) 0   200   400   600   800   1000

Exposure, in REM

FIGURE 18-5:
The logistic curve that fits the data from Table 18-1.

Calculating effective doses on a logistic curve

One point of special significance on a logistic curve with a numerical predictor is a *median effective dose*. This is a dose (X) that produces a 50 percent response, meaning where $Y = 0.5$, and is designated ED_{50}. Similarly, the X value that makes $Y = 0.8$ is called the *80 percent effective dose* and is designated ED_{80}, and so on. You can calculate these dose levels from the a and b parameters of the fitted logistic model in the preceding section.

Using your high-school algebra, you can solve the logistic formula $Y = 1/\left(1 + e^{-(a+bX)}\right)$ for X as a function of Y. If you don't remember how to do that, don't worry, here's the answer:

$$X = \frac{\log\left(\frac{Y}{1-Y}\right) - a}{b}$$

where *log* stands for natural logarithm. If you substitute 0.5 for Y in the preceding equation because you want to calculate the ED_{50}, the answer is $-a/b$. Similarly, substituting 0.8 for Y gives the ED_{80} as $\dfrac{1.39 - a}{b}$.

Imagine a logistic regression model based on a study of participants taking a drug at different doses where the predictor is level of drug dose, and the outcome is that it produces a therapeutic response. The model has $a = -3.45$ and $b = 0.0204$ mg/dL. In this case, the ED_{80} (or 80 percent effective dose) would be equal to $(1.39 - (-3.45))/0.0234$, which works out to about 207 mg/dL.

Calculating lethal doses on a logistic curve

When death is the outcome event, the corresponding terms are *median lethal dose* (abbreviated LD_{50}) and *80 percent lethal dose* (abbreviated LD_{80}), and so on. To calculated the LD_{50} using the data in Table 18-1, $a = -4.83$ and $b = 0.0115$, so $-a / b = -(-4.83) / 0.0115$, which works out to 420 REMs. An LD_{50} of 420 REMs dose of radiation means an individual has a 50 percent chance of dying shortly after being exposed to this level of radiation.

Making yes or no predictions

If you fit a logistic regression model, then learn of the value of predictor variables for an individual, you can plug them into the equation and calculate the predicted probability of the individual having the outcome. But sometimes, you are trying to actually predict the outcome — whether the event will happen or not, *yes* or *no* — to an individual. You can do this by setting a cut value on predicted probability. Imagine you select 0.5 as the cut value, and you make a rule that if the individual's predicted probability is 0.5 or greater, you'll predict *yes*; otherwise, you'll predict *no*.

In the following sections, we talk about *yes* or *no* predictions. We explain how they expose the ability of the logistic model to make predictions, and how you can strategically select the cut value that gives you the best tradeoff between wrongly predicting *yes* and wrongly predicting *no*.

Measuring accuracy, sensitivity, and specificity with classification tables

Software output for logistic regression provides several goodness-of-fit measures (see the earlier section "Assessing the adequacy of the model"). One intuitive indicator of goodness-of-fit is the extent to which your *yes* or *no* predictions from the logistic model match the actual outcomes. You can cross-tabulate the predicted and observed outcomes into a fourfold classification table. To do this, you would ask the software to generate a classification table for you from the data based on a cut value in the predicted probability. Most software assumes a cut value of 0.5 unless you tell it to use some other value. Figure 18-6 shows the classification table of observed versus predicted outcomes from radiation exposure, using a cut value of 0.5 predicted probability.

From the classification table shown in Figure 18-6, you can calculate several useful measures of the model's predicting ability for any specified cut value, including the following:

		Observed Outcome		
		Died	Lived	Total
Predicted Outcome from Logistic Model	Died	13	2	15
	Lived	2	13	15
	Total	15	15	30

© John Wiley & Sons, Inc.

FIGURE 18-6: The classification table for the radiation example.

>> **Overall accuracy:** This refers to the proportion of accurate predictions, as shown in the *concordant* cells, which are the upper-left and lower-right. Of the 30 individuals in the data set from Table 18-1, the logistic model predicted correctly $(13 + 13)/30 = 0.87$, or about 87 percent of the time. This means with the cut value where you placed it, the model would make a wrong prediction only about 13 percent of the time.

>> **Sensitivity:** This refers to the proportion of *yes* outcomes predicted accurately. As seen in the upper-left cell in Figure 18-6, with the cut value where it was placed, the logistic model predicted 13 of the 15 observed deaths (*yes* outcomes). So the sensitivity is $13 / 15 = 0.87$, or about 87 percent. This means the model would have a false-negative rate of 13 percent.

>> **Specificity:** This refers to the proportion of no outcomes predicted accurately. In the lower-right cell of Figure 18-6, the model predicted survival in 13 of the 15 observed survivors. So, the specificity is $13 / 15 = 0.87$, or about 87 percent. This means the model would have a false-positive rate of 13 percent.

Sensitivity and specificity are especially relevant to screening tests for diseases. An ideal test would have 100 percent sensitivity and 100 percent specificity, and therefore, 100 percent overall accuracy. In reality, no test could meet these standards, and there is a tradeoff between sensitivity and specificity.

REMEMBER

By judiciously choosing the cut value for converting a predicted probability into a *yes* or *no* decision, you can often achieve high sensitivity or high specificity, but it's hard to maximize both simultaneously. Screening tests are meant to detect disease, so how you select the cut value depends upon what happens if it produces a false-positive or false-negative result. This helps you decide whether to prioritize sensitivity or specificity.

WARNING

The sensitivity and specificity of a logistic model depends upon the cut value you set for the predicted probability. The trick is to select a cut value that gives the optimal combination of sensitivity and specificity, striking the best balance between false-positive and false-negative predictions, in light of the different consequences of the two types of false predictions. A false-positive screening result from a mammogram may mean the patient is worried until the negative diagnosis is confirmed by ultrasound, and a false-negative screening results from a prostate cancer screening may result in a delay in identifying the prostate tumor. To find this optimal cut value, you need to know precisely how sensitivity and specificity play against each other — that is, how they simultaneously vary with different cut values. There's a neat way to do that which we explain in the following section.

Rocking with ROC curves

The graph used to display the sensitivity/specificity tradeoff for any fitted logistic model is called the *Receiver Operator Characteristics* (ROC) graph. The name comes from its original use during World War II to analyze the performance characteristics of people who operated RADAR receivers, but the name has stuck, and now it is also referred to as an ROC curve.

REMEMBER

An ROC graph has a curve that shows you the complete range of sensitivity and specificity that can be achieved for any fitted logistic model based on the selected cut value. The software generates an ROC curve by effectively trying all possible cut values of predicted probability between 0 and 1, calculating the predicted outcomes, cross-tabbing them against the observed outcomes, calculating sensitivity and specificity, and then graphing sensitivity versus specificity. Figure 18-7 shows the ROC curve from the logistic model developed from the data in Figure 18-1 (using R software; see Chapter 4).

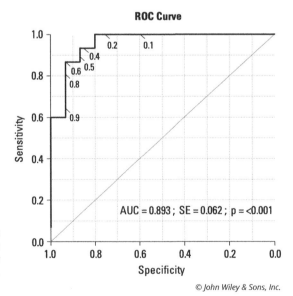

FIGURE 18-7: ROC curve from dose mortality data.

As shown in Figure 18-7, the ROC curve always starts in the lower-left corner of the graph, where 0 percent sensitivity intersects with 100 percent specificity. It ends in the upper-right corner, where 100 percent sensitivity intersects with 0 percent specificity. Most software also draws a diagonal straight line between the lower-left and upper-right corners because that represents the formula: sensitivity = 1 − specificity. If your model's ROC curve were to match that line, it would indicate the total absence of any predicting ability at all of your model.

Like Figure 18-7, every ROC graph has sensitivity running up the Y axis, which is displayed either as fractions between 0 and 1 or as percentages between 0 and 100. The X axis is either presented from left to right as 1 − specificity, or like it is in Figure 18-7, where specificity is labeled backwards — from right to left — along the X axis.

REMEMBER

Most ROC curves lie in the upper-left part of the graph area. The farther away from the diagonal line they are, the better the predictive model is. For a nearly perfect model, the ROC curve runs up along the Y axis from the lower-left corner to the upper-left corner, then along the top of the graph from the upper-left corner to the upper-right corner.

Because of how sensitivity and specificity are calculated, the graph appears as a series of steps. If you have a large data set, your graph will have more and smaller steps. For clarity, we show the cut values for predicted probability as a scale along the ROC curve itself in Figure 18-7, but unfortunately, most statistical software doesn't do this for you.

TIP

Looking at the ROC curve helps you choose a cut value that gives the best tradeoff between sensitivity and specificity:

>> **To have very few false positives:** Choose a higher cut value to give a high specificity. Figure 18-7 shows that by setting the cut value to 0.6, you can simultaneously achieve about 93 percent specificity and 87 percent sensitivity.

>> **To have very few false negatives:** Choose a lower cut value to give higher sensitivity. Figure 18-7 shows you that if you set the cut value to 0.3, you can have almost perfect sensitivity because you'll be at almost 100 percent, but your specificity will be only about 75 percent, meaning you'll have a 25 percent false positive rate.

The software may optionally display the *area under the ROC curve* (abbreviated AUC), along with its standard error and a p value. This is another measure of how good the predictive model is. The diagonal line has an AUC of 0.5, and there is a statistical test comparing your AUC to the diagonal line. Under $\alpha = 0.05$, if the p value < 0.05, it indicates that your model is statistically significantly better than the diagonal line at accurately predicting your outcome.

Heads Up: Knowing What Can Go Wrong with Logistic Regression

Logistic regression presents many of the same potential pitfalls as ordinary least-squares regression (see Chapters 16 and 17), as well as several that are specific to logistic regression. Watch out for some of the more common pitfalls:

>> **Don't fit a logistic function to non-logistic data:** Don't use logistic regression to fit data that doesn't behave like the logistic S curve. Plot your grouped data (as shown earlier in Figure 18-1b), and if it's clear that the fraction of positive outcomes isn't leveling off at $Y = 0$ or $Y = 1$ for very large or very small X values, then logistic regression is not the correct modeling approach. The H-L test described earlier under the section "Assessing the adequacy of the model" provides a statistical test to determine if your data qualify for logistic regression. Also, in Chapter 19, we describe a more generalized logistic model that contains other parameters for the upper and lower leveling-off values.

>> **Watch out for collinearity and disappearing significance:** When you are doing any kind of regression and two or more predictor variables are strongly related with each other, you can be plagued with problems of collinearity. We describe this problem in Chapter 17, and potential modeling solutions in Chapter 20.

>> **Check for inadvertent reverse-coding of the outcome variable:** The outcome variable should always be coded as 1 for a *yes* outcome and 0 for a no outcome (refer to Table 18-1 for an example). If the variable in the data set is coded using characters, you should recode an outcome variable using the 0/1 coding. It is important you do the coding yourself, and do not leave it to an automated function in the program, because it may inadvertently reverse the coding so that 1 = no and 0 = yes. This error of reversal won't affect any p values, but it will cause all your ORs and their CIs to be the reciprocals of what they would have been, meaning they will refer to the odds of no rather than the odds of *yes*.

>> **Don't misinterpret odds ratios for categorical predictors:** Categorical predictors should be coded numerically as we describe in Chapter 8. It is important to ensure that proper indicator variable coding is used, and these variables are introduced properly in the model, as described in Chapter 17.

Also, be careful not to misinterpret odds ratios for numerical predictors, and be mindful of the complete separation problem, as described in the following sections.

Don't misinterpret odds ratios for numerical predictors

WARNING

The OR always represents the factor by which the odds of getting the outcome event increases when the predictor increases by exactly one unit of measure, whatever that unit may be. Sometimes you may want to express the OR in more convenient units than what the data was recorded in. For the example in Table 18-1, the OR for dose as a predictor of death is 1.0115 per REM. This isn't too meaningful because one REM is a very small increment of radiation. By raising 1.0115 to the 100th power, you get the equivalent OR of 3.1375 per 100 REMs, and you can express this as, "Every additional 100 REMs of radiation more than triples the odds of dying."

The value of a regression coefficient depends on the units in which the corresponding predictor variable is expressed. So the coefficient of a height variable expressed in meters is 100 times larger than the coefficient of height expressed in centimeters. In logistic regression, ORs are obtained by exponentiating the coefficients, so switching from centimeters to meters corresponds to raising the OR (and its confidence limits) to the 100th power.

Beware of the complete separation problem

Imagine your logistic regression model perfectly predicted the outcome, in that every individual positive for the outcome had a predicted probability of 1.0, and every individual negative for the outcome had a 0 predicted probability. This is called *perfect separation* or *complete separation*, and the problem is called the *perfect predictor problem.* This is a nasty and surprisingly frequent problem that's unique to logistic regression, which highlights the sad fact that a logistic regression model will fail to converge in the software if the model fits perfectly!

WARNING

If the predictor variable or variables in your model completely separate the *yes* outcomes from the *no* outcomes, the maximum likelihood method will try to make the coefficient of that variable infinite, which usually causes an error in the software. If the coefficient is positive, the OR tries to be infinity, and if it is negative, it tries to be 0. The SE of the OR tries to be infinite, too. This may cause your CI to have a lower limit of 0, an upper limit of infinity, or both.

Check out Figure 18-8, which visually describes the problem. The regression is trying to make the curve come as close as possible to all the data points. Usually it has to strike a compromise, because there's a mixture of 1s and 0s, especially in the middle of the data. But with perfectly separated data, no compromise is necessary. As b becomes infinitely large, the logistic function morphs into a step function that touches all the data points (observe where $b = 5$).

WARNING

While it is relatively easy to identify if there is a perfect predictor in your data set by looking at frequencies, you may run into the perfect predictor problem as a result of a combination of predictors in your model. Unfortunately, there aren't any great solutions to this problem. One proposed solution called the Firth correction allows you to add a small number roughly equivalent to half an observation to the data set that will disrupt the complete separation. If you can do this correction in your software, it will produce output, but the results will likely be unstable (very near 0, or very near infinity). The approach of trying to *fix* the model by changing the predictors would not make sense, since the model fits perfectly. You may be forced to abandon your logistic regression plans and instead provide a descriptive analysis.

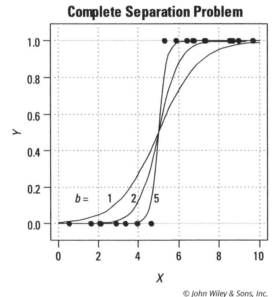

FIGURE 18-8: Visualizing the complete separation (or perfect predictor) problem in logistic regression.

© John Wiley & Sons, Inc.

Figuring Out the Sample Size You Need for Logistic Regression

Estimating the required sample size for a logistic regression can be a pain, even for a simple one-predictor model. You will have no problem specifying desired power and α level (see Chapter 3 for more about these items). And, you can state the effect size of importance as an OR.

REMEMBER

Assuming a one-predictor model, the required sample size for logistic regression also depends on the relative frequency of *yes* and *no* outcomes, and how the predictor variable is distributed. And with multiple predictors in the model, determining sample size is even more complicated. So for a rigorous sample-size calculation for a study that will use a logistic regression model with multiple predictors, you may have no choice but to seek the help of a professional statistician.

TIP

Here are two simple approaches you can use if your logistic model has only one predictor. In each case, you replace the logistic regression equation with another equation that is somewhat equivalent, and then do a sample-size calculation based on that. It's not an ideal solution, but it can give you an answer that's close enough for planning purposes.

>> **If the predictor is a dichotomous category** (a yes/no variable), logistic regression gives the same p value you get from analyzing a fourfold table. Therefore, you can use the sample-size calculations we describe in Chapter 12.

>> **If the predictor is a continuous numerical quantity** (like age), you can pretend that the outcome variable is the predictor, and age is the outcome. We realize this flips the cause-and-effect relationship backwards, but if you allow that conceptual flip, then you can ask whether the two different outcome groups have different mean values for the predictor. You can test that question with an unpaired Student t test, so you can use the sample-size calculations we describe in Chapter 11.

Chapter **19**

Other Useful Kinds of Regression

This chapter covers regression approaches you're likely to encounter in bio-statistical work that are not covered in other chapters. They're not quite as common as straight-line regression, multiple regression, and logistic regression (described in Chapters 16, 17, and 18, respectively), but you should be aware of them. We don't go into a lot of detail, but we describe what they are, the circumstances under which you may want to use them, how to execute the models and interpret the output, and special situations you may encounter with these models.

Note: We also don't cover survival regression in this chapter, even though it's one of the most important kinds of regression analysis in biostatistics. Survival analysis is the theme of Part 6 of this book, and is the topic of Chapter 23.

Analyzing Counts and Rates with Poisson Regression

Statisticians often have to analyze outcomes consisting of the number of occur-rences of an event over some interval of time, such as the number of fatal highway accidents in a city in a year. If the occurrences seem to be getting more common as time goes on, you may want to perform a regression analysis to see whether the upward trend is statistically significant (meaning not due to natural random fluctuations). If it is, you may want to create an estimate of the annual rate of increase, including a standard error (SE) and confidence interval (CI).

Some analysts use ordinary least-squares regression as described in Chapter 16 on such data, but event counts don't really meet the least-squares assumptions, so the approach is not technically correct. Event counts aren't well-approximated as continuous, normally-distributed data unless the counts are very large. Also, their variability is neither constant nor proportional to the counts themselves. So straight-line or multiple least-squares regression is not the best choice for event count data.

Because independent random events like highway accidents should follow a Poisson distribution (see Chapter 24), they should be analyzed by a kind of regression designed for Poisson outcomes. And — surprise, surprise — this type of specialized regression is called *Poisson regression.*

Introducing the generalized linear model

Most statistical software packages don't offer a command or function explicitly called Poisson regression. Instead, they offer a more general regression technique called the *generalized linear model* (GLM).

Don't confuse the *generalized* linear model with the very similarly named *general* linear model. It's unfortunate that these two names are almost identical, because they describe two very different things. Now, the *general* linear model is usually abbreviated LM, and the *generalized* linear model is abbreviated GLM, so we will use those abbreviations. (However, some old textbooks from the 1970s may use GLM to mean LM, because the generalized linear model had not been invented yet.)

GLM is similar to LM in that the predictor variables usually appear in the model as the familiar linear combination:

$$c_0 + c_1 x_1 + c_2 x_2 + c_3 x_3 + \ldots$$

where the x's are the predictor variables, and the c's are the regression coefficients (with c_0 being called a *constant term*, or *intercept*).

But GLM extends the capabilities of LM in two important ways:

> » With LM, the outcome is assumed to be a continuous, normally distributed variable. But with GLM, the outcome can be continuous or an integer. It can

follow one of several different distribution functions, such as normal, exponential, binomial (as in logistic regression), or Poisson.

>> With LM, the linear combination becomes the predicted value of the outcome, but with GLM, you can specify a *link function*. The link function is a transformation that turns the linear combination into the predicted value. As we note in Chapter 18, logistic regression applies exactly this kind of transformation: Let's call the linear combination *V*. In logistic regression, *V* is sent through the logistic function $1/\left(1+e^{-V}\right)$ to convert it into a predicted probability of having the outcome event. So if you select the correct link function, you can use GLM to perform logistic regression.

REMEMBER

GLM is the Swiss army knife of regression. If you select the correct link function, you can use it to do ordinary least-squares regression, logistic regression, Poisson regression, and a whole lot more. Most statistical software offers a GLM function; that way, other specialized regressions don't need to be programmed. If the software you are using doesn't offer logistic or Poisson regression, check to see whether it offers GLM, and if it does, use that instead. (Flip to Chapter 4 for an introduction to statistical software.)

Running a Poisson regression

Suppose that you want to study the number of fatal highway accidents per year in a city. Table 19-1 shows some made-up fatal-accident data over the course of 12 years. Figure 19-1 shows a graph of this data, created using the R statistical software package.

REMEMBER

Running a Poisson regression is similar in many ways to running the other common kinds of regression, but there are some differences. Here are the steps:

1. **As with any regression, prepare your predictor and outcome variables in your data.**

    For this example, you have a row of data for each year, so *year* is the experimental unit. For each row, you have a column containing the outcome values, which is number of accidents each year (*Accidents*). Since you have one predictor — which is year — you have a column for *Year*.

2. **Tell the software which variables are the predictor variables, and which one is the outcome.**

3. **Tell the software what kind of regression you want it to carry out by specifying the *family* of the dependent variable's distribution and the *link function*.**

Step 3 is not obvious, and you may have to consult your software's help file. In the R program, as an example, you have to specify both family and link in a single construction, which looks like this:

```
glm(formula = Accidents ~ Year, family = poisson(link = "identity"))
```

This code tells R that the outcome is the variable *Accidents,* the predictor is the variable *Year,* and the outcome variable follows the Poisson *family* of distributions. The code link = "identity" tells R that you want to fit a model in which the true event rate rises in a *linear* fashion, meaning that it increases by a constant amount each year.

4. **Execute the regression and obtain the output.**

The next step is to interpret the output.

TABLE 19-1

Yearly Data on Fatal Highway Accidents in One City

Calendar Year	Fatal Accidents
2010	10
2011	12
2012	15
2013	8
2014	8
2015	15
2016	4
2017	20
2018	20
2019	17
2020	29
2021	28

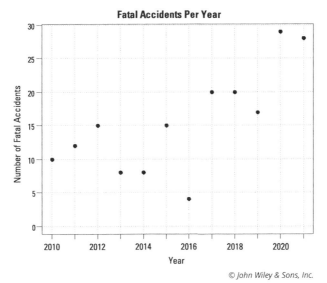

FIGURE 19-1:
Yearly data on fatal highway accidents in one city.

© John Wiley & Sons, Inc.

Interpreting the Poisson regression output

After you follow the steps for running a Poisson regression in the preceding section, the program produces output like that shown in Figure 19-2, which is the Poisson regression output from R's generalized linear model function (glm).

FIGURE 19-2:
Poisson regression output.

```
Call:
glm(formula=Accidents~Year,family=poisson(link="identity"))

Coefficients:
              Estimate  Std. Error    z value  Pr (>|z|)
(Intercept) -2651.4569    635.1064     -4.175  2.98e-05 ***
Year           1.3298       0.3169     -4.197  2.71e-05 ***

AIC: 81.72
```

This output has the same general structure as the output from other kinds of regression. The most important parts of it are the following:

>> In the coefficients table (labeled *Coefficients:*), the estimated regression coefficient for *Year* is 1.3298, indicating that the annual number of fatal accidents is increasing by an estimated 1.33 accidents per year.

>> The standard error (SE) is labeled *Std. Error* and is 0.3169, indicating the precision of the estimated rate increase per year. From the SE, using the rules given in Chapter 10, the 95 percent confidence interval (CI) around the estimated annual increase is approximately $1.3298 \pm 1.96 \times 0.3169$, which gives a 95 percent CI of 0.71 to 1.95 (around the estimate 1.33).

>> The column labeled *z value* contains the value of the regression coefficient divided by its SE. It's used to calculate the p value that appears in the last column of the table.

>> The last column, labeled $Pr(>|z|)$, is the p value for the significance of the increasing trend estimated at 1.33. The *Year* variable has a p value of 2.71 *e*-05, which is scientific notation (see Chapter 2) for 0.0000271. Using $\alpha = 0.05$, the apparent increase in rate over the 12 years would be interpreted as highly statistically significant.

>> AIC (Akaike's Information Criterion) indicates how well this model fits the data. The value of 81.72 isn't useful by itself, but it's very useful when choosing between two alternative models, as we explain later in this chapter.

R software can also provide the predicted annual event rate for each year, from which you can add a *trend line* to the scatter graph, indicating how you think the true event rate may vary with time (see Figure 19-3).

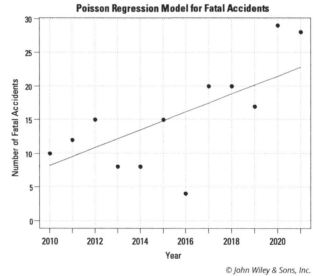

FIGURE 19-3: Poisson regression, assuming a constant increase in accident rate per year with trend line.

Discovering other uses for Poisson regression

The following sections describe other uses of R's GLM function in performing Poisson regression.

Examining nonlinear trends

The straight line in Figure 19-3 doesn't account for the fact that the accident rate remained low for the first few years and then started to climb rapidly after 2016. Perhaps the true trend isn't a straight line, where the rate increases by the same *amount* each year. It may instead be an *exponential* increase, where the rate increases by a certain *percentage* each year. You can have R fit an exponential increase by changing the link option from *identity* to *log* in the statement that invokes the Poisson regression:

glm(formula = Accidents ~ Year, family = poisson(link = "log"))

This produces the output shown in Figure 19-4 and graphed in Figure 19-5.

```
Call:
glm(formula=Accidents~Year,family=poisson(link="log"))

Coefficients:
                Estimate   Std. Error   z value  Pr (>|z|)
  (Intercept)  -206.18249    44.29432    -4.655  3.24e-06 ***
  Year            0.10414     0.02207    -4.718  2.38e-06 ***

AIC: 78.476
```

Because of the *log* link used in this regression run, the coefficients are related to the logarithm of the event rate. Thus, the relative rate of increase per year is obtained by taking the antilog of the regression coefficient for *Year*. This is done by raising *e* (the mathematical constant 2.718. . .) to the power of the regression coefficient for *Year*: $e^{0.10414}$, which is about 1.11. So, according to an exponential increase model, the annual accident rate increases by a factor of 1.11 each year — meaning there is an 11 percent increase each year. The dashed-line curve in Figure 19-4 shows this exponential trend, which appears to accommodate the steeper rate of increase seen after 2016.

Comparing alternative models

The bottom of Figure 19-4 shows the AIC value for the exponential trend model is 78.476, which is about 3.2 units lower than for the linear trend model in Figure 19-2 (AIC = 81.72). Smaller AIC values indicate better fit, so the true trend is more likely to be exponential rather than linear. But you can't conclude that the model with the lower AIC is really better unless the AIC is about six units better. So in this example, you can't say for sure whether the trend is linear or exponential, or potentially another distribution. But the exponential curve does seem to predict the high accident rates seen in 2020 and 2021 better than the linear trend model.

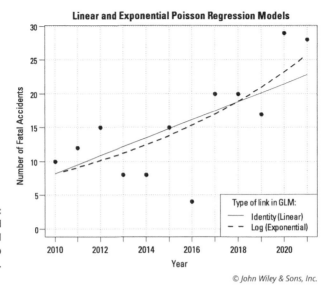

FIGURE 19-5:
Linear and exponential trends fitted to accident data.

Linear and Exponential Poisson Regression Models

Number of Fatal Accidents

Type of link in GLM:
— Identity (Linear)
– – Log (Exponential)

Year

© *John Wiley & Sons, Inc.*

Working with unequal observation intervals

In this fatal accident example, each of the 12 data points represents the accidents observed during a one-year interval. But imagine analyzing the frequency of emergency department visits for patients after being treated for emphysema, where there is one data point per patient. In that case, the width of the observation interval may vary from one individual in the data to another. GLM lets you provide an interval width along with the event count for each individual in the data. For arcane reasons, many statistical programs refer to this interval-width variable as the *offset.*

Accommodating clustered events

The Poisson distribution applies when the observed events are all independent occurrences. But this assumption isn't met if events occur in clusters. Suppose you count individual highway *fatalities* instead of fatal highway *accidents*. In that case, the Poisson distribution doesn't apply, because one fatal accident may kill several people. This is what is meant by *clustered* events.

TIP

The standard deviation (SD) of a Poisson distribution is equal to the square root of the mean of the distribution. But if clustering is present, the SD of the data is larger than the square root of the mean. This situation is called *overdispersion.* GLM in R can correct for overdispersion if you designate the distribution family *quasipoisson* rather than *poisson*, like this:

glm(formula = Accidents ~ Year, family = quasipoisson(link = "log"))

Anything Goes with Nonlinear Regression

Here, we finally present the potentially most challenging type of least-squares regression, and that's general nonlinear least-squares regression, or nonlinear curve-fitting. In the following sections, we explain how nonlinear regression is different from other kinds of regression. We also describe how to run and interpret a nonlinear regression using an example from drug research, and we show you some tips involving equivalent functions.

Distinguishing nonlinear regression from other kinds

In the kinds of regression we describe earlier in this chapter and in Chapters 16, 17, and 18, the predictor variables and regression coefficients always appear in the model as a linear combination: $c_0 + c_1x_1 + c_2x_2 + c_3x_3 + ... + c_nx_n$. But in nonlinear regression, the coefficients no longer have to appear paired up to be multiplied by predictor variables (like c_2x_2). In nonlinear regression, coefficients have a more independent existence, and can appear on their own anywhere in the formula. Actually, the term *coefficient* implies a number that's multiplied by a variable's value. This means that technically, you can't have a coefficient that isn't multiplied by a variable, so when this happens in nonlinear regression, they're referred to instead as *parameters*.

REMEMBER

The formula for a nonlinear regression model may be any algebraic expression. It can involve sums, differences, products, ratios, powers, and roots. These can be combined together in a formula with logarithmic, exponential, trigonometric, and other advanced mathematical functions (see Chapter 2 for an introduction to these items). The formula can contain any number of predictor variables, and any number of parameters. In fact, nonlinear regression formulas often contain many more parameters than predictor variables.

REMEMBER

Unlike other types of regression covered in this chapter and book, where a regression command and code are used to generate output, developing a full-blown nonlinear regression model is more of a do-it-yourself proposition. First, you have to decide what function you want to fit to your data, making this choice from the infinite number of possible functions you could select. Sometimes the general form of the function is determined or suggested by a scientific theory. Using a theory to guide your development of a nonlinear function means relying on a *theoretical* or *mechanistic* function, which is more common in the physical sciences than life sciences. If you choose your nonlinear function based on a function with a generally similar shape, you are using an *empirical* function. After choosing the function, you have to provide starting estimates for the value of each of the parameters appearing in the function. After that, you can execute the regression. The software tries to refine your estimates using an iterative process that may or may not converge to an answer, depending on the complexity of the function you're fitting and how close your initial estimates are to the truth. And in addition to attending to these unique issues, analysts running a nonlinear regression face all the other complications of multivariate regression, such as collinearity, as described in Chapter 17.

Checking out an example from drug research

One common nonlinear regression problem arises in drug development research. As soon as scientists start testing a promising new compound, they want to determine some of its basic pharmacokinetic (PK) properties. PK properties describe how the drug is absorbed, distributed, modified, and eliminated by the body. Typically, the earliest Phase I clinical trials attempt to obtain basic PK data as a secondary objective of the trial, while later-phase trials may be designed specifically to characterize the PKs of the drug accurately and in great detail.

Raw PK data often consist of the concentration level of the drug in the participant's blood at various times after a dose of the drug is administered. Consider a Phase I trial, in which 10,000 micrograms (μg) of a new drug is given as a single *bolus*, which is a rapid injection into a vein, in each participant. Blood samples are drawn at predetermined times after dosing and are analyzed for drug concentrations. Hypothetical data from one participant are shown in Table 19-2 and graphed in Figure 19-6. The drug concentration in the blood is expressed in units of μg per deciliter (*μg / dL*). Remember, a *deciliter* is one-tenth of a liter.

Several basic PK parameters, such as maximum concentration, time of maximum concentration, area under the curve (AUC), are usually calculated directly from the concentration-versus-time data, without having to fit any curve to the points. But two important parameters are usually obtained from a regression analysis:

>> **The volume of distribution (V_d):** This is the effective volume of fluid or tissue through which the drug is distributed in the body. This effective volume could be equal to the blood volume, but could be greater if the drug also spreads through fatty tissue or other parts of the body. If you know the dose of the drug infused *(Dose)*, and you know the blood plasma concentration at the moment of infusion (C_0), you can calculate the volume of distribution as $V_d = Dose / C_0$. But you can't directly measure C_0. By the time the drug has distributed evenly throughout the bloodstream, some of it has already been eliminated from the body. So C_0 has to be estimated by extrapolating the measured concentrations backward in time to the moment of infusion (Time = 0).

>> **The elimination half-life (λ):** The time it takes for half of the drug in the body to be eliminated.

TABLE 19-2

Blood Drug Concentration versus Time for One Participant

Time after Dosing (In Hours)	Drug Concentration in Blood (µg/dL)
0.25	57.4
0.5	54.0
1	44.8
1.5	52.7
2	43.6
3	40.1
4	27.9
6	20.6
8	15.0
12	10.0

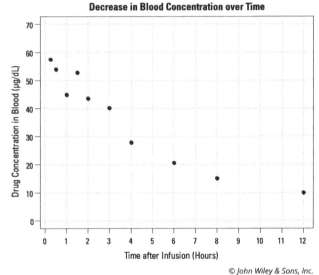

FIGURE 19-6: The blood concentration of an intravenous drug decreases over time in one participant.

© John Wiley & Sons, Inc.

PK theory is well-developed and predicts under a set of reasonable assumptions that the drug concentration *(Conc)* in the blood following a bolus infusion should vary with time *(Time)* according to the equation:

$$Conc = C_o e^{-keTime}$$

where k_e is the *elimination rate constant*. k_e is related to the elimination half-life (λ) according to the formula: $\lambda = 0.693 / k_e$, where 0.693 is the natural logarithm of 2. So, if you can fit the preceding equation to your *Conc*-versus-*Time* data in Table 19-2, you can estimate C_0, from which you can calculate V_d. You can also estimate k_e, from which you can calculate λ.

The preceding equation is nonlinear and includes parameters, with k_e appearing in the exponent. Before nonlinear regression software became widely available, analysts would take a shortcut by shoehorning this nonlinear regression problem into a straight-line regression by working with the logarithms of the concentrations. But that approach can't be generalized to handle more complicated equations that often arise.

Running a nonlinear regression

REMEMBER

Nonlinear curve-fitting is supported by many modern statistics packages, like SPSS, SAS, GraphPad Prism, and R (see Chapter 4). It is possible (though not easy) to set up calculations in Microsoft Excel. In addition, the web page `http://StatPages.info/nonlin.html` can fit any function you can write involving up to eight independent variables and up to eight parameters. Here are the steps we use to do nonlinear regression in R:

1. **Create a vector of time data, and a vector of concentration data.**

   In R, you can develop arrays called *vectors* from data sets, but in this example, we create each vector manually, naming them *Time* and *Conc*, using the data from Table 19-2:

   `Time=c(0.25, 0.5, 1, 1.5, 2, 3, 4, 6, 8, 12)`

   `Conc=c(57.4, 54.0, 44.8, 52.7, 43.6, 40.1, 27.9, 20.6, 15.0, 10.0)`

   In the two preceding equations, *c* is a built-in R function for *combine* that creates an array (see Chapter 2) as a vector from the lists of numbers.

2. **Specify the equation to be fitted to the data, using the algebraic syntax your software requires.**

   We write the equation using R's algebraic syntax this way: *Conc ~ C0 * exp(– ke * Time)*, where *Conc* and *Time* are your vectors of data, and *C0* and *ke* are parameters you set.

3. **Tell the software that C_0 and k_e are parameters to be fitted, and provide initial estimates for these values.**

   Nonlinear curve-fitting is a complicated task solved by the software through iteration. This means you give it some rough estimates, and it refines them into closer estimates to the truth, repeating this process until it arrives at the best-fitting, least-squares solution.

Coming up with starting estimates for nonlinear regression problems can be tricky. It's more of an art than a science. If the parameters have physiological meaning, you may be able to make a guess based on known physiology or past experience. Other times, your estimates have to be trial and error. To improve your estimates, you can graph your observed data in Microsoft Excel, and then superimpose a curve from values calculated from the function for various parameter guesses that you type in. That way, you can play around with the parameters until the curve is at least in the ballpark of the observed data.

In this example, C_0 (variable $C0$) is the concentration you expect at the moment of dosing (at $t = 0$). From Figure 19-6, it looks like the concentration starts out around 50, so you can use 50 as an initial guess for C_0. The k_e parameter (variable ke) affects how quickly the concentration decreases with time. Figure 19-6 indicates that the concentration seems to decrease by half about every few hours, so λ should be somewhere around 4 hours. Because $\lambda = 0.693 / k_e$, a little algebra gives the equation $ke = 0.693/X$. If you plug in 4 hours for X, you get $k_e = 0.693/4 = 0.2$, so you may try 0.2 as a starting guess for ke. You tell R the starting guesses by using the syntax: start=list(C0 = 50, ke = 0.2).

The statement in R for nonlinear regression is *nls*, which stands for *nonlinear least-squares*. The full R statement for executing this nonlinear regression model and summarizing the output is:

```
summary(nls(Conc ~ C0 * exp(-ke * Time), start = list(C0 = 50, ke = 0.2)))
```

Interpreting the output

As complicated as nonlinear curve-fitting may be, the output is actually quite simple. It is formatted and interpreted like the output from ordinary linear regression. Figure 19-7 shows the relevant part of R's output for this example.

```
Formula: Conc ~ C0 * exp ( -ke * Time)

Parameters:
    Estimate Std. Error t value  Pr (>|t|)
C0  59.46203    2.29329 25.929  5.25e-09 ***
ke   0.16330    0.01644  9.931  8.94e-06 ***

Residual std. err. :  3.556 on 8 deg.of freedom
```

FIGURE 19-7: Results of nonlinear regression in R.

In Figure 19-7, the output first restates the model being fitted. Next, what would normally be called the coefficients table is presented, only this time, it is labeled *Parameters*. It has a row for every adjustable parameter that appears in the function. Like other regression tables, it shows the fitted value for the parameter under *Estimate*, its standard error (SE) under *Std. Error*, and the p value under *Pr(>|t|)* indicating whether that parameter was statistically significantly different from zero. The output estimates C_0 at 59.5 ± 2.3 µg/dL and k_e at $0.163 \pm 0.0164 hr^1$ because first-order rate constants have units of *per time*. From these values, you can calculate the PK parameters you want:

» **Volume of distribution:** $V_d = \text{Dose} / C_0 = 10{,}000 \, \mu g / 59.5 \, \mu g / dL = 168 \, dL$, or 16.8 liters. Since this amount is several times larger than the blood volume of the average human, the results indicate that this drug is going into other parts of the body besides the blood.

» **Elimination half-time:** $\lambda = 0.693/ke = 0.693/0.163 hr^1$, or 4.25 hours. This result means that after 4.25 hours, only 50 percent of the original dose is left in the body. After twice as long, which is 8.5 hours, only 25 percent of the original dose remains, and so on.

How precise are these PK parameters? In other words, what is their SE? Unfortunately, uncertainty in any measured quantity will *propagate* through a mathematical expression that involves that quantity, and this needs to be taken into account in calculating the SE. To do this, you can use the online calculator at `https://statpages.info/erpropgt.html`. Choose the estimator designed for two variables, and enter the information from the output into the calculator. You can calculate that the $V_d = 16.8 \pm 0.65$ liters, and $\lambda = 4.25 \pm 0.43$ hours.

R can be asked to generate the predicted value for each data point, from which you can superimpose the fitted curve onto the observed data points, as in Figure 19-8.

R also provides the *residual standard error* (labeled *Residual std. err.* in Figure 19-7), which is defined as the standard deviation of the vertical distances of the observed points from the fitted curve. The value from the output of 3.556 means that the points scatter about 3.6 µg/dL above and below the fitted curve. Additionally, R can be asked to provide Akaike's Information Criterion (AIC), which is useful in selecting which of several possible models best fits the data.

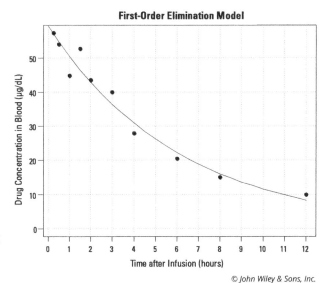

FIGURE 19-8: Nonlinear model fitted to drug concentration data.

First-Order Elimination Model

Drug Concentration in Blood (µg/dL)

Time after Infusion (hours)

Using equivalent functions to fit the parameters you really want

It's inconvenient, annoying, and error-prone to have to perform manual calculations on the parameters you obtain from nonlinear regression output. It's so much extra work to read the output that contains the estimates you need, like C_0 and the k_e rate constant, then manually calculate the parameters you want, like V_d and λ. It's even more work to obtain the SEs. Wouldn't it be nice if you could get V_d and λ and their SEs directly from the nonlinear regression program? Well, in many cases, you can!

Because nonlinear regression involves algebra, some fancy math footwork can help you out. Very often, you can re-express the formula in an equivalent form that directly involves calculating the parameters you actually want to know. Here's how it works for the PK example we use in the preceding sections.

Algebra tells you that because $V_d = Dose / C_0$, then $C_0 = Dose / V_d$. So why not use $Dose / V_d$ instead of C_0 in the formula you're fitting? If you do, it becomes $\mathrm{Conc} = \left(Dose \middle/ v_d \right) e^{-k_e Time}$. And you can go even further than that. It turns out that a first-order exponential-decline formula can be written either as $e^{-k_e Time}$ or as the algebraically equivalent form $2^{-\left(Time / t_{1/2} \right)}$.

Applying both of these substitutions, you get the equivalent model: $C = \left(\dfrac{Dose}{v_d}\right) 2^{-Time/\lambda}$, which produces exactly the same fitted curve as the original model. But it has the tremendous advantage of giving you exactly the PK parameters you want, which are V_d and λ, rather than C_0 and k_e which require post-processing with additional calculations.

From the original description of this example, you already know that $Dose = 10{,}000$ µg, so you can substitute this value for $Dose$ in the formula to be fitted. You've already estimated λ (variable $tHalf$) as 4 hours. Also, you estimated C_0 as about 50 µg/dL from looking at Figure 19-6, as we describe earlier. This means you can estimate V_d (variable Vd) as $10{,}000 / 50$, which is 200 dL. With these estimates, the final R statement is

```
summary(nls(Conc ~ (10000/Vd) * 2^(-Time/tHalf),
                start = list(Vd = 200, tHalf = 4)))
```

which produces the output shown in Figure 19-9.

```
Formula: Conc ~ (10000/Vd) * 2^( -Time / tHalf)

Parameters:
        Estimate Std. Error t value Pr (>|t|)
Vd      168.1745     6.4860  25.929 5.25e-09 ***
tHalf     4.2446     0.4274   9.931 8.94e-06 ***

Residual std. err. :  3.556 on 8 deg.of freedom
```

From Figure 19-9, you can see the direct results for Vd and $tHalf$. Using the output, you can estimate that the V_d is 168.2 ± 6.5 dL (or 16.8 ± 0.66 liters), and λ is 4.24 ± 0.43 hours.

Smoothing Nonparametric Data with LOWESS

Sometimes you want to fit a smooth curve to a set of points that don't seem to conform to a common, recognizable distribution, such as normal, exponential, logistic, and so forth. If you can't write an equation for the curve you want to fit, you can't use linear or nonlinear regression techniques. What you need is essentially a *nonparametric regression* approach, which would not try to fit any formula/model to the relationship, but would instead just try to draw a smooth line through the data points.

Several kinds of nonparametric data-smoothing methods have been developed. A popular one, called LOWESS, stands for Locally Weighted Scatterplot Smoothing. Many statistical programs can perform a LOWESS regression. In the following sections, we explain how to run a LOWESS analysis and adjust the amount of smoothing (*stiffness*) of the curve.

Running LOWESS

Suppose that you discover a new hormone called XYZ believed to be produced in women's ovaries throughout their lifetimes. Research suggests blood levels of XYZ should vary with age, in that they are low before going through puberty and after completing menopause, and high during child-bearing years. You want to characterize and quantify the relationship between XYZ levels and age as accurately as possible.

Suppose that for your analysis, you are allowed to obtain 200 blood samples drawn from consenting female participants aged 2 to 90 years for another research project, and analyze the specimens for XYZ levels. A graph of XYZ level versus age may look like Figure 19-10.

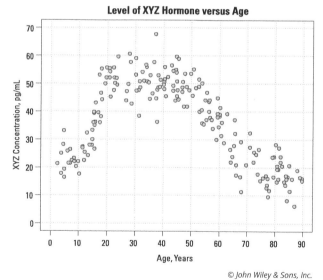

FIGURE 19-10: The relationship between age and hormone concentration doesn't conform to a simple function.

© *John Wiley & Sons, Inc.*

In Figure 19-10, you can observe a lot of scatter in these points, which makes it hard to see the more subtle aspects of the XYZ–age relationship. At what age does the hormone level start to rise? When does it peak? Does it remain fairly constant throughout child-bearing years? When does it start to decline? Is the rate of decline after menopause constant, or does it change with advancing age?

It would be easier to answer those questions if you had a curve that represented the data without all the random fluctuations of the individual points. How would you go about fitting such a curve to these data? LOWESS to the rescue!

Running LOWESS regression in R is similar to other regression. You need to tell R which variable represents x and which one represents y, and it does the rest. If your variables in R are actually named x and y, the R instruction to run a LOWESS regression is the following: lowess($x, y, f = 0.2$). (We explain the $f = 0.2$ part in the following section.)

Unlike other forms of regression, LOWESS doesn't produce a coefficients table. The only output is a table of smoothed y values, one for each data point, which you can save as a data file. Next, using other R commands, you can plot the x and y points from your data, and add a smoothed line superimposed on the scatter graph based on the smoothed y values. Figure 19-11 shows this plot.

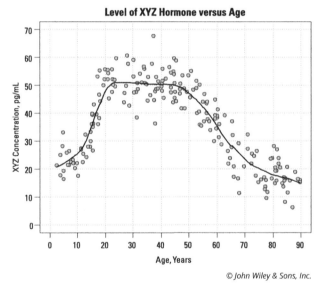

Level of XYZ Hormone versus Age

FIGURE 19-11: The fitted LOWESS curve follows the shape of the data, whatever it may be.

In Figure 19-11, the smoothed curve seems to fit the data quite well across all ages except the lower ones. The individual data points don't show any noticeable upward trend until age 12 or so, but the smoothed curve starts climbing right from age 3. The curve completes its rise by age 20, and then remains flat until almost age 50, when it starts declining. The rate of decline seems to be greatest between ages 50 to 65, after which it declines less rapidly. These subtleties would be very difficult to spot just by looking at the individual data points without any smoothed curve.

Adjusting the amount of smoothing

R's LOWESS program allows you adjust the *stiffness* of the fitted curve by specifying a *smoothing fraction*, called *f*, which is a number between 0 and 1. Figure 19-12 shows what the smoothed curve looks like using three different smoothing fractions.

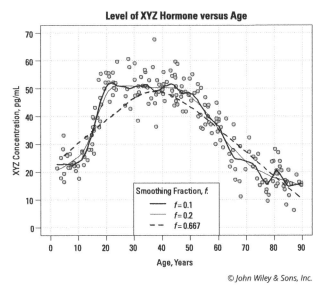

Level of XYZ Hormone versus Age

FIGURE 19-12: You can adjust the smoothness of the fitted curve by adjusting the smoothing fraction.

Looking at Figure 19-12, you can observe the following:

>> Setting *f* = 0.667 produces a rather *stiff* curve that rises steadily between ages 2 and 40, and then declines steadily after that (see dashed line). The value 0.667 represents 2/3, which is what R uses as the default value of the *f* parameter if you don't specify it. This curve misses important features of the data, like the low pre-puberty hormone levels, the flat plateau during child-bearing years, and the slowing down of the yearly decrease above age 65. You can say that this curve shows excessive *bias*, systematically departing from observed values in various places along its length.

>> Setting *f* = 0.1, which is at a lower extreme, produces a very jittery curve with a lot of up-and-down wiggles that can't possibly relate to actual ages, but instead reflect random fluctuations in the data (see dark, solid line). You can say that this curve shows excessive *variance*, with too many random fluctuations along its length.

>> Setting $f = 0.2$ produces a curve that's stiff enough not to have random wiggles (see medium, solid line). Yet, the curve is flexible enough to show that hormone levels are fairly low until age 10, reach their peak at age 20, stay fairly level until age 50, and then decline, with the rate of decline slowing down after age 70. This curve appears to strike a good balance, with low bias and low variance.

REMEMBER

Whenever you do LOWESS regression, you have to explore different smoothing fractions to find the sweet spot that gives the best tradeoff between bias and variance. You are trying to display real features of the curve while smoothing out the random noise. When used properly, LOWESS regression can be helpful as a way of gleaning insight from noisy data.

Chapter **20**

Getting the Hint from Epidemiologic Inference

I n Parts 5 and 6, we describe different types of regression, such as ordinary least-squares regression, logistic regression, Poisson regression, and survival regression. In each kind of regression we cover, we describe a situation in which you are performing *multivariable* or *multivariate* regression, which means you are making a regression model with more than one independent variable. Those chapters describe the mechanics of fitting these multivariable models, but they don't provide much guidance on *which* independent variables to choose to try to put in the multivariable model.

The chapters in Parts 5 and 6 also discuss model-fitting, which means the act of trying to refine your regression model so that it optimally fits your data. When you have a lot of *candidate* independent variables (or *candidate covariates*), part of model-fitting has to do with deciding which of these variables actually fit in the model and should stay in, and which ones don't fit and should be kicked out. Part of what guides this decision-making process are the mechanics of modeling and model-fitting. The other main part of what guides these decisions is the hypothesis you are trying to answer with your model, which is the focus of this chapter.

In this chapter, we revisit the concept of confounding from Chapter 7 and explain how to choose candidate covariates for your regression model. We also discuss modeling approaches and explain how to add interaction terms to your final model.

Staying Clearheaded about Confounding

Chapter 7 discusses study design and terminology in epidemiology. As a reminder, in epidemiology, *exposure* refers to a factor you hypothesize to cause a *disease* (or *outcome*). In your regression model, the outcome is the dependent variable. The exposure will be one of the covariates in your model. But what other covariates belong in the model? How do you decide on a collection of candidate-independent variables that you would even consider putting in a model with the exposure? The answer is that you choose them on the basis of their status as a potential confounder.

REMEMBER

A *confounder* is a factor that meets these three criteria:

>> It is associated with the exposure.

>> It is associated with the outcome.

>> It is *not* on the causal pathway between the exposure and outcome.

As an example, look at Figure 20-1, which illustrates a study of patients with Type II diabetes where there is a hypothesized causal relationship between the exposure of *having served in the military* and the negative outcome of *having an amputation due to diabetic complications*.

As shown Figure 20-1, *inability to exercise* and *low income* are both seen as potential confounders. That is because they are associated with both the exposure of military service and the outcome of amputation, and they are not on the causal pathway between military service and amputation. In other words, what is causing the outcome of amputation is not also causing the patient's inability to exercise, nor is it also causing the patient to have low income. But whatever is causing the patient's amputation is also causing the patient's retinopathy. That's because Type II diabetes causes poor circulation, which causes both retinopathy and amputation. This means that retinopathy and amputation are on the same causal pathway, and retinopathy cannot be considered a potential confounder.

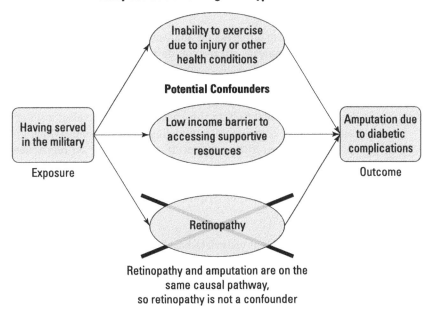

Study of Patients Living with Type II Diabetes

Inability to exercise due to injury or other health conditions

Potential Confounders

Having served in the military

Low income barrier to accessing supportive resources

Amputation due to diabetic complications

Exposure

Outcome

Retinopathy

Retinopathy and amputation are on the same causal pathway, so retinopathy is not a confounder

FIGURE 20-1: Example of how confounders are associated with exposure and outcome but are not on the causal pathway between exposure and outcome.

© John Wiley & Sons, Inc.

Avoiding overloading

You may think that choosing what covariates belong in a regression model is easy. You just put all the confounders and the exposure in as covariates and you're done, right? Well, unfortunately, it's not that simple. Each time you add a covariate to a regression model, you increase the amount of error in the model by some amount — no matter what covariate you choose to add. Although there is no official maximum to the number of covariates in a model, it is possible to add so many covariates that the software cannot compute the model, causing an error. In a logistic regression model as discussed in Chapter 18, each time you add a covariate, you increase the overall likelihood of the model. In Chapter 17, which focuses on ordinary least-squares regression, adding a covariate increases your sum of squares.

What this means is that you don't want to add covariates to your model that just increase error and don't help with the overall goal of model fit. A good strategy is to try to find the best collection of covariates that together deal with as much error as possible. For example, think of it like roommates who share apartment-cleaning duties. It's best if they split up the apartment and each clean different parts of it, rather than insisting on cleaning up the same rooms, which would be a waste of time. The term *parsimony* refers to trying to include the fewest covariates in your regression model that explain the most variation in the dependent variable. The modeling approaches discussed in the next section explain ways to develop such *parsimonious* models.

Adjusting for confounders

When designing a regression analysis, you first have to decide: Are you doing an exploratory analysis, or are you doing a hypothesis-driven analysis? If you are doing an *exploratory analysis,* you do not have a pre-supposed hypothesis. Instead, your aim is to answer the research question, "What group of covariates do I need to include as independent variables in my regression to predict the outcome and get the best model fit?" In this case, you need to select a set of candidate covariates and then come up with modeling rules to decide which groups of covariates produce the best-fitting model. In each chapter on regression in this book, we provide methods of comparing models using model-fit statistics. You would use those to choose your final model for your exploratory analysis. Exploratory analyses are considered descriptive studies, and are weak study designs (see Chapter 7).

But if you collected your data based on a hypothesis, you are doing a *hypothesis-driven analysis.* Epidemiologic studies require hypothesis-driven analyses, where you have already selected your exposure and outcome, and now you have to fit a regression model predicting the outcome, but including your exposure and confounders as covariates. You know you need to include the exposure and the outcome in every model you run. However, you may not know how to decide on which confounders stay in the model.

REMEMBER

Regardless of whether you are doing exploratory or hypothesis-driven modeling, you need to make rules before you start modeling that describe how you will make decisions about your final model and during your modeling process. You may make a rule that all the covariates in your final model must be associated with a p value that is statistically significant at $\alpha = 0.05$. You can make other stipulations about the final model, or the process of achieving the final model. What is important is that you make the modeling rules and write them down before you start modeling.

You then need to choose a modeling approach, which is the approach you will use to determine which candidate confounders stay in the model with the exposure and which ones are removed. There are three common approaches in regression modeling (although analysts have their customized approaches). These approaches don't have official names, but we will use terms that are commonly used. They are: forward stepwise, backward elimination, and stepwise selection.

>> **Forward stepwise:** This is where one confounder covariate at a time is added to the model in iterative models. If it does not meet rules to be kept in the model, it is removed and never considered again in the model. Imagine you were fitting a regression model with one exposure covariate and eight candidate confounders. Suppose that you add the first covariate with the exposure and it meets modeling rules, so you keep it. But when you add the second

covariate, it does not meet the rules, so you leave it out. You keep doing this until you run out of variables. Although forward stepwise can work if you have very few variables, most analysts do not use this approach because it has been shown to be sensitive to the order you choose in which to enter variables.

>> **Backward elimination:** In this approach, the first model you run contains all your potential covariates, including all the confounders and the exposure. Using modeling rules, each time you run the model, you remove or *eliminate* the confounder contributing the least to the model. You decide which one that is based on modeling rules you set (such as which confounder has the largest p value). Theoretically, after you pare away the confounders that do not meet the rules, you will have a final model. In practice, this process can run into problems if you have *collinear* covariates (see Chapters 17 and 18 for a discussions of collinearity). Your first model — filled with all your potential covariates — may error out for this reason, and not converge. Also, it is not clear whether once you eliminate a covariate you should try it again in the model. This approach often sounds better on paper than it works in practice.

>> **Stepwise selection:** This approach combines the best of forward stepwise and backward elimination. Starting with the same set of candidate covariates, you choose which covariate to introduce first into a model with the exposure. If this covariate meets modeling rules, it is kept, and if not, it is left out. This continues along as if you are doing forward stepwise — but then, there's a twist. After you are done trying each covariate and you have your forward stepwise model, you go back and try to add back the covariates you left out one by one. Each time one seems to fit back in, you keep it and consider it part of the *working model*. It is during this phase that collinearity between covariates can become very apparent. After you try back the covariates you originally left out and are satisfied that you were able to add back the ones that fit the modeling rules, you can declare that you have arrived at the final model.

Once you produce your final model, check the p value for the covariate or covariates representing your exposure. If they are not statistically significant, it means that your hypothesis was incorrect, and after controlling for confounding, your exposure was not statistically significantly associated with the outcome. However, if the p value is statistically significant, then you would move on to interpret the results for your exposure covariates from your regression model. After controlling for confounding, your exposure was statistically significantly associated with your outcome. Yay!

TIP

Use a spreadsheet to keep track of each model you run and a summary of the results. Save this in addition to your computer code for running the models. It can help you communicate with others about why certain covariates were retained and not retained in your final model.

WARNING

Computer software may include automated processes you can use for fitting models. We discourage you from using these in biostatistics because you want to have a lot of control over how a model is being fitted to make it possible for you to interpret the results. However, these processes can be used to create comparison models — or to simulate improved models — which are perfectly reasonable methods to explore ways to improve your model.

Understanding Interaction (Effect Modification)

In Chapter 17, we touch on the topic of interaction (also known as *effect modification*). This is where the relationship between an exposure and an outcome is strongly dependent upon the status of another covariate. Imagine that you conducted a study of laborers who had been exposed to asbestos at work, and you found that being exposed to asbestos at work was associated with three times the odds of getting lung cancer compared to not being exposed. In another study, you found that individuals who smoked cigarettes had twice the odds of getting lung cancer compared to those who did not smoke.

Knowing this, what would you predict are the odds of getting lung cancer for asbestos-exposed workers who also smoke cigarettes, compared to workers who aren't exposed to asbestos and do not smoke cigarettes? Do you think it would be *additive* — meaning three times for asbestos plus two times for smoking equals five times the odds? Or do you think it would be *multiplicative* — meaning three times two equals six times the odds?

Although this is just an example, it turns out that in real life, the effect of being exposed to both asbestos and cigarette smoking represents a greater than multiplicative synergistic interaction (meaning much greater than six) in terms of the odds for getting lung cancer. In other words, the risk of getting lung cancer for cigarette smokers is dependent upon their asbestos-exposure status, and the risk of lung cancer for asbestos workers is dependent upon their cigarette-smoking status. Because the factors work together to increase the risk, this is a synergistic interaction (with the opposite being an antagonistic interaction).

How and when do you model an interaction in regression? Typically, you first fit your final model using a multivariate regression approach (see the earlier section "Adjusting for confounders in regression" for more on this). Next, once the final model is fit, you try to interact the exposure covariate or covariates with a confounder that you believe is the other part of the interaction. After that, you look at the p value on the interaction term and decide whether or not to keep the interaction.

Imagine making a model for the study of asbestos workers, cigarette smoking, and lung cancer. The variable *asbestos* is coded 1 for workers exposed to asbestos and 0 for workers not exposed to asbestos, and the variable *smoker* is coded 1 for cigarette smokers and 0 for nonsmokers. The final model would already have *asbestos* and *smoker* in it, so the interaction model would add the additional covariate *asbestos* × *smoker*, which is called the higher order *interaction term*. For individuals who have a 0 for either *asbestos* or *smoker* or both, this term falls out of their individual predicted probability (because $1 \times 0 = 0$, and $0 \times 0 = 0$). Therefore, if this term is statistically significant, then individuals who qualify to include this term in their individual predicted probability have a statistically significantly greater risk of the outcome, and the interaction term should be kept in the model.

Getting Casual about Cause

Chapter 7 explains epidemiologic study designs and presents them in a pyramid format. The closer to the top of the pyramid, the better the study design is at providing evidence for causal inference, meaning providing evidence of a causal association between the exposure with the outcome (or in the case of a clinical trial of an intervention, the intervention and the outcome). At the top of the pyramid are systematic review and meta-analysis, where the results of similar studies are combined and interpreted. Because systematic reviews and meta-analyses combine results from other high-quality studies, they are at the very top of the pyramid — meaning they provide the strongest evidence of a causal association between the exposure or intervention and outcome.

TIP

An international organization called the Cochrane Collaboration organizes the production of systematic reviews and meta-analyses to help guide clinicians. Their reviews are internationally renowned for being high-quality and are available at www.cochrane.org.

The study designs on the evidence-based pyramid that could be answered with a regression model include clinical trial, cohort study, case-control study, and cross-sectional study. If in your final model your exposure is statistically significantly associated with your outcome, you now have to see how much evidence you have that the exposure caused the outcome. This section provides two methods by which to evaluate the significant exposure and outcome relationship in your regression: Rothman's causal pie and Bradford Hill's criteria of causality.

Rothman's causal pie

Kenneth Rothman described how causes of an outcome are not determinate. In other words, two people can have the same values of covariates and one will get the outcome, and the other will not. We can't say for sure what values of covariates will mean that you will for sure get the outcome. But that doesn't mean you can't make causal inferences. Rothman conceptualized *cause* as an empty pie tin, and when the pie tin is filled 100 percent with pieces of risk contributed by various causes, then the individual will experience the outcome. The exposure and confounders in your regression model represent these pieces.

For example, cigarette smoking is a very strong cause of lung cancer, as is occupational exposure to asbestos. There are other causes, but for each individual, these other causes would fill up small pieces of the causal pie for lung cancer. Some may have a higher genetic risk factor for cancer. However, if they do not smoke and stay away from asbestos, they will not fill up much of their pie tin, and may have *necessary but insufficient* cause for lung cancer. However, if they include both asbestos exposure and smoking in their tin, they are risking filling it up and getting the outcome.

Bradford Hill's criteria of causality

>> Sir Bradford Hill was a British epidemiologist who put forth criteria for causality that can be useful to consider when thinking of statistically significant exposure–outcome relationships from final regression models. Although there are more than the criteria we list here, we find the following criteria to be the most useful when evaluating potential exposure–outcome causal relationships in final models:

>> First, consider if the data you are analyzing are from a clinical trial or cohort study. If they are, then you will have met the criterion of *temporality,* which means the exposure or intervention preceded the outcome and is especially strong evidence for causation.

>> If the estimate for the exposure in your regression model is large, you can say you have a strong *magnitude* of association, and this is evidence of causation. This is especially true if your estimate is larger than those of the confounders in the model as well as similar estimates from the scientific literature.

>> If your exposure shows a *dose-response relationship* with the outcome, it is evidence of causation. In other words, if your regression model shows that the more individuals smoke, the higher their risk for lung cancer, this is evidence of causation (see Chapter 18 for more on dose-response relationships).

>> If the estimate is *consistent* in size and direction with other analyses, including previous studies you've done and studies in the scientific literature, there is more evidence for causation.

Analyzing Survival Data

6

Learn the definition of survival data and how to handle censored observations (where you do not observe the outcome as part of your study).

Prepare survival curves using the life-table and Kaplan-Meier methods.

Estimate median survival times and survival rates at specified times.

Compare survival curves between two or more groups using the log-rank test.

Analyze multiple predictors of survival using Cox proportional hazards regression.

Chapter **21**

Summarizing and Graphing Survival Data

T his chapter describes statistical techniques that deal with a special kind of numerical data called *survival data* or *time-to-event data*. These data reflect the interval from a particular starting point in time, such the date a patient receives a certain diagnosis or undergoes a certain procedure, to the first or only occurrence of a particular kind of event that represents an endpoint. Because these techniques are often applied to situations where the endpoint event is death, we usually call the use of these techniques *survival analysis,* even when the endpoint is something less drastic (or final) than death. Survival data could include time from resolution of a chronic illness symptom to its relapse, but it can also be a desirable endpoint, such as time to remission of cancer, or time to recovery from an acute condition. Throughout this chapter, we use terms and examples that imply that the endpoint is death, such as saying *survival time* instead of *time to event*. However, everything we say also applies to other kinds of endpoints.

You may wonder why you need a special kind of analysis for survival data in the first place. Why not just treat survival times as ordinary numerical variables? Why not summarize them as means, medians, standard deviations, and so on, and graph them as histograms and box-and-whiskers charts? Why not compare survival times between groups with t tests and ANOVAs? Why not use ordinary least-squares regression to explore how various factors influence survival time?

In this chapter, we explain how survival data aren't like ordinary numerical data and why you need to use specific techniques to analyze them properly. We describe two ways to construct survival curves: the life-table and the Kaplan–Meier methods. We guide you in preparing and interpreting survival curves and show you how to glean useful information from these curves, such as median survival time and five-year survival rates.

Understanding the Basics of Survival Data

To understand survival analysis, you first have to understand survival data. Survival times are *intervals* between a designated starting time point and the time point an event occurs. These intervals have can have a specific type of missing data due to a phenomenon called *censoring*. Because survival data usually include censored data, they must be analyzed in a very specific way to avoid generating biased estimates that lead to incorrect conclusions.

Examining how survival times are intervals

The techniques described in this chapter for summarizing, graphing, and comparing survival data deal with the time interval from a defined starting point to the first occurrence of an endpoint event. The event can be designated as death or a relapse of a particular condition, such as a recurrence of cancer. Or you could designate the event to be surgical removal (called an explant) of a failed mechanical component, such as an artificial heart valve. If a patient's heart valve was implanted on January 10 (beginning of time interval), but their body rejected it and the explant took place on January 30 (time of event), then the time interval from implant to explant is 30 − 10, or 20 days.

A person can die only once, so survival analysis can obviously be used for one-time events. But other endpoints can occur multiple times, such as having a stroke or having cancer go into remission. The techniques we describe in this chapter *only* analyze time to the first occurrence of the event. More advanced survival analysis methods are needed for models that can handle multiple occurrences of an event, and these are beyond the scope of this book.

REMEMBER

The starting point of the time interval is somewhat arbitrary, so it must be defined explicitly every time you do a survival analysis. Imagine that you're studying the progression of chronic obstructive pulmonary disease (COPD) in a group of patients. If you want to study the natural history of the disease, the starting point can be the diagnosis date. But if you're instead interested in evaluating the efficacy of a treatment, the starting point can be defined as the date the treatment began.

Recognizing that survival times aren't normally distributed

WARNING

Even though survival times are numerical quantities, they're almost never normally distributed. Because of this, it's generally *not* a good idea to use the following:

>> Means and standard deviations to describe survival times

>> T tests and ANOVAs to compare survival times between groups

>> Least-squares regression to investigate how survival time is influenced by other factors

If non-normality were the only problem with survival data, you'd be able to summarize survival times as medians and centiles instead of means and standard deviations. Also, you could compare survival between groups with nonparametric Mann-Whitney and Kruskal-Wallis tests instead of t tests and ANOVAs. But time-to-event data are susceptible to a specific type of missingness called *censoring.* Typical parametric and nonparametric regression methods are not equipped to deal with censoring, so we present survival analysis techniques in this chapter.

Considering censoring

Survival data are defined as the time interval between a selected starting point and an endpoint that represents an event. But unfortunately, the time the event takes place can be missing in survival data. This can happen in two general ways:

>> **You may not be able to observe all the participants in the data until they have the event.** Because of time constraints, at some point, you have to end the study and analyze your data. If your endpoint is death, hopefully at the end of your study, some of the participants are still alive! At that point, you would not know how much longer these participants will ultimately live. You only know that they were still alive up to the last date they were measured in the study as part of data collection, or the last date study staff communicated with them in some way (such as through a follow-up phone call). This date is called the *date of last contact* or the *last-seen date,* and would be the date that these participants would be censored in your data.

>> **You may lose track of some participants during the study.** Participants who enroll in a study may be *lost to follow-up* (LFU), meaning that it is no longer possible for study staff to locate them and continue to collect data for the study. These participants are also censored at their date of last contact, but in the case of LFU, this date is typically well before the observation period ends.

You can describe these two situations in one general way. You know that every participant in the study either died on a certain date (in which case they have the event), or was alive up to some last-seen date when they stopped being observed, in which case they are censored.

Figure 21-1 shows the results of a small study of survival in cancer patients after a surgical procedure to remove a tumor. Ten patients were recruited to participate in the study and were enrolled at the time of their surgery. The recruitment period went from Jan. 1, 2010, to the end of Dec. 31, 2011 (meaning a two-year enrollment period). All participants were then followed until they died, or until the conclusion of the study, on Dec. 31, 2016, which added five years of additional observation time after the last enrollment. Each participant has a horizontal timeline that starts on the date of surgery and ends with either the date of death or the censoring date.

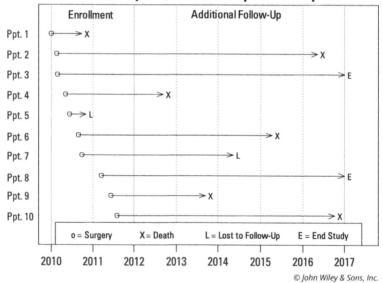

FIGURE 21-1: Survival of ten study participants following surgery for cancer.

© John Wiley & Sons, Inc.

In Figure 21-1, observe that each line ends with a code, and there's a legend at the bottom. Six of the ten participants (#'s 1, 2, 4, 6, 9, and 10, labeled X) died during the course of the follow-up study. Two participants (#5 and #7, labeled L) were LFU at some point during the study, and two participants (#3 and #8, labeled E) were still alive at the end of the study. So this study has four participants — the Ls and the Es — with censored survival times.

So, how do you analyze survival data containing censoring? The following sections explain the correct ways to proceed as well as mistakes to avoid.

Analyzing censored data properly

REMEMBER

Statisticians have developed techniques to utilize the partial information contained in censored observations. We describe two of the most popular techniques later in this chapter, which are the life-table method and the Kaplan-Meier (K-M) method. To understand these methods, you need to first understand two fundamental concepts — *hazard* and *survival*:

>> **The hazard rate** is the probability of the participant dying in the next small interval of time, assuming the participant is alive right now.

>> **The survival rate** is the probability of the participant living for a certain amount of time after some starting time point.

The first task when analyzing survival data is usually to describe how the hazard and survival rates vary with time. In this chapter, we show you how to estimate the hazard and survival rates, summarize them as tables, and display them as graphs. Most of the larger statistical packages (such as those described in Chapter 4) allow you to do the calculations we describe automatically, so you may never have to do them manually. But without first understanding how these methods work, it's almost impossible to understand any other aspect of survival analysis, so we provide a demonstration for instructional purposes.

Making mistakes with censored data

WARNING

Here are two mistakes you need to avoid when working with survival data:

>> You *shouldn't* exclude participants with a censored survival time from any survival analysis!

>> You *shouldn't* substitute the censored date with some other value, which is called *imputing*. When you impute numerical data to replace a missing value, it is common to use the last observed value for that participant (called *last observation carried forward,* or LOCF, imputation). However, you should not impute dates in survival analysis.

Exclusion and imputation don't work to fix the missingness in censored data. You can see why in Figure 21-2, where we've slid the timelines for all the participants over to the left as if they all had their surgery on the same date. The time scale shows survival time in years after surgery instead of chronological time.

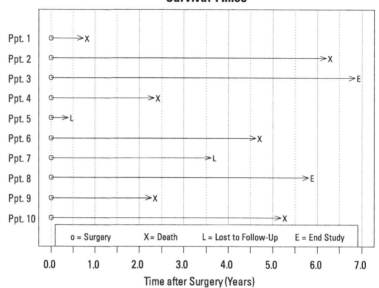

FIGURE 21-2:
Survival times
from the date of
surgery.

Survival Times

o = Surgery   X = Death   L = Lost to Follow-Up   E = End Study

© John Wiley & Sons, Inc.

If you exclude all participants who were censored in your analysis, you may be left with analyzable data on too few participants. In this example, there are only six uncensored participants, and removing them would weaken the power of the analysis. Worse, it would also bias the results in subtle and unpredictable ways.

Using the last-seen date in place of the death date for a censored observation may seem like a legitimate use of LOCF imputation, but because the participant did not die during the observation period, it is not acceptable. It's equivalent to assuming that all censored participants died immediately after the last-contact date. But this assumption isn't reasonable, because it would not be unusual for them to live on many years. This assumption would also bias your results toward artificially shorter survival times.

TIP

In your analytic data set, only include one variable to represent time observed (such as *Time* in days, months, or years), and one variable to represent event status (such as *Event* or *Death*), coded as 1 if they are have the event during the observation period, and 0 if they are censored. Calculate these variables from raw date variables stored in other parts of the data (such as date of death, date of visit, and so on).

Looking at the Life-Table Method

To estimate survival and hazard rates in a population from a set of observed survival times, some of which are censored, you must combine the information from censored and uncensored observations properly. How is this done? Well, it's *not* done by dividing the number of participants alive at a certain time point in the study by the total number of participants in the study, because this fails to account for censored observations.

Instead, think of the observation period in a study as a series of slices of time. Think about how each time a participant survives a slice of time and encounters the next one, they have a certain probability of surviving to the end of that slice and continuing on to encounter the next. The cumulative survival probability can then be obtained by successively multiplying all these individual time-slice survival probabilities together. For example, to survive three years, first the participant has to survive the first slice (Year 1), then survive the second slice (Year 2), and then survive the third slice (Year 3). The probability of surviving all three years is the product of the probabilities of surviving through Year 1, Year 2, and Year 3.

These calculations can be laid out systematically in a *life table,* which is also called an *actuarial life table* because of its early use by insurance companies. The calculations only involve addition, subtraction, multiplication, and division, so they can be done manually. They are easy to set up in a spreadsheet format, and there are many life-table templates available for Microsoft Excel and other spreadsheet programs that you can use.

Making a life table

To create a life table from your survival data, you should first break the entire range of survival times into convenient time slices. These can be months, quarters, or years, depending on the time scale of the event you're studying. Also, you have to consider the time increments in which you want to report your results. You should arrange to have at least five slices or else your survival and hazard estimates will be too coarse to show any useful features. Having many skinny slices doesn't disturb the calculations, but the life table will have many rows and may become unwieldy. For the survival times shown in Figure 21-2, a natural choice would be to use seven 1-year time slices.

Next, count how many participants experienced the event during each slice, and how many were *censored*, meaning they were last observed during this time slice and had not experienced the event. From Figure 21-2, you see that

>> During the first year after surgery, one participant died (#1), and one participant was censored (#5, who was LFU).

>> During the second year, no participants died or were censored.

>> During the third year, two participants died (#4 and #9), and none were censored.

Continue tabulating deaths and censored times for the fourth through seventh years, and enter these counts into the appropriate cells of a spreadsheet like the one shown in Figure 21-3.

A	B	C	D	E	F	G	H
Formula:	B – C – D in Prev Row	(data)	(data)	B – D/2	C/E	1 – F	Running Product of G
Time Slice	Alive at Start	Died	Last Seen Alive	At Risk	Probability of Dying	Probability of Surviving	Cumulative Survival
0–1 yr	10	1	1				
1–2 yr		0	0				
2–3 yr		2	0				
3–4 yr		0	1				
4–5 yr		1	0				
5–6 yr		1	1				
6–7 yr		1	1				

FIGURE 21-3: A partially completed life table to analyze the survival times shown in Figure 21-2.

© John Wiley & Sons, Inc.

To fill in the table shown in Figure 21-3:

>> Put the description of the time interval that defines each slice into Column A.

>> Enter the total number of participants alive at the start into Column B in the 0–1 yr row.

>> Enter the counts of participants who died within each time slice into Column C (labeled *Died*).

>> Enter the counts of participants who were censored during each time slice into Column D (labeled *Last Seen Alive*).

After you've entered all the counts, the spreadsheet will look like Figure 21-3. Then you perform the calculations shown in the *Formula* row at the top of the figure to generate the numbers in all the other cells of the table. (To see what it looks like when the table is completely filled in, take a sneak peek at Figure 21-4.)

Columns B, C, and D

Column B includes the number of participants known to be alive at the start of each year after surgery. This is equal to the number of participants alive at the start of the preceding year minus the number who died (Column C) or were censored (Column D) during the preceding year. Here's the formula, written in terms of the column letters: B for any year = B − C − D from the preceding year.

Here's how this process plays out in Figure 21-3:

>> Out of the ten participants alive at the start, one died and one was last seen alive during the first year. This means eight participants (10 − 1 − 1) are known to still be alive at the start of the second year. The missing participant is #5, who was LFU during the first year. They are censored and not counted in any subsequent years.

>> Zero participants died or were last seen alive during the second year. So, the same eight participants are still known to be alive at the start of the third year.

>> Calculations continue the same way for the remaining years.

Column E

Column E shows the number of participants *at risk for dying* during each year. You may guess that this is the number of participants alive at the start of the interval, but there's one minor correction. If any were censored during that year, then they weren't technically able to be observed for the entire year. Though they may die that year, if they are censored before then, the study will miss it. What if you don't know exactly when during that year they became censored? If you don't have the exact date, you can consider them being observed for half the time period (in this case, 0.5 years). So the number at risk can be estimated as the number alive at the start of the year, minus one-half of the number who became censored during that year, as indicated by the formula for Column E: E = B − D/2. (*Note:* To simplify the example, we are using years, but you could use months instead if you have exact censoring and death dates in your data to improve the accuracy of your analysis.)

Here's how this formula works in Figure 21-3:

>> Ten participants were alive at the start of Year 1, and one participant was censored during Year 1. To correct for censoring, divide 1 by 2, which is 0.5. Next, subtract 0.5 from 10 to get 9.5. After correcting for censoring, only 9.5 participants are at risk of dying during Year 1.

>> Eight participants were alive at the start of Year 2, and zero were censored during Year 2. So all eight participants continued to be at risk during Year 2.

>> Calculations continue in the same way for the remaining years.

Column F

Column F shows the *Probability of Dying* during each interval, assuming the participant has survived up to the start of that interval. To calculate this, divide the *Died* column by the *At Risk* column. This represents the fraction of those who were at risk of dying at the beginning of the interval who actually died during the interval. Formula for Column F: F = C/E.

Here's how this formula works in Figure 22-3:

>> For Year 1, the probability of dying is calculated by dividing the one death by the 9.5 participants at risk: 1/9.5, or 0.105 (10.5 percent).

>> Zero participants died in Year 2. So, for participants surviving Year 1 and alive at the beginning of Year 2, the probability of dying during Year 2 is 0. Woo-hoo!

>> Calculations continue in the same way for the remaining years.

Column G

Column G shows the *Probability of Surviving* during each interval for participants who have survived up to the start of that interval. Since surviving means not dying, the equation for this column is 1 − *Probability of Dying*, as indicated by the formula for Column G: G = 1 − F.

Here's how this formula works out in Figure 22-3:

>> The probability of dying in Year 1 is 0.105, so the probability of surviving in Year 1 is 1 − 0.105, or 0.895.

>> The probability of dying in Year 2 is 0.000, so the probability of surviving in Year 2 is 1 − 0.000, or 1.000.

>> Calculations continue in the same way for the remaining years.

Column H

Column H shows the cumulative probability of surviving from the time of surgery all the way through the end of this time slice. To survive from the start time through the end of any given year (year *N*), the participant must survive each of the years from Year 1 through Year N. Because surviving each year is an independent accomplishment, the probability of surviving all N of the years is the product of the individual years' probabilities. So Column H is a *running product* of Column G. In other words, the value of Column H for Year N is the product of the first N values in Column G.

Here's to fill in Figure 22-3 (with the results shown in Figure 22-4):

>> For Year 1, H is the same as G: a 0.895 probability of surviving one year.

>> For Year 2, H is the product of G for Year 1 times G for Year 2; that is, 0.895×1.000, or 0.895.

>> For Year 3, H is the product of the Gs for Years 1, 2, and 3; that is, $0.895 \times 1.000 \times 0.750$, or 0.671.

>> Calculations continue in the same way for the remaining years.

Putting everything together

Figure 21-4 shows the spreadsheet with the results of all the preceding calculations.

FIGURE 21-4:
Completed life
table to analyze
the survival
times shown in
Figure 22-2.

A	B	C	D	E	F	G	H
Formula:	B − C − D in Prev Row	(data)	(data)	B − D/2	C/E	1 − F	Running Product of G
Time Slice	Alive at Start	Died	Last Seen Alive	At Risk	Probability of Dying	Probability of Surviving	Cumulative Survival
0–1 yr	10	1	1	9.50	0.105	0.895	0.895
1–2 yr	8	0	0	8.00	0.000	1.000	0.895
2–3 yr	8	2	0	8.00	0.250	0.750	0.671
3–4 yr	6	0	1	5.50	0.000	1.000	0.671
4–5 yr	5	1	0	5.00	0.200	0.800	0.537
5–6 yr	4	1	1	3.50	0.286	0.714	0.383
6–7 yr	2	1	1	1.50	0.667	0.333	0.128

© *John Wiley & Sons, Inc.*

Interpreting a life table

REMEMBER

Figure 21-4 contains the hazard rates (in Column F) and the cumulative survival probabilities (in Column H) for each year following surgery, based on your sample of ten participants. Keep in mind these life-table features:

>> The hazard and survival values obtained from this life table are estimates from a sample of the true population hazard and survival functions (in this case, using one-year intervals).

>> The intervals are often the same size for all the rows in a life table like in the example, but they don't have to be. You may choose these on the basis of the probabilities in your data.

>> The hazard rate obtained from a life table for each time slice is equal to the *Probability of Dying* (Column F) divided by the width of the slice. Therefore, the hazard rate for the first year would be expressed as 0.105 per year, or 10.5 percent per year.

>> The *Cumulative Survival* probability, in Column H, is the probability of surviving from the start date through to the end of the interval. It has no units, and it can be expressed as a fraction or as a percentage. The value for any time slice applies to the moment in time at the end of the interval.

>> The cumulative survival probability is always 1.0 (or 100 percent) at time 0, whenever you designate that time 0 is (in the example, date of surgery), but it's not included in the table.

>> The cumulative survival function decreases only at the end of an interval that has at least one observed death, because censored observations don't cause a decrease in the estimated survival. Censored observations however influence the size of the decreases when subsequent events occur. This is because censoring reduces the number at risk, which is used in the denominator in the calculation of the death and survival probabilities.

>> If an interval contains no events and no censoring, like in the 1–2 years row in the table in Figure 21-4, it has no impact on the calculations. Notice how all subsequent values for Column B and for Columns E through H would remain identical if that row were removed.

Graphing hazard rates and survival probabilities from a life table

Graphs of hazard rates and cumulative survival probabilities (Columns F and H from Figure 21-4, respectively) can be prepared from life-table results using Microsoft Excel or another spreadsheet or statistical program with graphing capabilities. Figure 21-5 illustrates the way these results are typically presented.

>> **Figure 21-5a is a graph of hazard rates.** Hazard rates are often graphed as bar charts, because each time slice has its own hazard rate in a life table.

>> **Figure 21-5b is a graph of cumulative survival probabilities,** also known as the survival function. Survival values are usually graphed as *stepped line charts,*

where a horizontal line represents the cumulative survival probability during each time slice. The cumulative survival for the Year 0 to 1 time slice is 1.0 (100 percent), so the horizontal line stays at y = 1.0. But between Year 1 and Year 3, the cumulative survival probability drops to 0.895, so a vertical line is dropped from 1.0 to y = 0.895 at the time the Year 1 to Year 2 interval starts. It goes across both that interval and the next one because there are no deaths in these intervals. This stepped line continues downstairs and finally ends at the end of the last interval where the cumulative survival probability is 0.128.

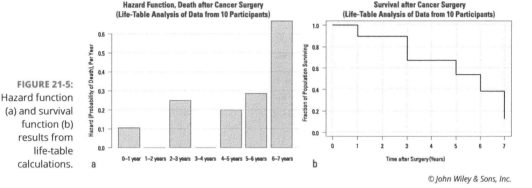

FIGURE 21-5: Hazard function (a) and survival function (b) results from life-table calculations.

© John Wiley & Sons, Inc.

Digging Deeper with the Kaplan-Meier Method

Using very narrow time slices doesn't hurt life-table calculations. In fact, you can define slices so narrow that each participant's survival time falls within its own private little slice. Imagine you had N participants. Your life table would have N rows with data from one participant each. You could theoretically add all rest of the rows to fill out the rest of the time slices. These would not have any data in them, and since empty rows don't affect the life-table calculations, you could just stick with your life table where each row has one participant's data. And if you happen to have two or more participants with exactly the same survival or censoring time, it's okay to put each one in their own row.

The life-table calculations work fine with only one participant per row and produce what's called *Kaplan–Meier (K–M) survival estimates*. You can think of the K–M method as a very fine-grained life table. Or, you can see a life table as a grouped K–M calculation.

A K–M worksheet for the survival times is shown in Figure 21-6. It is based on the one-participant-per-row idea and is laid out much like the usual life-table worksheet shown in Figure 22-4, but with a few differences in the raw data cells and minor differences in the calculations:

>> Instead of a column identifying the time slices, there are two columns identifying the individual participant (Column A) and their survival or censoring time (Column B). The table is ordered from the shortest time to the longest.

>> Instead of two columns containing the number who died and were censored in each interval, you need only one column indicating whether or not the participant in that row died (Column C). If they died during the observation period, use code 1, and if not and they were censored, use code 0.

>> These changes mean that Column D labeled *Alive at Start* now decreases by 1 for each subsequent row.

>> The *At Risk* column in Figure 21-4 isn't needed, because it can be calculated from the *Alive at Start* column. That's because if the participant is censored, the probability of dying is calculated as 0, regardless of the value of the denominator.

>> To calculate Column E, the *Probability of Dying*, divide the *Died* indicator by the number of participants alive for that time period in Column D, *Alive at Start*. Formula: E = C/D.

>> The probability of surviving (Column F) and the cumulative survival (Column G) are calculated the same way as in the life-table method.

A	B	C	D	E	F	G
Formula:	(data)	(data)	B – D/2	C/E	1 – E	Running Product of F
Ppt.	Death/Cens Time After Surgery (years)	Died	Alive at Start	Probability of Dying	Probability of Surviving	Cumulative Survival
5	0.40	0	10	0.000	1.000	1.000
1	0.74	1	9	0.111	0.889	0.889
9	2.27	1	8	0.125	0.875	0.778
4	2.34	1	7	0.143	0.857	0.667
7	3.61	0	6	0.000	1.000	0.667
6	4.62	1	5	0.200	0.800	0.533
10	5.18	1	4	0.250	0.750	0.400
8	5.80	0	3	0.000	1.000	0.400
2	6.21	1	2	0.500	0.500	0.200
3	6.85	0	1	0.000	1.000	0.200

FIGURE 21-6:
Kaplan-Meier
calculations.

© *John Wiley & Sons, Inc.*

Figure 21-7 shows graphs of the K-M hazard and survival estimates from Figure 21-6. These charts were created using the R statistical software. Most software that performs survival analysis can create graphs similar to this. The K-M survival curve in Figure 21-7b has smaller steps than the life-table survival curve in Figure 21-5b, so it's more fine-grained. This is because the step curve now decreases at every time point at which a participant died. You can tell from the figures where participant #1 died at 0.74 years, #9 died at 2.27 years, #4 died at 2.34 years, and so on.

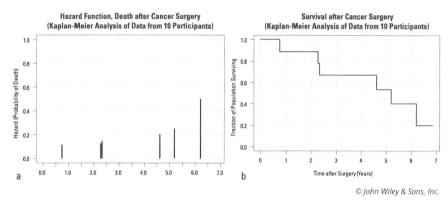

FIGURE 21-7: Kaplan-Meier estimates of the hazard (a) and survival (b) functions.

© John Wiley & Sons, Inc.

WARNING

While the K-M survival curve tends to be smoother than the life table survival curve, just the opposite is true for the hazard curve. In Figure 21-7a, each participant has their own very thin bar, and the resulting chart isn't easy to interpret.

Heeding a Few Guidelines for Life-Tables and the Kaplan-Meier Method

Most of the larger statistical packages (see Chapter 4) can perform life-table and Kaplan-Meier calculations for you and directly generate survival curves. You have to identify two variables for the software: one with the survival time for each participant, and a binary variable coded 1 if the survival time represents time to death or the event, and 0 if it represents censored time. It sounds simple, but it's surprisingly easy to mess up. Here are some pointers for setting up your data and interpreting the results properly.

Recording survival times correctly

REMEMBER

It is important to draw a distinction between data collection and data analysis. When recording the raw data, it's best to collect all the relevant dates for the study. Before the study starts, the dates of interest for data collection should be specified, which could include date of diagnosis, start of therapy, end of therapy, start of improvement or remission, date of relapse, or others. For events, you should record date of each event if it recurs, and even if death is not the event of interest, date of death should be recorded if available. For censoring purposes, ensure that you are collecting dates of contact so you can identify a last-seen date if needed. If you collect your data properly, you will later be able to calculate any time interval needed, as well as create an event status indicator needed.

Dates and times should be recorded to suitable precision. If your study timeline is years, it's best to keep track of dates to the day. In a Phase I clinical trial (see Chapter 5), participants may be studied for events that happen in a span of a few days. In those cases, it's important to record dates and times to the nearest hour or minute. You can even envision laboratory studies of intracellular events where time would have to be recorded with millisecond — or even microsecond — precision!

TECHNICAL STUFF

Dates and times can be stored in different ways in different statistical software (as well as Microsoft Excel). Designating columns as being in date format or time format can allow you to perform *calendar arithmetic*, allowing you to obtain time intervals by subtracting one date from another.

Miscoding censoring information

It can be surprisingly easy to miscode the event status indicator. If the name of the variable is *Death*, and is coded as 1 if the participant died during the observation period and 0 if they were censored, this seems intuitive. But analysts may want to identify all the censored observations in their data, so they may create a censored indicator named *Censored*, and code it as 1 if the participant is censored, and 0 if they are not. Because data may be used for different types of survival analyses, there could be other event indicators included in the data as well also coded as 1 and 0.

The problem is that if you accidentally use your censored indicator instead of your event indicator when running your survival analysis, you will unknowingly flip your analysis, and you won't get any warning or error message from the program. You'll only get incorrect results. Worse, depending on how many censored and uncensored observations you have, the survival curve may also not hint at any errors. It may look like a perfectly reasonable survival curve for your data, even though it's completely wrong.

REMEMBER

You have to read your software's documentation carefully to make sure you code your event variable correctly. Also, you should always check the program's output for the number of censored and uncensored observations and compare them to the known count of censored and uncensored participants in your data file.

Chapter **22**

Comparing Survival Times

The life table and Kaplan–Meier survival curves described in Chapter 21 are ideal for summarizing and describing the time to the first or only occurrence of a particular event based on times observed in a sample of individuals. They correctly incorporate data that reflect when an individual is observed during the study but does not experience the event, which is called *censored* data. Animal and human studies involving endpoints that occur on a short time-scale, like measurements taking during an experimental surgical procedure, may yield totally uncensored data. However, the more common situation is that during the observation period of studies, not all individuals experience the event, so you usually have censored data on your hands.

In biological research and especially in clinical trials (discussed in Chapter 5), you often want to compare survival times between two or more groups of individuals. In humans, this may have to do with survival after cancer surgery. In animals, it may have to do with testing the toxicity of a potential therapeutic. This chapter describes an important method for comparing survival curves between two groups called the *log-rank test*, and explains how to calculate the sample size you need to have sufficient statistical power for this test (see Chapter 3). The log-rank test can be extended to handle three or more groups, but this discussion is beyond the scope of this book.

REMEMBER

In this chapter, as in Chapters 21 and 23, we use the term *survival* in reference to the outcome of death. However, all the calculations pertain to any type of outcome event being studied, including good ones, such as cancer going into remission.

WARNING

There is some ambiguity associated with the name *log-rank test*. It has also been called different names (such as the Mantel-Cox test), and has been extended into variants such as the Gehan-Breslow test. You may also observe that different software may calculates the log-rank test slightly differently. In this chapter, we describe the most commonly used form of the log-rank test.

REMEMBER

If have no censored observations in your data, you can skip most of this chapter. This may happen if, for example, death is your outcome and at the end of your study period no individuals are alive anymore — they all have died in your study. As you may guess, this situation is much more common in animal studies than human studies. But if you have followed all the individuals in your data until they all experienced the outcome, and you have two or more groups of numbers indicating survival times that you want to compare, you can use approaches described in Chapter 11. One option is to use an unpaired Student t test to test whether one group has a statistically significantly longer mean survival time than the other. If you have three or more groups, you would use an ANOVA instead. But because survival times are very likely to be non-normally distributed, you may prefer to use a nonparametric test, such as the Wilcoxon Sum-of-Ranks test or Mann-Whitney U test, to compare the median survival time between two groups. With more than two groups, you would use the nonparametric Kruskal-Wallis test.

Suppose that you conduct a toxicity study with laboratory animals of a potential cancer drug. You obtain 90 experimental mice. The mice are randomly placed in groups such that 60 receive the drug in their food, and 30 are given control food with no drug. A laboratory worker observes them and records their vital status every day after the experiment starts, taking note of when each animal dies or is censored, meaning they are taken out of the study for another reason (such as not eating). You perform a life-table analysis on each group of mice — the drug compared to control — as described in Chapter 21, and graph the results. The graph displays the survival curves shown in Figure 22-1. As a bonus, the two life tables generated to support this display also provide the summary information needed the log-rank test.

The two survival curves in Figure 22-1 look different. The drug group seems to be showing better survival than the control group. But is this apparent difference real, or could it be the result of random fluctuations only? The log-rank test answers this question.

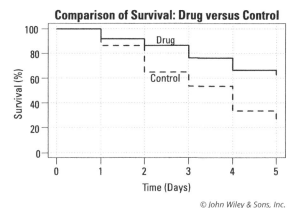

FIGURE 22-1:
Survival curves
for two groups of
laboratory
animals.

Comparing Survival between Two Groups with the Log-Rank Test

The log-rank test can be performed using individual-level data, or on data that has been summarized into a life-table format. In this section, we describe how to run a log-rank test with statistical software, which is how it is usually done. Next, to help you understand the underlying calculations, we describe the log-rank test calculations in detail using the life-table as you might carry them out manually using spreadsheet software such as Microsoft Excel.

Understanding what the log-rank test is doing

A two-group log-rank test asks whether events — which are deaths in our example — are split between the two groups in the same proportion as the number of at-risk individuals in the two groups. The computer selects a group and sums the difference between the observed and expected number of deaths in each time slice over all the time slices to get the total excess deaths for that group. The excess death sum is then *scaled down*, meaning it is divided by an estimate of its standard deviation. (Later in this chapter we describe how to calculate that standard deviation estimate.) The scaled-down excess deaths sum is a number whose random sampling fluctuations should follow a normal distribution, and from which a p value can be easily calculated. The null hypothesis of the log-rank test is that there is no difference in survival between the two groups, so a p value less than your selected α (usually 0.05) indicates a statistically significant difference.

Don't worry if the preceding paragraph makes your head spin. It is only meant to give you a general sense behind the calculations in the log-rank test.

Running the log-rank test on software

REMEMBER

Most commercial statistical software packages (like those described in Chapter 4) can perform a log-rank test. You first organize your data into a table that has one row per individual, and these three columns:

- » **Group:** The group variable contains a code indicating the individual's group. In this example, we could use the code Drug = 1 and Control = 2.

- » **Time:** A numerical variable containing the individual's survival time. For individuals experiencing the event during the study, it represents time to event. For censored individuals, it is time to the end of observation.

- » **Event status:** A variable that indicates the individual's status at the end of observation. If they got the event, it is usually coded as 1, and if not or they are censored, it is coded as 0.

To run the log-rank test, you tell your computer program which variable represents the group variable, which one means time, and which one contains the event status. The program should produce a p value for the log-rank test. If you set $\alpha = 0.05$ and the p value is less than that, you reject the null and conclude that the two groups have statistically significantly different survival curves.

In addition to the p value, the program may output median survival time for each group along with confidence intervals, and difference in median times between groups. If possible, you will also want to request graphs that show whether your data are consistent with the hazard proportionality assumption that we describe later in "Assessing the assumptions."

Looking at the calculations

The log-rank test should not be done manually because it is an error-prone task. But we believe you'll have a better appreciation of the log-rank test if you understand how it works, so we describe how the calculations could theoretically be carried out using a Microsoft Excel spreadsheet.

The log-rank test utilizes information from the life tables needed to produce the graph shown earlier in Figure 22-1. Figure 22-2 shows a portion of the life tables that produced the curves shown in Figure 22-1, with the data for the two groups displayed side by side.

FIGURE 22-2:
A portion of the
life-table
calculations for
two groups of
laboratory
animals.

A Formula:	B B − C − D in the Preceding Row	C (data)	D (data)	E B − D/2	F F − G − H in the Preceding Row	G (data)	H (data)	I F − H/2
	Group 1: Drug				Group 2: Control			
Time Slice	Alive at Start	Died	Last Seen Alive	At Risk	Alive at Start	Died	Last Seen Alive	At Risk
0–1 day	60	5	1	59.5	30	4	1	29.5
1–2 days	54	3	0	54.0	25	6	2	24.0
2–3 days	51	6	4	49.0	17	3	0	17.0
3–4 days	41	5	2	40.0	14	5	1	13.5
4–5 days	34	2	0	34.0	8	2	0	8.0

© John Wiley & Sons, Inc.

In Figure 22-2, the Drug group's results are in columns B through E, and the Control group's results are in columns F through I. The only measurements needed from Figure 22-2 for the log-rank test are *At risk* (columns E and I), meaning number at risk in each time slice for each group, and *Died* (columns C and G), meaning the number of observed deaths in that time slice for each group. The log-rank test calculations are in a second spreadsheet (shown in Figure 22-3).

FIGURE 22-3:
Basic log-rank
calculations done
manually (but
please use
software
instead!).

A Formula:	B	C	D	E	F B + D	G C + E	H B / F	I H * G	J C − I	K Complicated (See Text)
	Taken from Life Tables for Groups 1 & 2									
	Group 1: Drug		Group 2: Control		Groups 1 & 2 Combined		Comparison of Observed and Expected in Group 1			
Time Slice	At Risk	Died	At Risk	Died	At Risk	Died	% of At Risk	Expected Deaths	Excess Deaths	Variance
0–1 day	59.5	5	29.5	4	89.0	9	66.85%	6.02	−1.02	1.81
1–2 days	54.0	3	24.0	6	78.0	9	69.23%	6.23	−3.23	1.72
2–3 days	49.0	6	17.0	3	66.0	9	74.24%	6.68	−0.68	1.51
3–4 days	40.0	5	13.5	1	53.5	6	74.77%	4.49	0.51	1.02
4–5 days	34.0	2	8.0	2	42.0	4	80.95%	3.24	−1.24	0.57
							Sum:		−5.65	6.64

© John Wiley & Sons, Inc.

The spreadsheet shown in Figure 22-3 has the following columns:

>> Column A identifies the time slices, consistent with Figure 22-2.

>> Columns B and C pertain to the Drug group, and reprint the *At risk* and *Died* columns from Figure 22-2 for that group. Columns D and E pertain to the Control group and reprint the *At risk* and *Died* columns from Figure 22-2 for that group.

>> Columns F and G show the combined total number of individuals at risk and the total number of individuals who died, which is obtained by combining the corresponding columns for the two groups.

>> Column H, labeled *% At Risk*, shows Group 1's percentage of the total number of at-risk individuals per time slice.

>> Column I, labeled *Expected Deaths*, shows the number of deaths you'd expect to see in Group 1 based on apportioning the total number of deaths (in both groups) by Group 1's percentage of total individuals at-risk. For the 0–1 day row, Group 1 had about 2/3 of the 89 individuals at risk, so you'd expect it to have about 2/3 of the nine deaths.

>> Column J, labeled *Excess Deaths*, shows the excess number of actual deaths compared to the expected number for Group 1.

>> Column K shows the variance (equal to the square of the standard deviation) of the excess deaths. It's obtained from this complicated formula that's based on the properties of the binomial distribution (see Chapter 24):

$$V = D_T (N_1/N_T)(N_2/N_T)(N_T - D_T)/(N_T - 1)$$

For the first time slice (0–1 day), this becomes:
$V = 9(59.5/89)(29.5/89)(89 - 9)/(89 - 1)$, which equals approximately 1.813.

N refers to the number of individuals at risk, D refers to deaths, the subscripts 1 and 2 refer to groups 1 and 2, and T refers to the total of both groups combined.

Next, you add up the excess deaths in all the time slices to get the total number of excess deaths for Group 1 compared to what you would have expected if the deaths had been distributed between the two groups in the same ratio as the number of at-risk individuals.

Then you add up all the variances. You are allowed to do that, because the sum of the variances of the individual numbers is equal to the variance of the sum of a set of numbers.

Finally, you divide the total excess deaths by the square root of the total variance to get a test statistic called Z:

$$Z = \sum ExcessDeaths / \sqrt{\sum Variances}$$

The Z value is approximately normally distributed, so you can obtain a p value from a table of the normal distribution or from an online calculator. For the data in Figure 23-3, $z = -5.65/\sqrt{6.64}$, which is 2.19. This z value corresponds to a p value of 0.028, so the null hypothesis is rejected, and you can conclude that the two groups have a statistically significantly different survival curve.

Note: By the way, it doesn't matter which group you assign as Group 1 in these calculations. The final results come out the same either way.

Assessing the assumptions

Like all statistical tests, the log-rank test assumes that you studied an unbiased sample from the population about which you're trying to draw conclusions. It also assumes that any censoring that occurred was due to circumstances unrelated to the treatment being tested (for example, individuals didn't drop out of the study because the drug made them sick).

Also, the log-rank test looks for differences in *overall* survival time. In other words, it's not good at detecting differences in *shape* between two survival curves with similar overall survival time, like the two curves shown in Figure 22-4. These two curves actually have the same median survival time, but the survival experience is different, as shown in the graph. When two survival curves cross over each other, as shown in Figure 22-4b, the excess deaths are positive for some time slices and negative for others. This leads them to cancel out when they're added up, producing a smaller z value as a test statistic z value, which translates to larger, non-statistically significant p value.

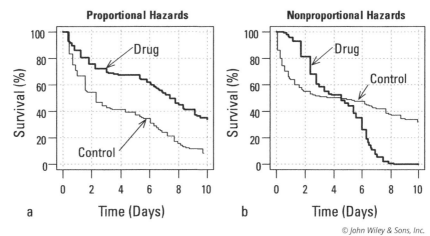

FIGURE 22-4: Proportional (a) and nonproportional (b) hazards relationships between two survival curves.

© John Wiley & Sons, Inc.

REMEMBER

Therefore, one very important assumption of the log-rank test is that the two groups have *proportional hazards,* which means the two groups must have generally similar survival shapes, as shown in Figure 22-4a. Flip to Chapter 21 for more about survival curves, and read about hazards in more detail in Chapter 23.

Considering More Complicated Comparisons

The log-rank test is good for comparing survival between two or more groups. But it doesn't extend well to more complicated situations. What if you want to do one of the following?

>> Test whether survival depends on age or some other continuous variable

>> Test the simultaneous effect of several variables, or their interactions, on survival

>> Correct for the presence of confounding variables or other covariates

In other areas of statistical testing, such situations are handled by regression techniques. *Survival analysis regression* uses survival outcomes with censored observations, and can accommodate these analyses. We describe survival regression in Chapter 23.

Estimating the Sample Size Needed for Survival Comparisons

We introduce power and sample size in Chapter 3. Calculating the sample size for survival comparisons is complicated by several factors:

>> **The need to specify an alternative hypothesis:** This hypothesis can take the form of a hazard ratio, described in Chapter 23, where the null hypothesis is that the hazard ratio = 1. Or, you can hypothesize the difference between two median survival times.

>> **The impact of censoring:** How censoring impacts sample size needed depends on the accrual rate, dropout rate, and the length of follow-up.

>> **The shape of the survival curves:** For sample-size calculations, it is often assumed that the survival curve is exponential, but that may not be realistic.

TIP

In Chapter 4, we recommend using free software G*Power for your sample-size calculations. However, because G*Power does not offer a survival sample-size estimator, for this, we recommend you use another free software package called PS (Power and Sample Size Calculation), which is available from Vanderbilt

University Medical Center (`https://biostat.app.vumc.org/wiki/Main/PowerSampleSize`).

After opening the PS program, choose the Survival tab, fill in the form, and click Calculate. The median survival times for the two groups are labeled m_1 and m_2, the accrual interval is labeled A, the post-accrual follow-up period is labeled F, and the group allocation proportion is labeled m. Note that the time variables must always be entered in the same units (days, in this example). You will also need to enter your chosen α and power.

Here is an example. Suppose that you're planning a study to compare an experimental drug for keeping cancer remission to placebo in two equal-sized groups of cancer patients whose cancer is in remission. You expect to observe participants for a total of three years to see whether their cancer returns (which is the outcome). From existing studies, you expect the median placebo time to be 20 months, and you think the drug should extend this to 30 months. If it truly does extend survival (time to remission) that much, you want to be able to detect this. You set $\alpha = 0.05$ and power at 80 percent so that you have an 80 percent chance of getting a p value of less than 0.05 when you compare drug to placebo using the log-rank test. If you fill in the PS form with these estimates and select Calculate, under Sample Size the software will say you need 170 participants in each group (a total of 340 participants).

Chapter **23**

Survival Regression

Survival regression is one of the most commonly used techniques in biostatistics. It overcomes the limitations of the log-rank test (see Chapter 22) and allows you to analyze how survival time is influenced by one or more predictors (the *X* variables), which can be categorical or numerical. In this chapter, we introduce survival regression. We specify when to use it, describe its basic concepts, and show you how to run survival regressions in statistical software and interpret the output. We also explain how to build prognosis curves and estimate the sample size you need to support a survival regression.

Note: Because time-to-event data so often describe actual survival, when the event we are talking about is death, we use the terms *death* and *survival time*. But everything we say about death applies to the first occurrence of any event, like pre-diabetes patients restoring their blood sugar to normal levels, or cancer survivors suffering a recurrence of cancer.

Knowing When to Use Survival Regression

In Chapter 21, we examine the special problems that come up when the researcher can't continue to collect data during follow-up on a participant long enough to observe whether or not they ever experience the event being studied. To recap, in this situation, you should *censor* the data. This means you should acknowledge the participant was only observed for a limited amount of time, and then was *lost to follow-up.* In that chapter, we also explain how to summarize survival data using life tables and the Kaplan-Meier method, and how to graph time-to-event data as survival curves. In Chapter 22, we describe the log-rank test, which you can use to compare survival among a small number of groups — for example, participants taking drug versus placebo, or participants initially diagnosed at four different stages of the same cancer.

But the log-rank test has limitations:

>> **The log-rank test doesn't handle numerical predictors well.** Because this test compares survival among a small number of categories, it does not work well for a numerical variable like age. To compare survival among different age groups with the log-rank test, you would first have to categorize the participants into age ranges. The age ranges you choose for your groups should be based on your research question. Because doing this loses the granularity of the data, this test may be less efficient at detecting gradual trends across the whole age range.

>> **The log-rank test doesn't let you analyze the simultaneous effect of different predictors.** If you try to create subgroups of participants for each distinct combination of categories for more than one predictor (such as three treatment groups and three diagnostic groups), you will quickly see that you have too many groups and not enough participants in each group to support the test. In this example — with three different treatment groups and three diagnostic groups — you would have 3×3 groups, which is nine, and is already too many for a log-rank test to be useful. Even if you have 100 participants in your study, dividing them into nine categories greatly reduces the number of participants in each category, making the subgroup estimate unstable.

REMEMBER

Use survival regression when the outcome (the Y variable) is a time-to-event variable, like survival time. Survival regression lets you do all of the following, either in separate models or simultaneously:

>> Determine whether there is a statistically significant association between survival and one or more other predictor variables

>> Quantify the extent to which a predictor variable influences survival, including testing whether survival is statistically significantly different between groups

>> Adjust for the effects of confounding variables that also influence survival

>> Generate a predicted survival curve called a *prognosis curve* that is customized for any particular set of values of the predictor variables

Grasping the Concepts behind Survival Regression

Note: Our explanation of survival regression has a little math in it, but nothing beyond high school algebra. In laying out these concepts, we focus on *multiple survival regression*, which is survival regression with more than one predictor. But everything we say is also true when you have only one predictor variable.

Most kinds of regression require you to write a formula to fit to your data. The formula is easiest to understand and work with when the predictors appear in the function as a *linear combination* in which each predictor variable is multiplied by a *coefficient*, and these terms are all added together (perhaps with another coefficient, called an *intercept*, thrown in). Here is an example of a typical regression formula: $y = c_0 + c_1 x_1 + c_2 x_2 + c_3 x_3$. Linear combinations (such as $c_2 x_2$ from the example formula) can also have terms with higher powers — like squares or cubes — attached to the predictor variables. Linear combinations can also have *interaction terms*, which are products of two or more predictors, or the same predictor with itself.

WARNING

Survival regression takes the linear combination and uses it to predict survival. But survival data presents some special challenges:

>> **Censoring:** Censoring happens when the event doesn't occur during the observation time of the study (which, in human studies, means during follow-up). Before considering using survival regression on your data, you need to evaluate the impact censoring may have on the results. You can do this using life tables, the Kaplan-Meier method, and the log-rank test, as described in Chapters 21 and 22.

>> **Survival curve shapes:** Some business disciplines develop models for estimating time to failure of mechanical or electronic devices. They estimate the times to certain kinds of events, like a computer's motherboard wearing out or the transmission of a car going kaput, and find that they follow

remarkably predictable *shapes* or *distributions* (the most common being the *Weibull distribution,* covered in Chapter 24). Because of this, these disciplines often use a *parametric* form of survival regression, which assumes that you can represent the survival curves by algebraic formulas. Unfortunately for biostatisticians, biological data tends to produce *nonparametric* survival curves whose distributions can't be represented by these parametric distributions.

As described earlier, nonparametric survival analyses using life tables, Kaplan-Meier plots, and log-rank tests are limiting. But as biostatisticians, we could not rely on using parametric distributions in our models; we wanted to use a hybrid, *semi-parametric* kind of survival regression. We wanted one that was partly *non-parametric,* meaning it didn't assume any mathematical formula for the shape of the overall survival curve, and partly *parametric,* meaning we could use some parameter (or predicted survival distribution shape) to guide our formulas the way other industries used the Weibull distribution. In 1972, a statistician named David Cox developed a workable method for doing this. The procedure is now called *Cox proportional hazards regression,* which we call *PH regression* for the rest of this chapter for brevity. In the following sections, we outline the steps of performing a PH regression.

WARNING

Since 1972, many issues have been identified when using survival regression for biological data, especially with respect to its appropriateness for the type of data. One way to examine this is by running a logistic regression model (see Chapter 18) with the same predictors and outcome as your survival regression model without including the time variable, and seeing if the interpretation changes.

The steps to perform a PH regression

You can understand PH regression in terms of several conceptual steps, although when using statistical software like is described in Chapter 4, it may appear that these steps take place simultaneously. That is because the output created is designed for you — the biostatistician — to walk through the following steps in your mind and make decisions. You must use the output to:

1. Determine the shape of the overall survival curve produced from the Kaplan-Meier method.

2. Estimate how your hypothesized predictor variables may impact the bends in this curve — in other words, in what ways your predictors may affect survival.

3. **Create a PH regression model that fits your data the best it can, and interpret the values of the regression coefficients so you can calculate predicted survival times.**

Determining the baseline in time-to-event analyses

Your software may define the baseline survival function in one of two ways:

>> **The survival curve of an *average participant*:** This curve is calculated as if the value of each predictor is equal to the group average value for that variable. The average-participant baseline is like the overall survival curve you get from a Kaplan-Meier calculation by using all the available participants.

>> **The survival curve of a hypothetical *zero participant*:** This curve is calculated assuming the value of each predictor is equal to 0. Some mathematicians prefer to use the *zero-participant* baseline because can make formulas simpler, but biostatisticians don't like it because it corresponds to a hypothetical participant who can't possibly exist in the real world. No actual person has an age equal to 0 years, or weighs 0 kilograms, and so on. The survival curve for this impossible person doesn't look like a regular survival curve, so as biostatisticians, we can't really use the zero-participant baseline survival function.

TIP

Luckily, the way your software defines its baseline function doesn't affect any of the calculated measures on your output, so you don't have to worry about it. But you should be aware of these definitions if you plan to generate prognosis curves, because the formulas to generate these are slightly different depending upon the way the computer calculates the baseline survival function.

Bending the baseline

REMEMBER

Now for the tricky part. How do you bend or *flex* this baseline curve to express how survival may increase or decrease for different predictor values? Survival curves always start at 1.0 at time 0, meaning 100 percent of the sample do not have the event at time 0. The bending process must preserve that time starts at 0, and maximum survival is 1.0. If you raise 0 or 1 to any power, you will find that they stay the same — 0 stays 0, and 1 stays 1. But, exponentiating any number between 0 and 1 smoothly raises or lowers all the values between 0 and 1.

We will demonstrate what we mean by imagining our baseline function was a straight line (even though no actual biological survival curve would ever be exactly a straight line). Look at Figure 23-1a, which is a graph of the equation $y = 1 - x$.

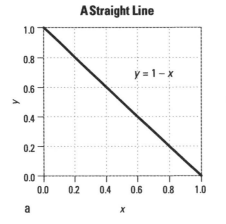

FIGURE 23-1:
Bending a straight line into different shapes by raising each point on the line to some power: *h*.

A Straight Line

$y = 1 - x$

a

Flexing a Straight Line by Raising It to a Power, *h*

$Y = (1 - x)^h$

$h = 0.2$

$h = 0.5$

$h = 1$

$h = 2$

$h = 5$

b

© John Wiley & Sons, Inc.

To understand the flex, look at what happens when you raise this straight line to various powers, which we refer to as *h* and illustrate in Figure 23-1b:

» **Squaring:** If you set *h* = 2, the *y* value for every point on the line always comes out smaller, because they are always less than 1. For example, 0.8^2 is 0.64.

» **Taking the square root:** If we set *h* = 0.05, the *y* value of every point on the line becomes larger. For example, the square root of 0.25 is 0.5.

Notice in Figure 23-1b, both 1^2 and $1^{0.5}$ remain 1, and 0^2 and $0^{0.5}$ both remain 0, so those two ends of the line don't change.

Does the same trick work for a survival curve that doesn't follow any particular algebraic formula? Yes, it does! Look at Figure 23-2.

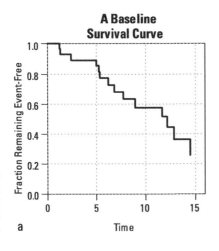
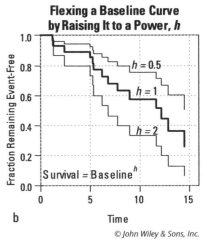

A Baseline Survival Curve

FIGURE 23-2:
Raising to a power works for survival curves, too.

a

Flexing a Baseline Curve by Raising It to a Power, *h*

$h = 0.5$

$h = 1$

$h = 2$

$Survival = Baseline^h$

b

© John Wiley & Sons, Inc.

Here are some important points about Figure 23-2:

>> Figure 23-2a shows a typical survival curve. It's not defined by any algebraic formula. It just graphs the table of values obtained by a life-table or Kaplan-Meier calculation.

>> Figure 23-2b shows how the baseline survival curve is flexed by raising every baseline survival value to a power. You get the lower curve by setting $h = 2$ and squaring every baseline survival value. You get the upper curve by setting $h = 0.05$ and taking the square root of every baseline survival value. Notice that the two flexed curves keep all the distinctive zigs and zags of the baseline curve, in that every step occurs at the same time value as it occurs in the baseline curve.

- The lower curve represents a group of participants who had a worse survival outcome than those making up the baseline group. This means that at any instant in time, they were somewhat more likely to die than a baseline participant at that same moment. Another way of saying this is that the participants in the lower curve have a higher *hazard rate* than the baseline participants.

- The upper curve represents participants who had better survival than a baseline person at any given moment — meaning they had a lower hazard rate.

Obviously, there is a mathematical relationship between the chance of dying at any instant in time, which is called *hazard,* and the chance of surviving up to some point in time, which we call *survival.* It turns out that raising the survival curve to the h power is exactly equivalent to multiplying the hazard curve by the natural logarithm of h. Because every point in the hazard curve is being multiplied by the same amount — by $Log(h)$ — raising a survival curve to a power is referred to as a *proportional hazards* transformation.

REMEMBER

But what should the value of h be? The h value varies from one individual to another. Keep in mind that the baseline curve describes the survival of a perfectly average participant, but no individual is completely average. You can think of every participant in the data as having her very own personalized survival curve, based on her very own h value, that provides the best estimate of that participant's chance of survival over time.

Seeing how predictor variables influence h

The final piece of the PH regression puzzle is to figure out how the predictor variables influence h, which influences survival. As you likely know, all regression procedures estimate the values of the coefficients that make the predicted values agree as much as possible with the observed values. For PH regression, the software estimates the coefficients of the predictor variables that make the predicted survival curves agree as much as possible with the observed survival times of each participant.

TECHNICAL STUFF

How does PH regression determine these regression coefficients? The short answer is, "You'll be sorry you asked!" The longer answer is that, like all other kinds of regression, PH regression is based on maximum likelihood estimation. The software uses the data to build a long, complicated expression for the probability of one particular individual in the data dying at any point in time. This expression involves that individual's predictor values and the regression coefficients. Next, the software constructs a longer expression that includes the likelihood of getting exactly the observed survival times for *all* the participants in the data set. And if this isn't already complicated enough, the expression has to deal with the issue of censored data. At this point, the software seeks to find the values of the regression coefficients that maximize this very long likelihood expression (similar to the way maximum likelihood is described with logistic regression in Chapter 18).

Hazard ratios

Hazard ratios (HRs) are the estimates of relative risk obtained from PH regression. HRs in survival regression play a similar role that odds ratios play in logistic regression. They're also calculated the same way from regression output — by exponentiating the regression coefficients:

» **In logistic regression:** $\text{Odds ratio} = e^{\text{Regression Coefficient}}$

» **In PH regression:** $\text{Hazard ratio} = e^{\text{Regression Coefficient}}$

REMEMBER

Keep in mind that *hazard* is the chance of dying in any small period of time. For each predictor variable in a PH regression model, a coefficient is produced that — when exponentiated — equals the HR. The HR tells you how much the hazard rate increases for the participants positive for the predictor compared to the comparison group when you increase the variable's value by exactly 1.0 unit. Therefore, a HR's numerical value depends on the units in which the variable is expressed in your data. And for categorical predictors, interpreting the HR depends on how you code the categories.

For example, if a survival regression model in a study of emphysema patients includes number of cigarettes smoked per day as a predictor of survival, and if the HR for this variable comes out equal to 1.05, then a participant's chances of dying at any instant increase by a factor of 1.05 (5 percent) for every additional cigarette smoked per day. A 5 percent increase may not seem like much, but it's applied for every additional cigarette per day. A person who smokes one pack (20 cigarettes) per day has that 1.05 multiplication applied 20 times, which is like multiplying by 1.05^{20}, which equals 2.65. One pack contains 20 cigarettes, so if you change the units in which you record smoking levels from *cigarettes* per day to *packs* per day, you would use units that are 20 times larger. In that case, the corresponding regression coefficient is 20 times larger, and the HR is raised to the 20th power (2.65 instead of 1.05 in this example).

And a two-pack-per-day smoker's hazard increases by a factor of 2.65 over a one-pack-per-day smoker. This translates to a 2.65^{2} increase (approximately sevenfold) in the chances of dying at any instant for the smoker compared to a nonsmoker.

Executing a Survival Regression

As with all statistical methods dealing with time-to-event data, your dependent variable is actually a pair of variables:

>> **Event status:** The event status variable is coded this way:

- Equal to 1 if the event was known to occur during the observation period *(uncensored)*

- Equal to 0 if the event didn't occur during the observation period *(censored)*

>> **Time-to-event:** In participants who experienced the event during the observation period, this is the time from the start of observation to the occurrence of the event. In participants who did not experience the event during the observation period, this is the time from the start of observation to the last time the participant was observed. We describe time-to-event data in more detail in Chapter 21.

And as with all regression methods, you designate one or more variables as the predictors. The rules for representing the predictor variables are the same as described in Chapter 18:

>> For continuous numerical variables, choose units of a convenient magnitude.

>> For categorical predictors, carefully consider how you recode the data, especially in terms of selecting a reference group. Consider a five-level age group variable. Would you want to model it as an ordinal categorical variable, assuming a linear relationship with the outcome? Or would you prefer using indicator variables, allowing each level to have its own slope relative to the reference level? Flip to Chapter 8 for more on recoding categorical variables.

You may not be sure which variables in your data to include as predictors in the regression. We provide advice on model-building in Chapter 17.

After you assemble and properly code the data, you execute the regression in statistical software using a similar approach as you use when doing ordinary least-squares or logistic regression. You need to specify the variables in the regression model:

1. **Specify the two outcome variables.**

   - The event status variable

   - The time-to-event variable

2. **Specify the predictor variables.**

   Make sure you are careful when you include categorical predictors, especially indicator variables. All the predictors you introduce should make sense together in the model.

REMEMBER

Most software also lets you specify calculations you want to see on the output. You should always request at least the following:

>> Coefficients table, including HRs and their confidence intervals

>> Tests of whether the hazard proportionality assumption is valid

You may also want to request the following output:

>> Summary descriptive statistics about the data. These can include number of censored and uncensored observations, median survival time, and mean and standard deviation for each predictor variable in the model

>> One or more measures of goodness-of-fit for the model

>> Baseline survival function, which outputs as a table of values and a survival curve

>> Baseline hazard function values, which output as a table and graph

After you specify all the input to the program, execute the code, retrieve the output, and interpret the results.

Interpreting the Output of
a Survival Regression

Suppose that you have conducted a long-term survival study of 200 Stage 4 cancer patients who were enrolled from four clinical centers (A, B, C, and D) and were randomized to receive either chemotherapy or radiation therapy. Participants were followed for up to ten years, after which the survival data were summarized by treatment (see Figures 23-3a and 23-3b for the two treatments) and by clinical center.

It would appear, from Figure 23-3, that radiation (compared to chemotherapy) and clinical centers A and B (compared to C and D) are associated with better survival. But are these apparent effects statistically significant? PH regression can answer these and other questions.

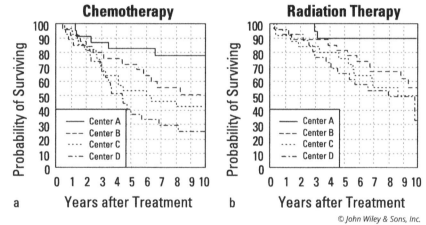

FIGURE 23-3:
Kaplan-Meier survival curves by treatment and clinical center.

To run a PH regression on the data from this example, you must indicate the following to the software in your code:

>> **The time-to-event variable.** We named this variable *Time,* and it was coded in years. For participants who died during the observation period, it was coded as the number of years from observation beginning until death. For participants who did not die during the observation period, it contains number of years they were observed.

>> **The event status variable.** We named this variable *Status,* and coded it as 1 if the participant was known to have died during the observation period, and 0 if they did not die.

>> **The treatment group variable.** In this case, we created the variable *Radiation*, and coded it as 1 if the participant was in the radiation group, and 0 if they were in the chemotherapy group. That way, the coefficient produced in the output will indicate the increase or decrease in proportional hazard associated with being in the radiation group compared to the chemotherapy group.

>> **The clinical center variable.** In this case, we choose to create an indicator variable called *CenterCD*, which is 1 if the participant is from Center C or Center D, and is 0 if they are from A or B. Alternatively, you could choose to create one indicator variable for each center, as described in Chapter 18.

REMEMBER

If you use a numerical variable such as age as a predictor and enter it into the model, the resulting coefficient will apply to increasing this variable by one unit (such as for one year of age).

Using the R statistical software, the PH regression can be invoked with a single command:

```
coxph(formula = Surv(Time, Status) ~ CenterCD + Radiation)
```

Figure 23-4 shows R's output, using the data that we graph in Figure 23-3. The output from other statistical programs won't look exactly like Figure 23-4, but you should be able to find the main components described in the following sections.

```
Call: coxph(formula = Surv(Time, Status) ~ CenterCD + Radiation

  n= 200, number of events= 92

              coef exp(coef) se(coef)       z Pr(>|z|)
CenterCD    0.4522    1.5717   0.1013  4.463 8.09e-06 ***
Radiation  -0.4323    0.6490   0.2116 -2.043   0.0411 *
---
Signif. codes:  0 '***' 0.001 '**' 0.01 '*' 0.05 '.' 0.1 ' ' 1

              exp(coef) exp(-coef) lower .95 upper .95
CenterCD        1.572     0.6362    1.2886    1.9170
Radiation       0.649     1.5407    0.4287    0.9826

Concordance= 0.642   (se = 0.031 )
Rsquare= 0.116    (max possible= 0.99 )
Likelihood ratio test= 24.64  on 2 df,    p=4.46e-06
Wald test            = 23.31  on 2 df,    p=8.67e-06
Score (logrank) test = 24.36  on 2 df,    p=5.124e-06
```

FIGURE 23-4: Output of a PH regression from R.

Testing the validity of the assumptions

When you're analyzing data using PH regression, you're assuming that your data are consistent with the idea of flexing a baseline survival curve by raising all the points in the entire curve to the same power (shown as h in Figures 23-1b and 23-2b). You're not allowed to *twist* the curve so that it goes higher than the baseline curve ($h < 1$) for small time values and lower than baseline ($h > 1$) for large time values. That would be a non-PH flexing of the curve.

One quick check to see whether a predictor is affecting your data in a non-PH way is to take the following steps:

1. **Split your data into two groups, based on the predictor.**

2. **Plot the Kaplan-Meier survival curve for each group (see Chapter 22).**

WARNING

If the two survival curves for a particular predictor display the slanted figure-eight pattern shown in Figure 23-5, either don't use PH regression on those data, or don't use that predictor in your PH regression model. That's because it violates the assumption of proportional hazards underlying PH regression.

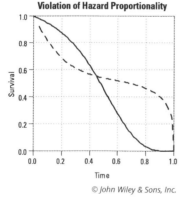

FIGURE 23-5:
Don't try PH regression on this kind of data because it violates the PH assumption.

© John Wiley & Sons, Inc.

TIP

Your statistical software may offer several options to test the hazard-proportionality assumption. Check your software's documentation to see what it offers and how to interpret the output. It may offer the following:

>> Graphs of the hazard functions versus time, which let you see the extent to which the hazards are proportional.

>> A statistical test for significant hazard non-proportionality. R provides a function called *cox.zph* for this purpose, and other packages may offer a comparable option.

Checking out the table of regression coefficients

A regression coefficients table in a survival regression looks very much like the tables produced by almost all kinds of regression: ordinary least-squares, logistic, Poisson, and so on. The survival regression table has a row for every predictor variable, usually containing the following items:

>> **The value of the *regression coefficient*.** This says how much the log of the HR increases when the predictor variable increases by exactly 1.0 unit. It's hard to interpret unless you exponentiate it into a HR. In Figure 23-4, the coefficient for *CenterCD* is 0.4522, indicating that every increase of 1 in *CenterCD* (which literally means comparing everyone at Centers A and B to those at Centers C and D), there is an increase the logarithm of the hazard by 0.4522. When exponentiated, this translates into a HR of 1.57 (listed on the output under *exp(coef)*). As predicted from looking at Figure 24-3, this indicates that those at Centers C and D together are associated with a higher hazard compared with those at Centers A and B together. For indicator variables, there will be a row in the table for each non-reference level, so in this case, you see a row for *Radiation*. The coefficient for *Radiation* is –0.4323, which when exponentiated, translates to an HR of 0.65 (again listed under *exp(coef)*). The negative sign indicates that in this study, radiation treatment is associated with less hazard and better survival than the comparison treatment, which is chemotherapy. Interpreting the HRs and their confidence intervals is described in the next section "Homing in on hazard ratios and their confidence intervals."

>> **The coefficient's *standard error* (SE),** which is a measure of the precision of the regression coefficient. The SE of the *CenterCD* coefficient is 0.1013, so you would express the *CenterCD* coefficient as 0.45 ± 0.10.

>> **The coefficient divided by its SE** often labeled *t* or *Wald*, but designated as z in Figure 23-4.

>> **The *p value*.** Under the assumption that $\alpha = 0.05$, if the p value is less than 0.05, it indicates that the coefficient is statistically significantly different from 0 after adjusting for the effects of all the other variables that may appear the model. In other words, a p value of less than 0.05 means that the corresponding predictor variable is statistically significantly associated with survival. The p value for *CenterCD* is shown as 8.09e–06, which is scientific notation for 0.000008, indicating that *CenterCD* is very significantly associated with survival.

>> **The *HR* and its confidence limits,** which we describe in the next section.

TIP

You may be surprised that no intercept (or constant) row is in the coefficient table in the output shown in Figure 23-4. PH regression doesn't include an intercept in the linear part of the model because the intercept is absorbed into the baseline survival function.

Homing in on hazard ratios and their confidence intervals

HRs from survival and other time-to-event data are used extensively as safety and efficacy outcomes of clinical trials, as well as in large-scale epidemiological studies. Depending on how the output is formatted, it may show the HR for each predictor in a separate column in the regression table, or it may create a separate table just for the HRs and their confidence intervals (CIs).

TIP

If the software doesn't output HRs or their CIs, you can calculate them from the regression coefficients and standard errors (SEs) as follows:

>> Hazard ratio $= e^{\text{Coef}}$

>> Lower 95 percent confidence limit $= e^{\text{Coef} - 1.96 \times SE}$

>> Upper 95 percent confidence limit $= e^{\text{Coef} - 1.96 \times SE}$

In Figure 23-4, the coefficients are listed under *coef*, and the SEs are listed under *se(coef)*. HRs are useful and meaningful measures of the extent to which a variable influences survival.

>> A HR of 1 corresponds to a regression coefficient of 0, and indicates that the variable has no effect on survival.

>> The CI around the HR estimated from your sample indicates the range in which the true HR of the population from which your sample was drawn probably lies.

In Figure 23-4, the HR for *CenterCD* is $e^{0.4522} = 1.57$, with a 95 percent CI of 1.29 to 1.92. This means that an increase of 1 in *CenterCD* (meaning being a participant at Centers A or B compared to being one at Centers C or D) is statistically significantly associated with a 57 percent increase in hazard. This is because multiplying by 1.57 is equivalent to a 57 percent increase. Similarly, the HR for *Radiation* (relative to the comparison, which is chemotherapy) is 0.649, with a 95 percent CI of 0.43 to 0.98. This means that those undergoing radiation had only 65 percent the hazard of those undergoing chemotherapy, and the relationship is statistically significant.

TIP

Risk factors, or predictors associated with increased risk of the outcome, have HRs greater than 1. *Protective factors*, or predictors associated with decreased risk of the outcome, have HRs less than 1. In the example, *CenterCD* is a risk factor, and *Radiation* is a protective factor.

Assessing goodness-of-fit and predictive ability of the model

There are several measures of how well a regression model fits the survival data. These measures can be useful when you're choosing among several different models:

>> Should you include a possible predictor variable (like *age*) in the model?

>> Should you include the squares or cubes of predictor variables in the model (meaning including age^2 or age^3 in addition to *age*)?

>> Should you include a term for the interaction between two predictors?

Your software may offer one or more of the following goodness-of-fit measures:

>> A measure of agreement between the observed and predicted outcomes called *concordance* (see the bottom of Figure 23-4). Concordance indicates the extent to which participants with higher predicted hazard values had shorter observed survival times, which is what you'd expect. Figure 23-4 shows a concordance of 0.642 for this regression.

>> An *r* (or r^2) value that's interpreted like a correlation coefficient in ordinary regression, meaning the larger the r^2 value, the better the model fits the data. In Figure 23-4, r^2 (labeled *Rsquare*) is 0.116.

>> A likelihood ratio test and associated p value that compares the full model, which includes all the parameters, to a model consisting of just the overall baseline function. In Figure 23-4, the likelihood ratio p value is shown as $4.46e-06$, which is scientific notation for $p = 0.00000446$, indicating a model that includes the *CenterCD* and *Radiation* variables can predict survival statistically significantly better than just the overall (baseline) survival curve.

>> *Akaike's Information Criterion* (AIC) is especially useful for comparing alternative models but is not included in Figure 23-4.

Focusing on baseline survival and hazard functions

The *baseline survival function* is represented as a table with two columns — time and predicted survival — and a row for each distinct time at which one or more events were observed.

TIP

The baseline survival function's table may have hundreds of rows for large data sets, so instead of printing it, you should save the table as a data file. Then, you can use it to generate a customized prognosis curve (described in the next section) for any specific set of values for the predictor variables.

The software may also offer a graph of the baseline survival function. If your software is using an average-participant baseline (see the earlier section, "The steps to perform a PH regression"), this graph is useful as an indicator of the entire group's overall survival. But if your software uses a zero-participant baseline, the curve is not helpful.

How Long Have I Got, Doc? Constructing Prognosis Curves

A primary reason to use regression analysis is to predict outcomes from any particular set of predictor values. For survival analysis, you can use the regression coefficients from a PH regression along with the baseline survival curve to construct an *expected survival (prognosis)* curve for any set of predictor values.

Suppose that you're survival time (from diagnosis to death) for a group of cancer patients in which the predictors are age, tumor stage, and tumor grade at the time of diagnosis. You'd run a PH regression on your data and have the program generate the baseline survival curve as a table of times and survival probabilities. After that, whenever a patient is newly diagnosed with cancer, you can take that person's age, stage, and grade, and generate an expected survival curve tailored for that particular patient. (The patient may not want to see it, but at least it could be done.)

TIP

You'll probably have to do these calculations outside of the software that you use for the survival regression, but the calculations aren't difficult and can be done in a Microsoft Excel spreadsheet. The example in the following sections uses the small set of sample data that's preloaded into the online calculator for PH regression at `https://statpages.info/prophaz.html`. This particular example has only one predictor, but the basic idea extends to multiple predictors.

Obtaining the necessary output

Figure 23-6 shows the output from the built-in example (omitting the Iteration History and Overall Model Fit sections). Pretend that this model represents survival, in years, as a function of age for patients just diagnosed with some particular disease. In the output, the age variable is called Variable 1.

```
Descriptive Stats...


Variable          Avg            SD
    1           51.1818      10.9778


Coefficients, Std Errs, Signif, and Conf Intervs...
    Var         Coeff.    StdErr       p        Lo95%      Hi95%
     1          0.3770    0.2542     0.1379    -0.1211     0.8752


Risk Ratios and Confidence Intervs...
    Var      Risk Ratio      Lo95%      Hi95%
     1         1.4580       0.8859     2.3993
```

```
Baseline Survivor Function (at predictor means)...
    2.0000      0.9979
    7.0000      0.9820
    9.0000      0.9525
   10.0000      0.8310
```

Looking at Figure 23-6, first consider the table in the Baseline Survivor Function section, which has two columns: time in years, and predicted survival expressed as a fraction. It also has four rows — one for each time point in which one or more deaths was actually observed. The baseline survival curve for the example data starts at 1.0 (100 percent survival) at time 0, as survival curves always do, but this row isn't shown in the output. The survival curve remains flat at 100 percent until year two, when it suddenly drops down to 99.79 percent, where it stays until year seven, when it drops down to 98.20 percent, and so on.

In the Descriptive Stats section near the start of the output in Figure 23-6, the average age of the 11 patients in the example data set is 51.1818 years, so the baseline survival curve shows the predicted survival for a patient who is exactly 51.1818 years old. But suppose that you want to generate a survival curve that's customized for a patient who is a different age — like 55 years old. According to the PH model, you need to raise the entire baseline curve to some power h. This means you have to exponentiate the four tabulated points by h.

REMEMBER

In general, h depends on two factors:

>> The value of the predictor variable for that patient. In this example, the value of age is 55.

>> The values of the corresponding regression coefficients. In this example, in Figure 23-6, you can see 0.3770 labeled as *Coeff.* in the regression table.

Finding h

To calculate the *h* value, do the following for each predictor:

1. **Subtract the average value from the patient's value.**

In this example, you subtract the average age, which is 51.18, from the patient's age, which is 55, giving a difference of +3.82.

2. **Multiply the difference by the regression coefficient and call the product *v*.**

In this example, you multiply 3.82 from Step 1 by the regression coefficient for age, which is 0.377, giving a product of 1.44 for *v*.

3. **Calculate the *v* value for each predictor in the model.**

4. **Add all the *v* values, and call the sum of the individual *v* values *V*.**

This example has only one predictor variable, which is age, so *V* equals the *v* value you calculate for age in Step 2, which is 1.44.

5. **Calculate e^V.**

This is the value of *h*. In this example, $e^{1.44}$ gives the value 4.221, which is the *h* value for a 55-year-old patient.

6. **Raise each of the baseline survival values to the power of *h* to get the survival values for the prognosis curve.**

In this example, you have the following prognosis:

- For year-zero survival $1.000^{4.221} = 1.000$, or 100 percent
- For two-year survival: $0.9979^{4.221} = 0.9912$, or 99.12 percent
- For seven-year survival $0.9820^{4.221} = 0.9262$, or 92.62 percent
- For nine-year survival $0.9525^{4.221} = 0.8143$, or 81.43 percent
- For ten-year survival $0.8310^{4.221} = 0.4578$, or 45.78 percent

You then graph these calculated survival values to give a customized survival curve for this particular patient. And that's all there is to it!

TIP

Here's a short version of the procedure:

1. *V* = sum of [(patient value – average value) * coefficient] *summed over all the predictors*

2. $h = e^V$

3. Customized survival = (baseline survival)^h

REMEMBER

Some points to keep in mind:

>> If your software outputs a zero-based baseline survival function, you don't subtract the average value from the patient's value. Instead, calculate the *v* term as the product of the patient's predictor value multiplied by the regression coefficient.

>> If a predictor is a categorical variable, you have to code the levels as numbers. If you have a dichotomous variable like *pregnancy status,* you could code not pregnant = 0 and pregnant = 1. Then, if in a sample only including women, 47.2 percent of the sample is pregnant, the *average pregnancy status* is 0.472. If the patient is not pregnant, the subtraction in Step 1 is 0 – 0.472, giving –0.472. If the patient is pregnant, you would use the equation 1 – 0.472, giving 0.528. Then you carry out all the other steps exactly as described.

>> It's even a little trickier for multivalued categories (such as different clinical centers) because you have to code each of these variables as a set of indicator variables.

Estimating the Required Sample Size for a Survival Regression

Note: Elsewhere in this chapter, we use the word *power* in its algebraic sense, such as in x^2 is x to the power of 2. But in this section, we use *power* in its statistical sense to mean the probability of getting a statistically significant result when performing a statistical test.

Except for straight-line regression discussed in Chapter 16, sample-size calculations for regression analysis tend not to be straightforward. If you find software that will calculate sample-size estimates for survival regression, it often asks for inputs you don't have.

TIP

Very often, sample-size estimates for studies that use regression methods are based on simpler analytical methods. We recommend that when you're planning a study that will be analyzed using PH regression, you base your sample-size estimate on the simpler log-rank test, described in Chapter 22. The free PS program handles these calculations very well.

You still have to specify the following:

>> **Desired α level:** We recommend 0.05

>> **Desired power:** We usually use 80 percent

>> **Effect size of importance:** This is typically expressed as a HR or as the difference in median survival time between groups

You also need estimates of the following:

>> **Anticipated enrollment rate:** How many participants you hope to enroll per time period

>> **Planned duration of follow-up:** How long you plan to continue following all the participants after the last participant has been enrolled before ending the study and analyzing your data

TIP

If you are uncomfortable with estimating sample size for a large study that will be evaluated with a regression model, consult a statistician with experience in developing sample-size estimates for similarly-designed studies. They will be able to guide you in the tips and tricks they use to arrive at an adequate sample-size calculation given your research question and context.

7

The Part of Tens

Chapter **24**

Ten Distributions Worth Knowing

This chapter describes ten statistical distribution functions you'll probably encounter in biological research. For each one, we provide a graph of what that distribution looks like, as well as some useful or interesting facts and formulas. You find two general types of distributions here:

» **Distributions that describe random fluctuations in observed data:** Your study data will often conform to one of the first seven common distributions. In general, these distributions have one or two adjustable parameters that allow them to *fit* the fluctuations in your observed data.

» **Common test statistic distributions:** The last three distributions don't describe your observed data. Instead, they describe how a test statistic that is calculated as part of a statistical significance test will fluctuate if the null hypothesis is true. The Student t, chi-square, and Fisher F distributions allow you to calculate test statistics to help you decide if observed differences between groups, associations between variables, and other effects you want to test should be interpreted as due to random fluctuations or not. If the apparent effects in your data are due only to random fluctuations, then you will fail to reject the null hypothesis. These distributions are used with the test statistics to obtain p values, which indicate the statistical significance of the apparent effects. (See Chapter 3 for more information on significance testing and p values.)

This chapter provides a very short table of critical values for the t, chi-square, and F distributions. A *critical value* is the value that your calculated test statistic must exceed in order for you to declare statistical significance at the $\alpha = 0.05$ level. For example, the critical value for the normal distribution is 1.96 at $\alpha = 0.05$.

The Uniform Distribution

The uniform distribution is the simplest distribution. It's a continuous number between 0 and 1. To generalize, it is a continuous number between a and b, with all values within that range equally likely (see Figure 24-1). The uniform distribution has a mean value of $(b+a)/2$ and a standard deviation of $(b-a)/\sqrt{12}$. The uniform distribution arises in the following contexts:

>> Round-off errors are uniformly distributed. For example, a weight recorded as 85 kilograms (kg) can be thought of as a uniformly distributed random variable between $a = 84.5$ kg and $b = 85.5$ kg. This causes the mean to be $(84.5 + 85.5)/2 = 85$ kg, with a standard error of $(84.4 - 84.5)/\sqrt{12}$, which is $1/3.46 = 0.29$ kg.

>> In the case the null hypothesis is true, the p value from any exact significance test is uniformly distributed between 0 and 1.

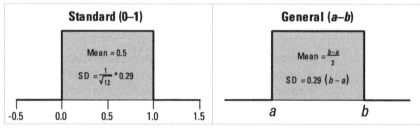

FIGURE 24-1: The uniform distribution.

The Microsoft Excel formula $= \text{RAND}()$ generates a random number drawn from the standard uniform distribution.

The Normal Distribution

The most popular and widely-used distribution is the normal distribution (also called the *Gaussian distribution* and the *probability bell curve*). It describes variables whose fluctuations are the combined result of many independent causes. Figure 24-2 shows the shape of the normal distribution for various values of the mean and standard deviation. Many other distributions (binomial, Poisson, Student t, chi-square, Fisher F) become nearly normal-shaped for large samples.

TIP

The Microsoft Excel statement $= \text{NORMSINV}(\text{RAND}())$ generates a normally distributed random number, with mean $= 0$ and SD $= 1$.

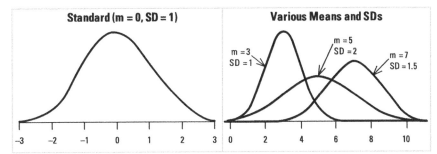

FIGURE 24-2:
The normal distribution at various means and standard deviations.

© John Wiley & Sons, Inc.

The Log-Normal Distribution

This distribution is also called *skewed*. If a set of numbers is log-normally distributed, then the logarithms of those numbers will be normally distributed (see the preceding section "The normal distribution"). Laboratory values such as enzyme and antibody concentrations are often log-normally distributed. Hospital lengths of stay, charges, and costs are also approximately log-normal.

You should suspect log-normality if the standard deviation of a set of numbers is so big it's in the ballpark of the size of the mean. Figure 24-3 shows the relationship between the normal and log-normal distributions.

If a set of log-normal numbers has a mean A and standard deviation D, then the natural logarithms of those numbers will have a standard deviation $s = Log\left[1 + (D/A)^2\right]$, and a mean $m = Log(A) - s^2/2$.

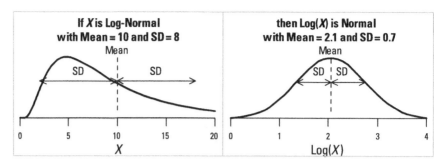

FIGURE 24-3:
The log-normal
distribution.

© John Wiley & Sons, Inc.

The Binomial Distribution

The binomial distribution helps you estimate the probability of getting x successes out of N independent tries when the probability of success on one try is p. (See Chapter 3 for an introduction to probability.) A common example of the binomial distribution is the probability of getting x heads out of N flips of a coin. If the coin is fair, p = 0.5, but if it is lopsided, p could be greater than or less than 0.5 (such as p = 0.7). Figure 24-4 shows the frequency distributions of three binomial distributions, all having $p = 0.7$ but having different N values.

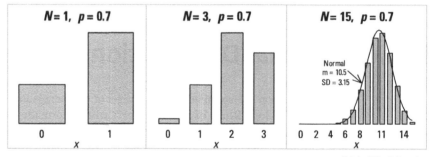

FIGURE 24-4:
The binomial
distribution.

© John Wiley & Sons, Inc.

The formula for the probability of getting x successes in N tries when the probability of success on one try is p is $\Pr\left(x, N, p\right) = p^{x}\left(1-p\right)^{N-x} N! / \left[x!(N-x)!\right]$.

Looking across Figure 24-4, you might have guessed that as N gets larger, the binomial distribution's shape approaches that of a normal distribution with mean $= Np$ and standard deviation $= \sqrt{Np(1-p)}$.

The arc-sine of the square root of a set of proportions is approximately normally distributed, with a standard deviation of $1/\sqrt{4N}$. Using this *transformation*, you can analyze data consisting of observed proportions with t tests, ANOVAs, regression models, and other methods designed for normally distributed data. For example, using this transformation, you could use these methods to statistically compare proportions of participants who responded to treatment in two different treatment groups in a study. However, whenever you transform your data, it can be challenging to back-transform the results and interpret them.

The Poisson Distribution

The Poisson distribution gives the probability of observing exactly N independent random events in some interval of time or region of space if the mean event rate is m. The Poisson distribution describes fluctuations of random event occurrences seen in biology, such as the number of nuclear decay counts per minute, or the number of pollen grains per square centimeter on a microscope slide. Figure 24-5 shows the Poisson distribution for three different values of m.

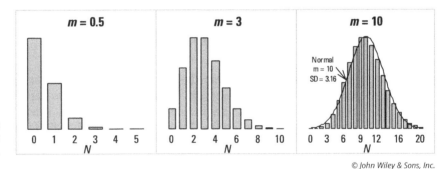

FIGURE 24-5:
The Poisson distribution.

The formula to estimate probabilities on the Poisson distribution is $\Pr(N, m) = m^N e^{-m} / N$.

Looking across Figure 24-5, you might have guessed that as m gets larger, the Poisson distribution's shape approaches that of a normal distribution, with mean $= m$ and standard deviation $= \sqrt{m}$.

The square roots of a set of Poisson-distributed numbers are approximately normally distributed, with a standard deviation of 0.5.

The Exponential Distribution

If a set of events follows the Poisson distribution, the *time intervals* between consecutive events follow the exponential distribution, and vice versa. Figure 24-6 shows the shape of two different exponential distributions.

The Microsoft Excel statement $= -\text{LN}(\text{RAND}())$ makes exponentially distributed random numbers with mean $= 1$.

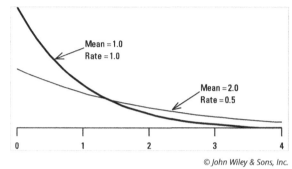

FIGURE 24-6:
The exponential distribution.

© John Wiley & Sons, Inc.

The Weibull Distribution

This distribution describes *failure* times for devices (such as light bulbs), where the failure rate can be constant, or can change over time depending on the *shape parameter, k*. It is also used in human survival analysis, where failure is an outcome (such as death). In the Weibull distribution, the failure rate is proportional to time raised to the $k - 1$ power, as shown in Figure 24-7a.

>> If $k <$ 1, the failure rate has a lot of early failures, but these are reduced over time.

>> If $k =$ 1, the failure rate is constant over time, following an exponential distribution.

>> If $k >$ 1, the failure rate increases over time as items wear out.

Figure 24-7b shows the corresponding cumulative survival curves.

The Weibull distribution shown in Figure 24-7 leads to survival curves of the form *Survival* $= 1 - e^{-\text{Time}^k}$, which are widely used in industrial statistics. But survival methods that don't assume a distribution for the survival curve are more common in biostatistics (we cover examples in Chapters 21, 22, and 23).

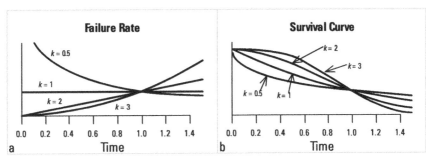

FIGURE 24-7:
The Weibull
distribution.

The Student t Distribution

This family of distributions is most often used when comparing means between two groups, or between two paired measurements. Figure 24-8 shows the shape of the Student t distribution for various degrees of freedom. (See Chapter 11 for more info about t tests and degrees of freedom.)

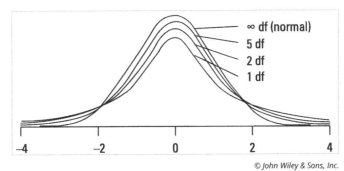

FIGURE 24-8:
The Student t
distribution.

In Figure 24-8, as the degrees of freedom increase, the shape of the Student t distribution approaches that of the normal distribution.

Table 24-1 shows the *critical* t value for various degrees of freedom at $\alpha = 0.05$.

TIP

Under $\alpha = 0.05$, random fluctuations cause the t statistic to exceed the critical t value only 5 percent of the time. This 5 percent includes exceeding t on either the positive or negative side. From the table, if you determine your critical t is 2.01 at 50 df, and your test statistic is 2.45, it exceeds the critical t, and is statistically significant at $\alpha = 0.05$. But this would also be true if your test statistic was −2.45, because the table only presents absolute values of critical t.

TABLE 24-1

Critical Values of Student t for $\alpha = 0.05$

Degrees of Freedom	t_{crit}
1	12.71
2	4.30
3	3.18
4	2.78
5	2.57
6	2.45
8	2.31
10	2.23
20	2.09
50	2.01
∞	1.96

For other α and df values, the Microsoft Excel formula =T.INV.2T(α, df) gives the critical Student t value.

TIP

The Chi-Square Distribution

This family of distributions is used most commonly for two purposes: testing goodness-of-fit between observed and expected event counts, and for testing for association between categorical variables. Figure 24-9 shows the shape of the chi-square distribution for various degrees of freedom.

As you look across Figure 24-9, you may notice that as the degrees of freedom increase, the shape of the chi-square distribution approaches that of the normal distribution. Table 24-2 shows the *critical* chi-square value for various degrees of freedom at $\alpha = 0.05$.

Under $\alpha = 0.05$, random fluctuations cause the chi-square statistic to exceed the critical chi-square value only 5 percent of the time. If the chi-square value from your test exceeds the critical value, the test is statistically significant at $\alpha = 0.05$.

TIP

For other α and df values, the Microsoft Excel formula = CHIINV(α, df) gives the critical χ^2 value.

TIP

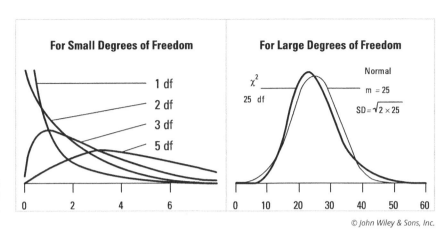

FIGURE 24-9:
The chi-square
distribution.

TABLE 24-2

Critical Values of Chi-Square for $\alpha = 0.05$

Degrees of Freedom	$\chi^2 Crit$
1	3.84
2	5.99
3	7.81
4	9.49
5	11.07
6	12.59
7	14.07
8	15.51
9	16.92
10	18.31

The Fisher F Distribution

This family of distributions is frequently used to obtain p values from an analysis of variance (ANOVA). Figure 24-10 shows the shape of the Fisher F distribution for various degrees of freedom.

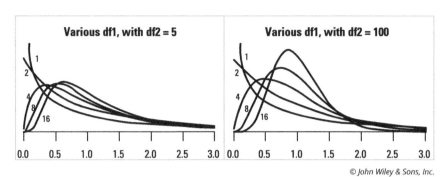

FIGURE 24-10:
The Fisher F
distribution.

© John Wiley & Sons, Inc.

TIP

Random fluctuations cause F to exceed the critical F value only 5 percent of the time. If the F value from your ANOVA exceeds this value, the test is statistically significant at $\alpha = 0.05$. For other values of α, df_1, and df_2, the Microsoft Excel formula $= FINV(\alpha, df_1, df_2)$ will give the critical F value.

Chapter **25**

Ten Easy Ways to Estimate How Many Participants You Need

Sample-size calculations (also called *power calculations*) tend to frighten researchers and send them running to the nearest statistician. But if you you need a ballpark idea of how many participants are needed for a new research project, you can use these ten quick and dirty rules of thumb.

TIP

Before you begin, take a look at Chapter 3 — especially the sections on hypothesis testing and the power of a test. That way, you'll refresh your memory about what power and sample-size calculations are all about. For your study, you will need to select the *effect size of importance* that you want to detect. An effect size could be the difference of at least 10 mmHg in mean systolic blood-pressure lowering between groups on two different hypertension drugs, or it could be having the degree of correlation between two laboratory values of at least 0.7. Once you select your effect size and compatible statistical test, look in this chapter for the rule for the statistical test you selected to calculate the sample size.

The first six sections tell you how many participants you need to provide complete data for you to analyze in order to have an 80 percent chance of getting a p value that's less than 0.05 when you run the test if a true difference of your effect size does indeed exist. In other words, we are setting the parameters 80 percent power at $\alpha = 0.05$, because they are widely used in biological research. The remaining four sections tell you how to modify your estimate for other power or α values, and how to adjust your estimate for unequal group size and dropouts from the study.

Comparing Means between Two Groups

» **Applies to:** Unpaired Student t test, Mann-Whitney U test, and Wilcoxon Sum-of-Ranks test.

» **Effect size (E):** The difference between the means of two groups divided by the standard deviation (SD) of the values within a group.

» **Rule:** You need $16/E^2$ participants in each group, or $32/E^2$ participants altogether.

For example, say you're comparing two hypertension drugs — Drug A and Drug B — on lowering systolic blood pressure (SBP). You might set the effect size of 10 mmHg. You also know from prior studies that the SD of the SBP change is known to be 20 mmHg. Then the equation is $E = 10/20$, or 0.5, and you need $16/(0.5)^2$, or 64 participants in each group (128 total).

Comparing Means among Three, Four, or Five Groups

» **Applies to:** One-way Analysis of Variance (ANOVA) or Kruskal-Wallis test.

» **Effect size (E):** The difference between the largest and smallest means among the groups divided by the within-group SD.

» **Rule:** You need $20/E^2$ participants in each group.

Continuing the example from the preceding section, if you're comparing three hypertension drugs — Drug A, Drug B, and Drug C — and if any mean difference of 10 mmHg in SBP between any pair of drug groups is important, then E is still $10/20$, or 0.5, but you now need $20/(0.5)^2$, or 80 participants in each group (240 total).

Comparing Paired Values

>> **Applies to:** Paired Student t test or Wilcoxon Signed-Ranks test.

>> **Effect size (_E_):** The average of the paired differences divided by the SD of the paired differences.

>> **Rule:** You need $8/E^2$ participants (pairs of values).

Imagine that you're studying test scores in struggling students before and after tutoring. You determine a six-point improvement in grade points is the effect size of importance, and the SD of the changes is ten points. Then $E = 6/10$, or 0.6, and you need $8/(0.6)^2$, or about 22 students, each of whom provides a _before_ score and an _after_ score.

Comparing Proportions between Two Groups

>> **Applies to:** Chi-square test of association or Fisher Exact test.

>> **Effect size (_D_):** The difference between the two proportions (P_1 and P_2) that you're comparing. You also have to calculate the average of the two proportions: $P = (P_1 + P_2)/2$.

>> **Rule:** You need $16 \times P \times (1 - P)/D^2$ participants in each group.

For example, if a disease has a 60 percent mortality rate, but you think your drug can cut this rate in half to 30 percent, then $P = (0.6 + 0.3)/2$, or 0.45, and $D = 0.6 - 0.3$, or 0.3. You need $16 \times 0.45 \times (1 - 0.45)/(0.3)^2$, or 44 participants in each group (88 total).

Testing for a Significant Correlation

>> **Applies to:** Pearson correlation test. It is also a good approximation for the non-parametric Spearman correlation test.

>> **Effect size:** The correlation coefficient (r) you want to be able to detect.

>> **Rule:** You need $8/r^2$ participants (pairs of values).

Imagine that you're studying the association between weight and blood pressure, and you want the correlation test to come out statistically significant if these two variables have a true correlation coefficient of at least 0.2. Then you need to study $8/(0.2)^2$, or 200 participants.

Comparing Survival between Two Groups

>> **Applies to:** Log-rank test or Cox proportional-hazard regression.

>> **Effect size:** The hazard ratio (*HR*) you want to be able to detect.

>> **Rule:** The required *total* number of observed deaths/ events = $32/(\text{natural log of } HR)^2$.

Here's how the formula works out for several values of *HR* greater than 1:

Hazard Ratio	Total Number of Events
1.1	3,523
1.2	963
1.3	465
1.4	283
1.5	195
1.75	102
2.0	67
2.5	38
3.0	27

WARNING

Your enrollment must be large enough and your follow-up must be long enough to ensure that the required number of events take place during the observation period. This may be difficult to estimate beforehand as it involves considering recruitment rates, censoring rates, the shape of the survival curve, and other factors difficult to forecast. Some research protocols provide only a tentative estimate of the expected enrollment for planning, budgeting, and ethical purposes. Many state that enrollment and/or follow-up will continue until the required number of events has been observed. Even with ambiguity, it is important to follow conventions described in this book when designing to avoid criticism for departing from good general principles.

Scaling from 80 Percent to Some Other Power

Here's how you take a sample-size estimate that provides 80 percent power from one of the preceding rules and scale it up or down to provide some other power:

>> **For 50 percent power:** Use only half as many participants — multiply the estimate by 0.5.

>> **For 90 percent power:** Increase the sample size by 33 percent — multiply the estimate by 1.33.

>> **For 95 percent power:** Increase the sample size by 66 percent — multiply the estimate by 1.66.

For example, if you know from doing a prior sample size calculation that a study with 70 participants provides 80 percent power to test its primary objective, then a study that has 1.33×70, or 93 participants will have about 90 percent power to test the same objective. The reason to consider power of levels other than 80 percent is because of limited sample. If you know that 70 participants provides 80 percent power, but you will only have access to 40, you can estimate maximum power you are able to achieve.

Scaling from 0.05 to Some Other Alpha Level

Here's how you take a sample-size estimate that was based on testing at the $\alpha = 0.05$ level, and scale it up or down to correspond to testing at some other α level:

>> **For $\alpha = 0.10$:** Decrease the sample size by 20 percent — multiply the estimate by 0.8.

>> **For $\alpha = 0.025$:** Increase the sample size by 20 percent — multiply the estimate by 1.2.

>> **For $\alpha = 0.01$:** Increase the sample size by 50 percent — multiply the estimate by 1.5.

For example, imagine that you've calculated you need a sample size of 100 partici-pants using α = 0.05 as your criterion for significance. Then your boss says you have to apply a two-fold Bonferroni correction (see Chapter 11) and use α = 0.025 as your criterion instead. You need to increase your sample size to 100 x 1.2, or 120 participants, to have the same power at the new α level.

Adjusting for Unequal Group Sizes

When comparing means or proportions between two groups, you usually get the best power for a given sample size — meaning it's more *efficient* — if both groups are the same size. If you don't mind having unbalanced groups, you will need more participants overall in order to preserve statistical power. Here's how to adjust the size of the two groups to keep the same statistical power:

>> **If you want one group twice as large as the other:** Increase one group by 50 percent, and reduce the other group by 25 percent. This increases the total sample size by about 13 percent.

>> **If you want one group three times as large as the other:** Reduce one group by a third, and double the size of the other group. This increases the total sample size by about 33 percent.

>> **If you want one group four times as large as the other:** Reduce one group by 38 percent and increase the other group by 250 percent. This increases the total sample size by about 56 percent.

Suppose that you're comparing two equal-sized groups, Drug A and Drug B. You've calculated that you need two groups of 32, for a total of 64 participants. Now, you decide to randomize group assignment using a 2:1 ratio for A:B. To keep the same power, you'll need 32 × 1.5, or 48 for Drug A, an increase of 50 percent. For B, you'll want 32 × 0.75, or 24, a decrease of 25 percent, for an overall new total 72 participants in the study.

Allowing for Attrition

Sample size estimates apply to the number of participants who give you complete, analyzable data. In reality, you have to increase this estimate to account for those who will drop out of the study, or provide incomplete data for other reasons (called *attrition*). Here's how to scale up your sample size estimate to develop an enrollment target that compensates for attrition, remembering longer duration studies may have higher attrition:

Enrollment = Number Providing Complete Data × 100/(100 – *%Attrition*)

Here are the enrollment scale-ups for several attrition rates:

Expected Attrition	Increase the Enrollment by
10%	11%
20%	25%
25%	33%
33%	50%
50%	100%

If your sample size estimate says you need a total of 60 participants with complete data, and you expect a 25 percent attrition rate, you need to enroll 60 × 1.33, or 80 participants. That way, you'll have complete data on 60 participants after a quarter of the original 80 are removed from analysis.

Index

Symbols

α (alpha)
  Bonferroni, 153–154
  definition of, 41
  level, 206
  relation to sample sizes, 365–366
  setting, 43
* (asterisk), 155
β (beta), 41
λ (half-life), 280–282
κ (kappa), 189–190
μg (micrograms), 280–282
Π (pi), 27–28
√ (radical sign), 21
Σ (sigma), 27–28
γ (skewness coefficient), 121

A

absolute values, 23
accuracy, 37, 38, 262–264
active group, 187
actuarial life tables, 307, 311–316, 320–321
addition, 18–19
additive, 296
administrative measurements, 63
adverse events, 70
agriculture, 1
Akaike's Information Criterion (AIC), 259, 276–277, 342
alcohol intake, 94–98
alpha (α)
  Bonferroni, 153–154
  definition of, 41
  level, 206
  relation to sample sizes, 365–366
  setting, 43

alternative hypothesis, 40, 43, 144, 150–151, 324
Alzheimer's disease, 91, 146
amputation, 292–293
analysis of variance (ANOVA)
  assessing, 152–157
  introduction to, 11, 47–49
  using, 143–145, 158
analytic dataset, 76
analytic research, 88–90
analytic study designs, 91
analytic suite, 57–58
analyzing data, 7, 9–10, 74–76
and rule, 31
animal research, 1
ANOVA (analysis of variance)
  assessing, 152–157
  introduction to, 11, 47–49
  using, 143–145, 158
anticipated enrollment rate, 347
antilogarithm, 22, 118–119
anti-synergy, 245–247
area under the ROC curve (AUC), 265, 280
arguments, 23
arithmetic mean, 115–116
arrays, 25–27
asbestos, 296–298
asymptomatic confidence limits, 134
attrition, 366–367
average values, 11, 39–40, 141–158

B

background information, 69
backward elimination approach, 295
bad fit line, 215–216
balanced groups, 154
bar charts, 113, 126

D

data. *See also* cross-tabulated data
  analyzing and collecting, 1, 7, 9–10, 74–76, 101–110
  categorical, 112–114
  free-text, 103
  interval and ordinal, 102
  ratio, 102, 107–108
  skewed and unskewed, 11, 114, 121, 353
  survival, 208, 301–306, 337, 343
  time, 108–110
data close-out, 76
data dictionary, 110
data safety monitoring board (DSMB), 73, 76
data safety monitoring committee (DSMC), 73
data snapshot, 76
date data, 108–110
date of last contact, 303
DBP (diastolic blood pressure), 116–117
deciliter (dL), 280
decision theory, 10, 39–40
degrees of freedom (df)
  calculating, 147–148, 152–153
  for chi-square tests, 166–167, 358–359
dementia, 91, 146, 187–188
denominator, 41–42
dependent variable, 208, 213, 235–245
descriptive research, 88–90
descriptive study designs, 91
desired power, 347
desired α level, 347
determinants, 191
deviation, 119, 258–259
df (degrees of freedom)
  calculating, 147–148
  for chi-square test, 166–167, 358–359
  numerator and denominator, 152
diabetes, 135–136, 236–240. *See also* Type II diabetes
diagnostic procedures, 183–188
diastolic blood pressure (DBP), 116–117, 123–124
dichotomous variables, 173–174, 249, 269

difference, 147–148, 163
difference table, 163
disease, 191, 193–194
dispersion, 115, 119
distribution center, 115
distributions
  bimodal (two-peaked), 114–117
  binomial, 36, 354–355
  chi-square, 165–166, 358–359
  exponential, 356
  Fisher F, 152, 359–360
  frequency, 47–48
  leptokurtic and platykurtic, 122
  normal, 13, 36, 114, 353
  probability, 35–37
  sampling, 38
  statistical, 13
  student t, 357–358
  weibull, 330, 356–357
District of Columbia, 34–35
division, 20
dL (deciliter), 280
dose-response relationship, 298
double-blinding, 66, 97
double-precision numbers, 107
drug description, 70
drug development research, 280–282
DSMB (data safety monitoring board), 73, 76
DSMC (data safety monitoring committee), 73
Dupont, William D. (biostatistician), 60

E

ECG (electrocardiogram), 188
ecologic fallacy, 93
ecologic studies, 91–93
effect modification, 296–297
effect size
  compared to power and sample size, 45–47
  definitions of, 362–364
  example of, 39
  of importance, 158, 206, 361

GLM (generalized linear model), 272–278

glucose values, 25–26, 153

gold standard test, 183–184

good fit line, 215–216

goodness of fit, 227–228, 258–259

G*Power

  description of, 59–60, 68

  using, 158, 198, 207, 324–325

graphing. *See also* charts and charting

  categorical data, 112–114

  correlation coefficients, 202–203

  hazard rates and survival probabilities, 312–315

  multiple regression, 243–245

  numerical data, 124–128

  Poisson regression, 273–276

  Receiver Operator Characteristics (ROC), 264–265

  residuals, 222–223

  software for, 57–58

  s-shaped data, 252–256

  student t test, 45–47

GraphPad, 67

Greek letters, 17

GUI (guided user interface), 56, 58

H

h value, 344–346

half-life (λ), 280–282

hazard rate

  definition of, 305

  from life tables, 311–315

  relation to survival rate, 333

hazard ratios (HR), 334–335, 340, 364

health insurance, 112–114

healthcare, 9–10

highway accidents, 274–278

Hill, Bradford (epidemiologist)

  Bradford Hills' criteria of causality, 297–298

histogram, 34–35, 124–125

historical control, 142

H-L test, 259

homogeneity of variances, 155

hormone concentration, 287–290

Hosmer-Lemeshow Goodness of Fit test, 259

HR (hazard ratios), 334–335, 340

HTN (hypertension), 90, 94–98, 177–178

human health research, 88

human subjects protection certification, 73

hyperplane, 234

hypertension (HTN), 90, 94–98, 177–178

hypothesis, 40–47, 63, 94, 247. *See also* null hypothesis

hypothesis-driven analysis, 294

hypothesized cause, 83, 175, 178, 193, 292

I

ICF (Informed Consent Form), 72–73

ICH (International Conference on Harmonization), 72

icons explained, 3

identification (ID) numbers, 104

identity line, 245

imputation, 75

incidence, 191–198

incidence rate, 192–198

inclusion criteria, 64

independent t test, 148

independent variable, 208–210, 213, 215, 291–294

indicator variables, 237–238

indices, 174

individual-level data, 160

inferential statistics, 34, 77

inferring, 10

infinity, 33

influenza, 192

Informed Consent Form (ICF), 72–73

inner mean, 118

integers, 107

LOWESS (locally weighted scatterplot smoothing) curve-fitting, 12, 286–290

lung cancer, 296–298

M

Mann, Henry (professor), 141

Mann-Whitney U test, 47–49, 143, 362

Mantel-Cox test. *See* log-rank test

Mantel-Haenszel chi-square test, 168

margin of error (ME), 134

marginal totals, 160

masking, 66, 70, 171

mathematical expressions, 15

mathematical operations, 18–25

matrix, 26

matrix algebra, 26

maximum value, 222

ME (margin of error), 134

mean

arithmetic, 115–116

compared to other values, 142–157, 362

confidence limits, 134–135

mean square (mean Sq), 155

measurements, 63-64, 102–103

mechanical function, 279

median, 116–117, 123, 222

meta-analyses, 97–98

metadata, 110

mice, 1, 318

micrograms (µg), 280–282

Microsoft Excel

for data collection, 103, 105, 107–110

functions of, 57

for log-rank tests, 319–320

for randomization, 67

for straight-line regression, 217

for survival regressions, 343

millimeters of mercury (mmHg), 218–226, 229, 239

minimum value, 222

missing data, 74–75

Mitra, Amal K. (author)

Epidemiology for Dummies, 92

mmHg (millimeters of mercury), 218–226, 229, 239

mode, 117

model building, 246

model fit statistics, 242

models

generalized linear (GLM), 272–278

linear, 272–273

null, 228, 242, 259

parsimonious, 293

predictive, 228–229

regression, 68, 208–209

molecular biology, 7

multicollinearity, 246–247

multi-dimensional arrays, 26–27

multilevel variable, 236

multiple regression

basics of, 234–235

introduction to, 26

sample size for, 247–248

special considerations, 245–247

using, 236–245

multiple R-squared, 242

multiplication, 18–20

multiplicative, 296

multiplicity, 75–76

multi-site study, 104

multi-stage sampling, 85–86

multivariable regression, 291

multivariate analysis, 128, 145, 291

N

Nagelkerke R-square, 259

National Health and Nutrition Examination Survey (NHANES), 82, 86, 93, 148–157

National Institutes of Health (NIH), 72–73

natural logarithms, 22

negative predicted value (NPV), 187

negatively skewed data, 121

NHANES (National Health and Nutrition Examination Survey), 82, 86, 93, 148–157

NIH (National Institutes of Health), 72–73

nominal variables, 102

non-code-based methods, 60

nonlinear function, 211

nonlinear least-squares regression, 12

nonlinear regression, 279–286

nonlinear trends, 277

nonparametric regression, 286–290

nonparametric tests, 48–49, 157

non-proportional hazards, 323

non-sampling error, 78

non-steroidal anti-inflammatory drugs (NSAIDS), 159–166

normal distribution, 13, 36, 114, 353

normal Q-Q graph, 222–223

normal-based confidence intervals, 134

normal-based confidence limits, 134

normality assumption, 143

not rule, 31

notches, 128

NPV (negative predicted value), 187

NSAIDs (non-steroidal anti-inflammatory drugs), 159–166

nuisance variables, 145

null hypothesis
  definition of, 40
  evaluating, 42–43, 150, 152–153, 322, 351–352
  example of, 161–165, 319

null model, 228, 242, 259

numerator, 41–42

numerical data, 107–109, 114–123

O

obesity, 177–178, 182–183

observational research, 88–90

observed count, 164

observed *versus* predicted graph, 245

ODA (SAS OnDemand for Academics), 55–56

odds, 32–33, 181

odds ratio (OR), 94–96, 181–183, 266–267

Office for Human Research Protections (OHRP), 72

one-dimensional arrays, 25

one-group t test, 148

one-sided confidence interval, 133

one-way ANOVA, 144

open-source software, 58–59

OpenStat, 59

OR (odds ratio), 94–96, 181–183, 266–267

or rule, 31

order of operation, 24

ordinal data, 102

ordinary multiple linear regression model. *See* multiple regression

ordinary regression, 210

outcome, 208

outcome-related measurements, 64

outliers, 229

overall accuracy, 185

P

p value
  definition of, 41, 242
  determining, 165–167
  evaluating, 42, 144, 147–157, 226–227, 340
  from the H-L test, 259

paired t test, 148

paired values, 363

parabolic relationship, 214, 252–253

parallel design, 65

parameters, 33–34, 77, 208, 279

parametric tests, 48–49

parsimonious models, 293

parsimony, 293

participant identification (ID), 240

participant study identifier, 104

participants. *See also* sample size; samples
  enrolling, 68
  protection for, 71–73
  selecting, 64–65, 236–237
PatSat, 106
PCR (polymerase chain reaction), 184
Pearson, Karl (biostatistician), 161
Pearson Correlation test, 47–49, 227
Pearson kurtosis index, 122
percentile, 120
perfect predictor problem, 267–268
perfect separation, 267–268
periodicity, 83
PH (proportional hazards regression), 330–331, 333–334
pharmacokinetic (PK) properties, 280–282
pi (П), 27–28
pie charts, 113
pilot study, 230
placebo, 66–67, 171, 187–188
placebo effect, 66, 187–188
plain text format, 16, 24
platykurtic distribution, 122
Plummer, Walton D. (biostatistician), 60
pointy-topped distribution, 114
poisson distribution, 36, 355
poisson regression
  definition of, 12, 210
  using, 271–278
polymerase chain reaction (PCR), 184
populations, 33–37, 175
positive predictive value (PPV), 187
positively skewed data, 121
post-hoc tests, 143, 152–157
potential confounding variables, 64
Power and Sample Size Calculation (PS)
  for chi-square and Fisher exact tests, 171–172
  definition of, 60
  for survival comparisons, 324–325
power calculations, 47, 171–172, 361, 365
powers, 20–21, 41, 44, 45–47, 206

PPV (positive predictive value), 187
precision, 37, 38, 147
predicted values, 242
predictive model, 228–229
predictive value negative, 187
predictive value positive, 187
predictors
  introduction to, 208, 233
  in iterative models, 246–247
  in logistic models, 255–256
  in regression models, 273–274, 279
  relation to the outcome, 242, 245–246, 250
  types of, 209, 235–236
pregnancy, 171, 185–187
prevalence, 179, 186, 191–194
prevalence ratio, 179
primary diagnosis (PrimaryDx), 236–238
primary efficacy objective, 62
primary objectives, 62
primary sampling units (PSU), 86
privacy, 71
probability, 30–33
probability bell curve, 353
probability distributions, 35–37
probability of independence, 166
procedural descriptions, 70
product, of an array, 27
prognosis curves, 329, 331, 343–346
proportional hazards (PH) regression, 330–331, 333–334
proportions, 11, 135–136, 363
protective factor, 178
protractor, 113
PS (Power and Sample Size Calculation)
  for chi-square and Fisher exact tests, 171–172
  definition of, 60
  for survival comparisons, 324–325
pseudo-r-squared values, 259
PSU (primary sampling units), 86
Python, 58

R

R (software)
  description of, 58
  nonlinear regression, 282–286
  odds ratio calculation, 183
  risk ratio calculation, 180–181
  straight-line regression, 221
r value, 203–206
radiation exposure, 251–256, 260–263, 267,
    337–338
radical sign ($\sqrt{}$), 21
random number generator (RNG), 80–81
random shuffling, 67
random variability, 158
randomization, 97, 171
randomized controlled trials (RCTs), 65–67, 98
randomness, 33
range, 120
ranks, 49
rate ratio (RR), 195–196
ratio data, 102, 107–108
rationale, 69
RCTs (randomized controlled trials), 65–67, 98
Receiver Operator Characteristics (ROC), 257,
    264–265
reference level, 237
regression
  logistic
    basics of, 251–254
    definition of, 12, 210
    disadvantages of, 266–268
    evaluating, 257–265
    sample size for, 268–269
    using, 249–250, 255–257
  multiple
    basics of, 234–235
    introduction to, 26
    sample size for, 247–248
    special considerations, 245–247
    using, 236–245
  multivariable, 291
  ordinary, 210

  straight-line
    basics of, 215–216
    disadvantages of, 229–231
    evaluating, 220–224
    using, 216–220
    when to use, 213–215
  survival
    concepts of, 329–335
    definition of, 210
    evaluating, 337–343
    sample size for, 346–347
    using, 335–336
    when to use, 328–329, 343
  univariate, 209
regression analysis, 12, 207–208
regression models, 68, 208–209
relative frequency, 30
relative risk, 95, 178–181
REM (Roentgen Equivalent Man), 251–254,
    260–262, 267
research
  analytic, descriptive and observational, 88–90
  animal, 1
  epidemiological, 1, 9–12
  experimental, 61, 88–90, 97–98
  human health, 88
  longitudinal, 90
research studies, 1
residual information, 242
residual standard error, 222, 242
residuals, 222–224, 242–245
residuals *versus* fitted graph, 222–223
retinopathy, 292–293
right skewed data, 121
risk ratio, 96, 178–181
RMS (root-mean-square), 222
RNG (random number generator), 80–81
ROC (Receiver Operator Characteristics), 257,
    264–265
Roentgen Equivalent Man (REM), 251–254,
    260–262, 267
Roman letters, 17

About the Authors

Monika M. Wahi, MPH, CPH, is a well-published data scientist with more than 20 years of experience, and president of the public health informatics and education firm DethWench Professional Services (DPS) (www.dethwench.com). She is the author of *Mastering SAS Programming for Data Warehousing* and has coauthored over 35 peer-reviewed scientific articles. After obtaining her master of public health degree in epidemiology from the University of Minnesota School of Public Health, she has served many roles at the intersection of study design, biostatistics, informatics, and research in the public and private sectors, including at Hennepin County Department of Corrections in Minneapolis, the Byrd Alzheimer's Institute in Tampa, and the U.S. Army. After founding DPS, she worked as an adjunct lecturer at Laboure College in the Boston area for several years, teaching about the U.S. healthcare system and biostatistics in their bachelor of nursing program. At DPS, she helps organizations upgrade their analytics pipelines to take advantage of new research approaches, including open source. She also coaches professionals moving into data science from healthcare and other fields on research methods, applied statistics, data governance, informatics, and management.

John C. Pezzullo, PhD, spent more than half a century working in the physical, biological, and social sciences. For more than 25 years, he led a dual life at Rhode Island Hospital as an information technology programmer/analyst (and later director) while also providing statistical and other technical support to biological and clinical researchers at the hospital. He then joined the faculty at Georgetown University as informatics director of the National Institute of Child Health and Human Development's Perinatology Research Branch. He created the StatPages website (https://statpages.info), which provides online statistical calculating capability and other statistics-related resources.

Dedication

This book is dedicated to my favorite "dummy," my dear old dad, Bhupinder Nath "Ben" Wahi. He is actually a calculus whiz. He used to point to the For Dummies books when we'd see them at the bookstore and say, "Am I a dummy?" Of course, I won't answer that! — Monika

Author's Acknowledgments

First and foremost, I want to acknowledge and honor the late Dr. John Pezzullo, the original author of this work. It has been a pleasure to revise his thorough and interesting writing, delivered with the enthusiasm of a true educator. I am also extremely grateful for Matt Wagner of Fresh Books, who opened the doors necessary for my coauthorship of this book. Further, I am indebted to editor Katharine Dvorak for her constant support, guidance, and helpfulness through the writing process. Additionally, I want to extend a special "thank you" to my amazing colleague, Sunil Gupta, who provided his typically excellent technical review. Finally, I want to express my appreciation for all the other members of the For Dummies team at Wiley who helped me along the way to make this book a success. Thank you for helping me be the best writer I can be! — Monika

Publisher's Acknowledgments

Executive Editor: Lindsay Berg

Managing Editor: Murari Mukundan

Project Editor: Katharine Dvorak

Technical Editor: Sunil K. Gupta, Founder of R-Guru.com and SASSavvy.com

Production Editor: Pradesh Kumar

Cover Image: © ArtemisDiana/Shutterstock

Printed and bound by CPI Group (UK) Ltd, Croydon, CR0 4YY

16/07/2024

14529212-0001